33-00
Woods

Adult Abnormal Psychology

Adult Abnormal Psychology

EDITORS

Edgar Miller PhD FBPsS
District Psychologist,
Cambridge Health Authority

Peter J. Cooper DPhil DipPsych
Lecturer in Psychopathology,
University of Cambridge

CHURCHILL LIVINGSTONE
EDINBURGH LONDON MELBOURNE AND NEW YORK 1988

CHURCHILL LIVINGSTONE
Medical Division of Longman Group UK Limited

© Longman Group UK Limited 1988

All rights reserved; no part of this publication may be reproduced, stored in a retrieval system, or transmitted in any form or by any means, electronic, mechanical, photocopying, recording, or otherwise without either the prior written permission of the Publishers (Churchill Livingstone, Robert Stevenson House, 1–3 Baxter's Place, Leith Walk, Edinburgh EH1 3AF) or a licence permitting restricted copying in the United Kingdom issued by the Copyright Licensing Agency Ltd, 33–34 Alfred Place, London, WC1E 7DP.

First published 1988

ISBN 0-443-03513-X

British Library Cataloguing in Publication Data
Adult abnormal psychology
 1. Psychology, Pathological
 I. Miller, Edgar, II. Cooper, Peter J.
 157   RC454

Library of Congress Cataloging in Publication Data
Adult abnormal psychology / editors, Edgar Miller, Peter J. Cooper.
 Includes index.
 ISBN 0-443-03513-X
 1. Psychology, Pathological.   I. Miller, Edgar.   II. Cooper, Peter J.
 [DNLM: 1. Mental Disorders – in adulthood.   2. Psychopathology. WM 100 A2415]
 RC454.A318   1988
 616.89 – dc19

Produced by Longman Singapore Publishers (Pte) Ltd
Printed in Singapore

Preface

Although there are currently a number of texts on Abnormal Psychology, these are almost all of an introductory nature and only suitable for use by undergraduate students. There is little available for those seeking a more advanced treatment of the material. This volume is intended to fill that gap. The book should be of particular use to postgraduate students training in Clinical Psychology. It is hoped that it will also be of value to other postgraduate students working in the general field of Abnormal Psychology; as well as to others in related disciplines, such as Psychiatry, who might wish to be informed of a psychological perspective on particular topics.

Cambridge, 1987   E. M.
                                                                                                                      P. J. C.

Contributors

G E Berrios MA(Oxon) DPhilSci(Oxon) MD FRCPsych
University Lecturer and Consultant in Psychiatry, University of Cambridge; Director of Medical Studies and Fellow, Robinson College, Cambridge

Ivy M Blackburn PhD MA DipClinPsychol FBPsS
Top Grade Clinical Psychologist, MRC Brain Metabolism Unit, Royal Edinburgh Hospital

Ronald Blackburn MS(Cantab) MSc PhD FBPsS
Chief Psychologist, Park Lane Hospital, Maghull, Liverpool

Peter Geoffrey Britton BSc PhD
Senior Lecturer in Applied Psychology, University of Newcastle upon Tyne; Honorary Clinical Psychologist, Newcastle Health Authority

Elizabeth A Campbell MA MPhil DPhil
Lecturer in Clinical Psychology, University of Surrey; Honorary Clinical Psychologist, Mid-Downs Health Authority

Peter J Cooper DPhil DipPsych
Lecturer in Psychopathology, University of Cambridge

Zafra Cooper DPhil DipPsych
Clinical Psychologist, Fulbourn Hospital, Cambridge

Colin MacLeod BSc DPhil MPhil
Senior Research Worker, Psychology Department, St George's Hospital Medical School, Tooting, London

Keith Hawton DM MRCPsych DPM
Consultant Psychiatrist and Clinical Lecturer, Warneford Hospital and University Department of Psychiatry, Oxford

David R Hemsley MA MPhil PhD
Senior Lecturer in Psychology, Institute of Psychiatry, London University; Honorary Top Grade Clinical Psychologist, Bethlem-Maudsley Special Health Authority, London

Ray Hodgson BA DipPsych PhD
Head of Clinical Psychology Department, South Glamorgan Health Authority, Wales

Liz Kuipers BSc MSc PhD
Lecturer in Clinical Psychology, Institute of Psychiatry, London; Honorary Principal Clinical Psychologist, Maudsley Hospital, London

Andrew Miles Mathews BSc DipPsych PhD
Professor of Psychology, St George's Hospital Medical School; Department of Psychology, University of London, London

Edgar Miller PhD FBPsS
District Psychologist, Cambridge Health Authority

Padmal de Silva BA MA MPhil
Lecturer in Psychology, Institute of Psychiatry, University of London; Principal Clinical Psychologist, Maudsley and Bethlem Royal Hospital, London

Contents

Preface	v
1 Introduction *Edgar Miller and Peter J. Cooper*	1
2 Classification and diagnosis *Zafra Cooper and Peter J. Cooper*	6
3 Historical background to abnormal psychology *German E. Berrios*	26
4 Methodological issues in abnormal psychology *Edgar Miller*	52
5 Social perspectives on depression and schizophrenia *Elizabeth A. Campbell and Liz Kuipers*	67
6 Psychological models of schizophrenia *David R. Hemsley*	101
7 Psychological processes in depression *Ivy M. Blackburn*	128
8 Current perspectives on anxiety *Andrew Mathews and Colin MacLeod*	169
9 Obsessive-compulsive disorder *Padmal de Silva*	194
10 Psychopathy and personality disorder *Ronald Blackburn*	218
11 Hysteria *Edgar Miller*	245
12 Eating disorders *Peter J. Cooper and Zafra Cooper*	268
13 Alcohol and drug dependence *Ray J. Hodgson*	299

14 Sexual dysfunctions *Keith Hawton*	318
15 Abnormalities in the elderly *Peter J. Britton*	336
Name Index	365
Subject Index	376

1   Edgar Miller and Peter J. Cooper

Introduction

Abnormal psychology is a rapidly expanding field with many facets and which incorporates many widely differing theoretical approaches to its subject matter. No text can be entirely comprehensive in covering all aspects of abnormal psychology and from all conceivable theoretical orientations. Some selection of both material and approaches to understanding that material is essential. As an introduction to this volume it is appropriate therefore to give some justification for its form and content.

In general the focus of this book is on abnormal rather than clinical psychology. The primary concern is with the nature of abnormal behaviour and the ways in which such behaviour can be explained and understood. This book is not concerned directly with issues of clinical practice, such as the ways in which disorders can be assessed or evaluated as a part of clinical work, or with the treatment or management of clinical problems. These questions are considered to be part of the practice of clinical psychology. To some extent, the distinction between abnormal and clinical psychology is an artificial one. One important reason for studying abnormal behaviour, but by no means the only reason, is the potential contribution that understanding underlying mechanisms may have for clinical practice. Similarly, clinical practice raises issues that have a bearing on the understanding of the phenomena of abnormal behaviour. Despite these connections between abnormal and clinical psychology, the two may still be viewed as conceptually distinct; and the emphasis in this volume is on the former rather than the latter.

A major assumption underlying this volume is that abnormal behaviour is best understood in terms of a broadly empirical approach. The entire field is therefore viewed through the general framework of experimental psychology. Thus the very extensive and complex approach to behavioural abnormality based on psychodynamic theories is in the main ignored, because this approach does not derive from, or relate easily to, experimental psychology. Similarly, attention will not be devoted to work within the framework of humanistic psychology and certain other theoretical positions which do not readily lend themselves to the generation of testable hypotheses.

The present volume is further limited in that it only considers the problems of abnormal psychology that arise in what might loosely be termed adult psychiatric patients. Other manifestations of abnormal behaviour which occur, for example, in children, in the mentally handicapped and those with neurological disease, are traditionally considered separately. They constitute areas of study large enough to justify volumes of their own and are not covered here.

Having settled on the general approach and the limits of the subject matter, this still leaves other issues to be considered. For some who are familiar with the field of abnormal psychology, the organization of material in this book may seem outmoded. For the most part, it is structured around the familiar Kraepelinian psychiatric classificatory system. This way of dividing and classifying material has, with some justification, been the subject of much criticism in the past. The use of this means of dividing the subject matter has several important implications, which are taken up in the next chapter. Briefly, and in relation to present concerns, it is necessary to have some way of breaking up the material to be considered into manageable sections, preferably on the basis of some system which is readily comprehensible to the reader. Two main alternative approaches can be suggested and neither is wholly ideal. The first, which is adopted here, is to base the material around the Kraepelinian clinical categories (depression, schizophrenia, hysteria, etc.). The second is to classify the material in terms of deficits in specific psychological functions (disorders of attention, mood, memory, etc.). This latter alternative of building the text around disturbed psychological functions has been used by some editors (e.g. Costello 1970, Eysenck 1973). It has the advantage of classifying material in terms of essentially psychological rather than psychiatric concepts. Thus the kinds of subdivisions which psychologists have found useful in studying normal behaviour are the fundamental units of analysis. The major limitation of this approach is that research in abnormal psychology is largely based on the use of clinical categories. As a result, a chapter on, say, disturbances in attention inevitably divides the material into sections concerned with attentional abnormalities in schizophrenia, the mentally handicapped, and so on. Thus the clinical categories have a habit of creeping back into a major place in the discussion.

Despite the apparent inevitability of ending up by dividing the material in terms of clinical categories, there are three possible disadvantages that this brings. One has already been alluded to: namely, that the classification of material by clinical disorders is essentially to use the concepts and terminology of another discipline as a fundamental unit of analysis. This is not a substantial criticism. If a useful means of subdividing manifest psychological phenomena has been produced, then it is patently foolish to reject the system simply because it arose within the medical profession or, indeed, any other profession or discipline. Its acceptance should be predicated solely on its reliability and validity.

The second criticism of using the clinical classificatory system is potentially more serious and much more fundamental. This is that the system is too unreliable to offer a sound basis for subdividing abnormal behaviour. It is certainly true that many early studies of the agreement between diagnosticians revealed reliability to be very low However, as discussed in the next chapter, recent years have seen considerable effort put into improving the reliability of psychiatric diagnoses by the introduction of standardized interviews, such as the Present State Examination (Wing et al 1974), and formalized diagnostic systems such as the Research Diagnostic Criteria (Spitzer et al 1978). These improvements have led to the achievement of quite impressive levels of inter-rater reliability. Whilst further improvements in reliability might be desirable, current levels now usually offer a perfectly adequate basis for research. It should also be noted that categorizing abnormal behaviour in terms of impairments in psychological functions also raises a problem of reliability. For example, the failure of a person with lowered or depressed mood to remember things adequately is not always readily ascribed to an impairment in memory *per se*, as opposed to decreased attention causing a failure to register what is to be remembered, or a biasing effect of low mood on the kind of material that is most readily recalled. The reliability with which phenomena like this can be classified according to the nature of the psychological function primarily involved could well be appreciably lower than the assignment of individuals to clinical categories.

The final problem in using a classificatory system based on clinical categories is that labels like 'mania', 'depression' and 'schizophrenia' may not actually be analogous to the familiar diagnostic concepts from general medicine which carry specific implications for aetiology, treatment and prognosis. To say that a medical patient has pulmonary tuberculosis carries very strong and specific implications about the microorganism that caused the problem, the underlying mechanisms of action, how the disorder will progress, and what kinds of drugs will be effective in combating the disease. To say that a psychiatric patient has an 'anxiety state' carries a much weaker set of implications. In particular, it says little, if anything, about the aetiology of the problem. Nevertheless, as argued in the next chapter, the validity of such psychiatric concepts stands or falls by their usefulness. They are useful precisely because to say that one person is suffering from a major depressive disorder and another from phobic anxiety does indicate something about the likely course that these disorders will follow and their response to specific treatments. Of course, this phenomenologically based system will require perpetual revision and adaptation as further knowledge is acquired.

A number of issues recur in the chapters of this book reflecting current debates in abnormal psychology. One of these concerns the issue of classification itself. Once it is accepted that it is useful to think in terms of distinct groups of disorders, it is necessary to specify the criteria which have to be met for any individual's behaviour to fall within a given category or class. This fundamental issue remains a problem for many aspects of abnormal psychology and most of the contributors to this volume have found it necessary to specify criteria for membership of a given group. The most extreme case, discussed in Chapter 10, is the field of personality disorders where specifying the necessary and sufficient conditions for the particular categories remains the dominant question in this field.

Three other fundamental issues have been thought important enough to warrant chapters of their own at the beginning of this book. The terminology that is used in the study of psychopathology and abnormal behaviour is often ill-understood and poorly defined. One important way of coming to grips with this terminology is to examine its historical development. This text is believed to be unique amongst books of its kind in including a chapter on the historical aspects of the subject. A second basic issue is that of methodology. Work in abnormal psychology raises a number of methodological problems which are largely peculiar to this field and which have attracted particular solutions. A chapter on methodology has therefore been included to describe these problems and evaluate attempts to overcome them. Finally, an important area of development over recent years has been the investigation of the role of social factors in the development and maintenance of psychological disorders. Since there is now much research in this area, an entire chapter is devoted to the role of social factors in depression and schizophrenia. It seems likely that future developments will reveal that social factors are of fundamental importance in other areas of abnormal psychology.

Psychological accounts of abnormal behaviour may attempt to explain the development of the disorder, the maintenance of features of that disorder, or how various aspects of the disorder may relate together. It is apparent from a number of chapters in this volume that psychological accounts have been much more successful in achieving the latter two objectives than they have been in explaining the development of disorders in the first place. In part this is often because aetiology is complex, with a number of different factors probably playing a role in producing any particular disorder. The problem of determining aetiology then obviously revolves around teasing out the separate effects of the different factors. Some of these may be directly causal whilst others may exercise only an indirect effect, as when they merely act to increase the vulnerability of the person to the influence of factors which act more directly. There has been little work of this kind.

Although this book is not directly concerned with clinical practice, the clinical problem of what to do about the abnormal phenomena discussed still remains below the surface. It is a fundamental assumption of the editors that an effective clinical psychology can be built only on a firm and detailed understanding of the basic psychological mechanisms involved in abnormal behaviour. Clearly, clinical practice is not always based on a sound empirical foundation because practising clinicians cannot ignore distressing problems simply because of insufficient knowledge. Nevertheless, further advances in the understanding of abnormal behaviour offer the only firm basis on which clinical practice can be substantially developed and improved.

REFERENCES

Costello C G 1970 Symptoms of psychopathology. Wiley, New York
Eysenck H J 1973 Handbook of abnormal psychology. 2nd edn. Pitman, London
Spitzer R L, Endicott J, Robins E 1978 Research diagnostic criteria: rationale and reliability. Archives of General Psychiatry 35: 773–782
Wing J K, Cooper J E, Sartorius N 1974 The measurement and classification of psychiatric symptoms. Cambridge University Press, Cambridge

Classification and diagnosis

THE NATURE AND IMPORTANCE OF CLASSIFICATION

Classification, the dividing of a given set of objects or abstract entities into subclasses, is a fundamental activity of any science. The dividing of its subject matter or universe of discourse in this way is fundamental in two respects: by permitting adequate description of the objects of scientific investigation it enables communication between scientists and practitioners; and by grouping together objects or entities with common characteristics it allows the possibility of establishing general theories or laws by means of which these particular phenomena can be explained and understood.

Clearly, communication is hardly possible without some form of classification of objects. Indeed, language itself is based on classification. The words we use to name objects and entities all refer to and thus presuppose the existence of a class of objects with certain characteristics in common. It is also clear that the assumptions underlying the grouping together of objects and entities, which are reflected in the criteria used to classify, will, in part, determine the development of subsequent explanatory theories. The accurate assumptions underlying the classification of plants developed by Linnaeus and the classification of chemical elements developed by Mendeleev greatly enhanced the subsequent development of knowledge in these scientific disciplines; whereas the understanding of diseases was hindered by their classification as deficiencies or excesses of one of the four galenical humours (Kendell 1983). It is therefore of the utmost importance that any system for the classification of psychological disorders identifies, describes, and distinguishes the disorders it is concerned to understand as accurately as possible. It is clear that it will only be possible to gain an understanding of the psychological and physiological processes involved in, for example, schizophrenia, if it is possible to identify schizophrenia accurately and to distinguish it from other forms of psychiatric disorder. Similarly, the development of effective treatments depends on being able to identify accurately the disorder one wishes to treat. These points are well illustrated by Kendell (1982) with several examples from the history of medicine. He points out that Noguchi could not have elucidated the syphilitic origin of general paresis had Bayle and Calmiel not previously distinguished the syndrome of general paresis from other forms of mental disorder; and that Lejeune would not have discovered the chromosomal abnormality responsible for Down's syndrome had Langdon Down not previously distinguished what he called mongolism from other forms of mental handicap.

Given the fundamental importance of classification, it is helpful to examine the logical characteristics underlying the classificatory procedure in general before discussing the particular problems raised by classification and diagnosis in the realm of psychological or psychiatric disorder.[1] Classification, as stated above, involves dividing a given set or class of objects into subclasses. The objects of a classification system may be concrete things, such as plants, elements or books; or they may be abstract entities, such as numbers, religions or philosophical doctrines. The ideal classification system divides its subject matter into a set of mutually exclusive and collectively exhaustive subclasses. Each subclass is then defined by the specification of necessary and sufficient conditions for membership; that is, it states certain characteristics which all and only members of a particular class must possess. Each subclass may then be defined by a certain concept which represents the characteristics necessary for membership in that class. Thus, for example, in the division of positive integers into prime and composite numbers, the condition of membership in the class of prime numbers is that the particular number one wishes to assign to a subclass be greater than one, and an integral multiple of only one and itself. This condition of membership then defines the concept of a prime number, and the actual class of numbers picked out by this definition is the extension of the concept of a prime number (Hempel 1961). Clearly, on this view of classification, the assignment of an individual object to its appropriate subclass involves simply determining the attributes of the individual and knowing the defining attributes of all classes in the particular universe of discourse.

This process of the assignment of objects or individual cases to classes in a taxonomic system appears to describe, if in somewhat ideal form, what is involved in diagnosis. Diagnosis means, literally, to distinguish or differentiate and, as such, refers to the process of applying a given classificatory system. When the term diagnosis is used in the medical context, it describes the process by which an individual is assigned to a particular class in a

---

[1] In this chapter no distinction is made between psychological and psychiatric disorder. It seems that, if such a distinction were to be drawn, it must rest on some theoretical knowledge about the nature of the fundamental abnormality or disturbance thought to underlie these disorders. Since our knowledge about such matters is at present limited, it is impossible to decide *a priori* whether any given disorder will turn out to be psychological or psychiatric in these terms. Furthermore, since it seems likely that all such disorders will be capable of being described at both a physiological and psychological level, this distinction may not be a useful one.

taxonomic system of diseases or disorders on the basis of some relevant attributes. Medical diagnosis has a crucial and self-evident function because of its relation to treatment and prognosis.

As described above, each class in a classificatory system is in fact the extension of a concept; that is, it consists of those objects, entities, or individuals in the universe of discourse which conform to the specific characteristics which the concept defines. Thus the establishment of a classificatory system involves the formation of a number of classificatory concepts; and it is necessary for these concepts to meet certain conditions if they are to perform their intended function. Clearly, to realize the first objective of classication, that of adequate description, it is necessary that the terms used to refer to classificatory concepts have clearly specified meanings and are understood in the same way by all who use them. One way of achieving this is the use of so-called operational definitions for scientific terms. The term 'operational definition' was introduced by Bridgman (1927) and defined as follows: 'an operational definition of a scientific term S is a stipulation to the effect that S is to apply to all and only those cases for which performance of test operation T yields the specified outcome O.' While the emphasis in this definition on clear and precise publicly usable criteria for the application of scientific terms is clearly desirable, this rather extreme formulation of the notion of an operational definition requires certain qualifications. First, operational definitions of terms are often less than full definitions of the concepts for which they stand. They do indeed provide criteria of application for a given term and its corresponding concept which enables an investigator to fix the reference of the term or concept. However, this process can often be achieved by specifying only a partial definition of the concept under consideration. One may identify water in a clear and precise way by its characteristic look and feel and also by many of its other observable phenomenal properties, and thereby provide criteria for application for the term water. This does not, however, reflect the full meaning of the term water, which requires crucially that it be defined in terms of its molecular structure, in terms of its links with the theoretical structure within which it is understood (Putnam 1975). Second, unless the idea of an operation is taken rather liberally, the requirement of operational definitions of scientific terms may become unduly restrictive. The liberal interpretation of operation that Hempel (1961) suggests, and one that seems most reasonable to adopt, does not require actual manipulation of the objects under consideration, but merely their observation. Thus, the requirement of operational definitions for scientific terms becomes a requirement merely that a term may be applied to all those objects and only those objects which meet a certain specified criteria O, where O is clearly specified and inter-subjectively certifiable.

However important clear and objective criteria are for the application of scientific terms, these criteria alone will not ensure that the resulting concepts will provide a means of realizing the second objective to be met by the classificatory concept, that of lending themselves to the formulation of general theories or laws. This is what Hempel (1961) has termed the requirement of 'systematic import'. This requires that classifications are 'natural' rather than 'artificial'. This rather vague requirement needs clarification. Simply stated, classifications which are natural are those in which those characteristics which determine class membership are associated either universally or, more likely, probabilistically, with other important characteristics. An example of such a classification is the division of humans into males and females on the basis of primary sexual characteristics. These characteristics are related to a large number of concomitant physical, physiological, and possibly psychological traits (Hempel 1961). Similarly, in the area of medicine, the division of patients exhibiting, amongst others, the symptoms of a cough and blood-stained sputum, into those who have pulmonary tuberculosis and those who have a bronchial carcinoma, is natural in the sense that those characteristics which determined their diagnosis are, at least practically or functionally, related to a number of other important characteristics of the patient, such as the drugs to which they will respond and the likely prognosis of their illness. Of course, if classificatory concepts are to retain their systematic import, they must be open to revision so that they can change if need be with systematic advances made in the field of which they are a part.

The application of the logical structure described above to the existing essentially Kraepelinian system of taxonomy of psychiatric disorders raises a number of problems. It is not possible to specify necessary and sufficient conditions for most psychiatric disorders. Rather, they are generally defined by the presence of some or most of a number of characteristic features, none of which is either necessary or sufficient for class membership. Thus, schizophrenia may be defined by the presence of some of the 'first rank' symptoms of schizophrenia (Schneider 1959) without it being necessary that the patient either exhibits all of these symptoms, or, indeed, any one of them. As a result, a diagnosis of schizophrenia is not simply a straightforward process of determining the attributes of the individual patient concerned and assigning them to the appropriate class of other individuals who possess the same known attributes. The process whereby an individual is assigned a diagnosis is complicated by the fact that a decision has to be made as to whether the combination of symptoms exhibited is sufficient for a diagnosis. In addition, the process is further complicated by the problem of deciding whether the symptoms exhibited are severe enough for them to qualify as such. Thus, attributes for class membership may not be merely absent or present, but subject to quantitative variation.

The difficulties with establishing class membership in the classification of psychological or psychiatric disorders lead directly to problems in both defining the corresponding classificatory concepts to be used and in determining their extension. Thus, the term schizophrenia may appear not to be very clearly defined and the class of those individuals who may be said to suffer from schizophrenia may have an indeterminate reference. As a result, psychiatrists disagree amongst themselves about the definition of this term and they may also disagree about whether a given individual is suffering from schizophrenia or some other disorder. Given that the terms used to refer to classificatory concepts are neither clearly specified nor used in the same way by all practitioners, clearly the classificatory system does not fulfil its first function of allowing adequate description and communication.

A further perhaps even more serious problem with the traditional psychiatric classificatory system is that, even if agreement could be achieved about the definition of the various disorders it attempts to classify, it is not clear that this classificatory scheme has 'systematic import'. Although the system distinguishes between, say, schizophrenia and affective disorder, those characteristics which determine that someone may be said to be suffering from schizophrenia as opposed to an affective disorder do not always appear to be appropriately related to important characteristics, such as the prognosis of the disorder and the most effective form of treatment. Thus, as Kendell (1975) notes, if someone is diagnosed as suffering from schizophrenia they are likely to be treated with phenothiazines and to recover completely, incompletely, or continue to have a chronic form of the disorder. If, on the other hand, a depressive disorder is diagnosed, the person is more likely to be treated with electroconvulsive therapy or tricyclic medication and to recover completely, incompletely, or not at all. However, whichever diagnosis is made, the treatment may involve phenothiazines or electroconvulsive therapy or tricyclic medication or even all three. It appears, therefore, that the traditional system of classification used in psychiatry does not even have systematic import in the sense of its classificatory concepts being systematically related to functional and practical considerations such as modes of treatment and likely prognosis. It certainly does not, with its symptom-based method of classification, appear to lend itself to the formulation of theoretical principles expressed in theoretical terms for the explanation and understanding of the disorders it classifies.

The existing system of psychiatric classification, therefore, seems to fail to meet the conditions necessary for it to perform the two most fundamental functions of a classificatory scheme. For this reason, it has attracted a great deal of criticism from both psychologists and psychiatrists, prompting Eysenck (1986) to write that 'psychiatry deals with disorders of unknown origin, treated by different psychiatrists in different ways, but hardly ever with much success'. Generally those who have raised objections against the existing Kraepelinian symptom-based classification system have argued that it should be abandoned altogether. These arguments are sometimes accompanied by a suggestion that it be replaced by a system based on some other criteria for classification.

There are essentially three related arguments which have been advanced in support of abandoning the traditional system of classification. First, it has been argued that this system of classification implies the notion of 'disease entities' which do not actually exist, and that the resulting 'medical model' is therefore misleading. Second, it has been argued that the system is neither reliable nor valid. Finally, it has been argued that the present method of classification assumes, wrongly, that psychiatric disorders are categorical rather than dimensional. Each of these arguments will be discussed in turn. This discussion will attempt to demonstrate that, although the existing classificatory system has shortcomings, these are not an intrinsic defect of classification as such; that some of the undoubted shortcomings of this system can be overcome; and that at present the existing system with all its problems is all that we have.

THE MEDICAL MODEL: SYMPTOMS, DISEASES AND DISEASE ENTITIES

One of the major criticisms that have been levelled at the Kraepelinian symptom-based classification system is that it assumes a traditional medical model (e.g. Menninger 1948, Szasz 1960, Eysenck & Rachman 1965, Kanfer & Saslow 1969, Rachman & Philips 1978, Rachman & Wilson 1980, Watts 1983). It is argued that this medical model is totally inappropriate for psychological or psychiatric disorders. Essentially, this model involves the recognition of what Ledley & Lusted (1959) have called a 'disease complex' and a 'symptom complex'. The disease complex refers to known or postulated pathological processes, while the symptom complex refers to the signs present in the individual patient which are thought to be the result of the underlying pathological process. This is the view which is embodied in the essentially rationalistic system of classification developed by Kraepelin, which assumes a finite number of disease entities, each with a distinct cause, psychological form or symptom pattern, outcome and cerebral pathology. Despite some opposition to this view from those adhering to a Hippocratic or empirical tradition, the rationalist position is the one which has prevailed.

Before considering the application of the rationalist view to psychological or psychiatric disorders, or indeed to modern medicine, it is necessary briefly to clarify the notion of disease itself. Clearly the notion of disease or illness is fundamental in medicine; yet, although familiar, it is rarely adequately defined. It is often pointed out that those definitions which have been offered are either hopelessly vague, or tautologous. In addition, they either exclude those who are generally regarded as ill, or include those who are not commonly regarded as such (Kendell 1975). Dictionary definitions, both medical and otherwise, tend to define disease in terms of sickness or impaired health, which is not very helpful; or in terms of a disturbance of function, leaving it unclear what would constitute such a disturbance. One view of disease or illness which was dominant until quite recently is that of disease as a demonstrable physical abnormality of some sort. This view probably originated from anatomical and histological evidence that illness was often accompanied by structural damage to the body, a view easily extended to the idea that physiological and biochemical abnormalities might also constitute illness. This concept of illness as some physical abnormality offered some objective criterion for establishing its presence, and also provided an explanation of the patient's symptoms. The problems with this view, however, are that it assumes that what defines abnormality is simply any departure from a clear, well-defined pattern of normality. However, the physical variability of human beings is such that it is not always obvious at what point such departure from normality begins. Hypertension is a good example of a condition where there is no sharp discontinuity between what is regarded as normal and what is regarded as abnormal. Even when such a discontinuity exists, as with certain congenital abnormalities, it is not always clear that one would wish to regard them as diseases. A further problem, and one which is particularly pertinent in the case of psychological or psychiatric disorders, is that many diseases or illnesses are initially defined by their characteristic symptoms and only later is the underlying physical abnormality identified. Thus, according to this view of diseases, at least in the early stages of knowledge, such conditions are not diseases; but these conditions may later come to be regarded as diseases when a corresponding physical abnormality is identified. Thus, defining disease in terms of demonstrable pathology results in a notion of disease which varies subject to the current state of knowledge. This means that one would have to say that Parkinson's disease used not to be a disease but now is one.

One way of dealing with the problem of what constitutes normality is to use a statistical concept (Cohen 1943). According to this view, a disease is a deviation from normality defined statistically. The problem with this view is that it fails to distinguish between harmful deviation from the norm and those deviations which are either neutral or beneficial. Scadding (1967) has attempted to overcome this problem by requiring that the deviation from normality must place the individual at a biological disadvantage; that is, reducing their chances for procreation or survival. Scadding offers the following formal definition of disease: 'the sum of the abnormal phenomena displayed by a group of living organisms in association with a specified common characteristic or set of characteristics by which they differ from the norm for their species in such a way as to place them at a biological disadvantage'. This definition explicitly stresses the statistical nature of abnormality, thus recognizing that the boundary between normality and abnormality is arbitrary; and it attempts to restrict such deviations to those which are harmful by the notion of biological disadvantage. However, biological disadvantage is itself far from clear. In these terms, homosexuality is a biological disadvantage; but few would wish to regard it as a disease. Also, biological disadvantage may not be as universal as it may at first seem. A characteristic may be biologically advantageous or otherwise, depending on the environmental circumstances. Kendell (1975) cites the example of the sickle cell trait, which in most environments would be disadvantageous, but is an advantage in one where malaria is endemic. Even the apparently clear notion of statistical normality may present problems when so little is known about normal functioning. For example, the distinction between normal and pathological grief may be difficult to draw, as may be the distinction between normal cleanliness and pathological cleaning rituals.

It appears, therefore, even from this brief discussion, that despite its importance in the medical model there is no clear or adequate definition for disease. The situation is not improved by a consideration of individual diseases in the field of general medicine, which reveals that they are defined in a variety of ways (Kendell 1975). Sometimes they are defined in terms of symptoms or constellations of symptoms (e.g. senile pruritus and migraine); sometimes in terms of morbid anatomy (e.g. mitral stenosis); sometimes in terms of bacteriological findings (e.g. tuberculosis and syphilis); and sometimes in terms of chromosomal architecture (e.g. Down's syndrome).

The above considerations support the view that Kraepelin's notion of disease entities, each with a single discrete cause, whose presence invariably produced the disease with its distinctive clinical picture, distinctive course, and distinctive neuropathology, is naive, even when applied to present-day general medicine. The notion of a single cause has given way to ideas about a complex chain or sequence of interacting events; and to the idea of there being a diversity of defining characteristics for individual diseases reflecting the diversity of their conceptual bases. Different diseases may thus be defined at different levels of analysis: for example, at the level of symptomatology, the level of a disorder of function, the level of morbid anatomy, and so on. Clearly, the naive Kraepelinian notion of disease fits the case of psychological or psychiatric disorders even less well than it fits the case of physical disorders. Most psychological or psychiatric disorders are defined at a descriptive clinical level in terms of their symptoms, or simply in terms of manifest abnormal behaviour and experiences. This is necessarily the case, as little is known about the antecedents of these phenomena or about any more fundamental dysfunction, be it psychological or physical. Indeed, critics of the use of the medical model in psychiatry have argued that in many disorders, such as anxiety, depression, and obsessive–compulsive disorders, in which abnormal behaviour and experience are a fundamental feature, there is little reason to assume an underlying pathology. This argument was advanced by Rachman & Philips (1978), who also pointed out that it is rare to find a single cause or a physical basis for psychological problems of this kind. They concluded from these arguments that these disorders are unlikely to be symptoms of an illness. They contrast disorders of this kind with general paresis and Korsakoff's syndrome, which they regard as fitting well into the medical model. Although they do not elaborate this argument, they appear to be claiming that general paresis and

Korsakoff's psychosis, unlike most psychological or psychiatric disorders, can legitimately be considered illnesses because in both cases there is demonstrable brain pathology, with a known cause, which produces the abnormal behaviour and experiences. Similar assumptions as to the nature of disease entities appear to have prompted Szasz (1960) and others to claim that disorders like schizophrenia do not exist.

Besides the fact that the medical model, at least as narrowly conceived, does not appear to fit the case of psychological or psychiatric disorders, critics of the model have also pointed to a number of practical implications of regarding someone as ill or having a disease. Briefly, if someone is ill a diagnosis of the illness or disease is likely to be considered appropriate and may be thought to help determine appropriate treatment. It is argued, however, that diagnosis is not particularly helpful in determining interventions in the field of psychological or psychiatric disorders (Menninger 1948, Kanfer & Saslow 1969, Rachman & Philips 1978, Watts 1983); and, furthermore, that it results in people being 'labelled' as patients. This process of labelling may, it is argued, have harmful and long-lasting effects on people's behaviour towards the patient so labelled, especially as many psychiatric diagnoses have strong pejorative connotations (Rosenhan 1973, Rachman & Wilson 1980).

The problems with the medical model have led critics to suggest that classification and diagnosis based on this model should be abandoned altogether (Menninger 1948, Kanfer & Saslow 1969, Rachman & Wilson 1980, Watts 1983). Traditional classification and diagnosis, it has been suggested by some, should be replaced with a lengthy and detailed formulation of each patient's predicament (Menninger 1963); while others suggest a detailed functional analysis of the antecedents and consequences of carefully defined problem behaviours (Kanfer & Saslow 1969). Both suggestions, although very different in content, emphasize the uniqueness of both the individual and the presenting problem; and they prescribe a formulation of the problem in a way which it is believed would be more directly related to treatment.

Although there are undoubted problems with the medical model in the understanding of psychological and psychiatric disorders, it is not justified to conclude that classification and diagnosis of these disorders should therefore be abandoned altogether. None of the arguments advanced points to intrinsic defects in classification as such, but merely to problems in one rather narrow interpretation of the medical model. Indeed, this interpretation is no longer even acceptable in general medicine. Both the notion of a formulation and that of a functional analysis which, it has been suggested, should replace classification and diagnosis, sacrifice the advantages of taxonomy for an approach which emphasizes the uniqueness of the individual. However, in so doing, it is implicitly assumed that in the case of psychological or psychiatric disorders, those characteristics which are unique to individuals are more important than those that they share with some others; and that classification is, therefore, of little value. In as much as this view denies the value of classification altogether, it implies that it is not possible to generalize from experiences with one individual to the case of another. Thus, if there are not significant similarities between individuals with psychological or psychiatric disorders, learning about such disorders from experience is not possible; nor, indeed, is it possible to communicate about these disorders. If this were so, it would not be possible to accumulate any scientific knowledge or understanding about psychopathology. However, such knowledge is clearly required in order to arrive at useful formulations or relevant functional analyses of an individual's presenting problems. Without classification, not only would research and communication not be possible, but it would also be impossible to plan rational psychiatric and psychological services.

While it is clear that comprehensive formulations or individual functional analyses cannot replace classification and diagnosis, this is not to deny the value of such individual approaches. Diagnosis, in the sense of assigning someone to one of the categories of a classification system of psychological disorders, is almost never adequate on its own for planning a treatment programme. Diagnosis does, however, set limits on what it is possible to achieve in treatment, and it does point to certain forms of treatment which are most likely to be successful while excluding others from consideration. It needs, however, to be supplemented with additional information about the individual. It is apparent, therefore, that in the case of psychological or psychiatric disorders, both diagnosis and a detailed analysis of the person's unique situation are required rather than one or the other.

If classification is inevitable, and the shortcomings of diagnosis discussed above are in fact problems with a rather rigid interpretation of the medical model underlying the existing classification system, then perhaps there is some other interpretation of the requirements of this model which better accord with the case of psychological or psychiatric disorders. It is of the utmost importance that such an interpretation can be defended because at present there simply does not seem to be an alternative to the existing classificatory system. Although there have been suggestions that the classificatory system based on symptoms should be replaced by one based on scores on cognitive or other psychological tests, by accounts of defence mechanisms, or by comprehensive analyses of behaviour, none of these suggestions has resulted in a novel system of classification (Kendell 1983).

Kendell (1975) has suggested that the traditional symptom-based classification system can be retained if diseases or disorders are regarded, not as entities which have a single discrete cause or underlying pathology, but as useful concepts. Such concepts are abstractions justified by their convenience, and they are liable to change when they no longer perform their intended function. The role of such concepts is to demarcate a group of people who manifest certain anomalous behaviour, have certain unusual experiences, have a relatively homogeneous response to certain treatments which do not have an analogous effect on others, and whose disorder has a relatively homogeneous outcome. Thus, Kendell has argued that the usefulness of the concept of schizophrenia is at present amply justified by the universal occurrence of the behavioural and experiential anomalies to which this term refers, by the biological disadvantage associated with these anomalies, by the evidence that these abnormalities are, at least in part, genetically determined, and by the influence on them of certain drugs which do not have similar effects on others. He argues, further, that the term may well be replaced if, as a result of further research, it loses its usefulness. It will not, however, be replaced because it is suddenly realized that it does not exist.

Whether, in the future, the symptom-based classificatory system will be replaced by classification in terms of some more fundamental abnormality, be it physiologically or psychologically defined, is entirely dependent upon whether such abnormalities are identified by future research. This is an entirely empirical matter and not one which can be decided *a priori*. In the case of Korsakoff's psychosis and general paresis a fundamental abnormality has been identified; and, as a result, Rachman & Philips (1978) see these disorders as quite consistent with the medical model. However, as noted earlier, in the case of other psychological or psychiatric disorders, they argue *a priori* that the medical model is inappropriate. It is not clear how these psychological disorders differed from the case of Korsakoff's psychosis or general paresis before their fundamental abnormalities were identified. It must remain an open question whether equivalent fundamental abnormalities, be they physiological or psychological, may be found in the case of these psychological or psychiatric disorders. Indeed, a two-process learning theory account of phobic anxiety and, some would argue, obsessive–compulsive neurosis, is an attempt to specify just such an underlying abnormality. Any change from a symptom-based classificatory scheme to one based, for example, on the specification of underlying abnormalities will not be the result of discovering an entity but of it becoming apparent that it is more useful, or has greater systematic import, to classify in terms of such abnormalities.

Such a Kendellian interpretation of the medical model appears quite consistent with what is at present known about psychological or psychiatric disorders. Furthermore, adopting such an interpretation of the model does not appear to involve a commitment to any view about how such disorders will be defined or understood in the future.

RELIABILITY AND VALIDITY

As discussed earlier, if a classificatory concept is to perform its intended function, it must be capable of being used reliably in order to identify valid classes of whatever is being classified. Reliability is concerned with the accuracy and repeatability of the defining characteristics of a particular concept and its corresponding class; while validity concerns the extent and importance of the correlates of such class membership. These notions of reliability and validity are obviously related to one another: while low reliability necessarily leads to low validity, high levels of reliability clearly do not ensure high levels of validity. Both reliability and validity are crucial to the classification of psychological or psychiatric disorders. A diagnosis is of little value unless assigning someone to a diagnostic group has certain useful implications; and, if assignment to a group is itself the subject of disagreement, the usefulness of these implications will inevitably be reduced. Given the importance of these two notions, it is necessary before advocating the continued use of the existing system of classification to assess whether it can be defended against charges that it cannot meet acceptable standards of reliability and validity.

Reliability

Empirical evidence suggesting that psychiatric diagnosis was not reliable first began emerging in the 1930s (Masserman & Carmichael 1938). Beck (1962) reviewed a series of eight studies concerning reliability carried out in the intervening years and concluded that, if organic cases were excluded, none of these studies achieved an overall inter-judge agreement rate for specific diagnoses higher than 42%. He drew attention in this review to a number of methodological problems in the studies which, he argued, made it impossible to draw any firm conclusions about the reliability of psychiatric diagnoses. Others have been less cautious in their conclusions and have questioned the entire enterprise of diagnosis and classification in psychiatry on the grounds of poor reliability (e.g. Passamanick 1963).

It is apparent from the early studies that lack of agreement between observers can arise from at least two sources. First, poor reliability may be the result of observers not using a standard nomenclature or not using a nomenclature which is sufficiently clearly defined for it to be applicable in a standard way. Thus, there may not be a consensus on the criteria to be employed in deciding, for example, whether someone is to be diagnosed as suffering from schizophrenia; nor even a consensus on the actual categories which comprise the classificatory system. Second, reliability may be low because the diagnoses of various observers are not made under the same standard conditions. Diagnoses may thus be made on the basis of varying amounts of information elicited in a variety of ways.

An attempt was made to minimize at least one of these potential sources of unreliability in a study conducted by Beck et al (1962). The nomenclature of the first edition of the *Diagnostic and Statistical Manual* of the American Psychiatric Association (1952) was used as the basis for classification. This was further supplemented by working definitions regarding specific criteria for each diagnostic category. All interviews were carried out by experienced psychiatrists. Thus, while considerable effort was made to ensure a standard nomenclature, rather less effort was directed at ensuring that information was gained in a standard way. A similar study, conducted by Kreitman et al (1961) in Britain, also made considerable attempts to agree on working definitions for key terms, while similarly paying rather less attention to the elicitation of information. Although in both studies overall agreement between raters was higher than the level previously estimated by Beck, the overall agreement rates on specific diagnoses in the two studies was still disappointingly low: 54% for the American study and 63% for the British study.

The widespread evidence that the reliability of psychiatric diagnosis was low, together with the demonstration of serious international differences in the usage of key diagnostic terms (Cooper et al 1972), resulted in a general recognition of the need both for unambiguous rules for applying diagnostic terms and for standardized methods of eliciting information from patients. The need to use a standardized, well-defined nomenclature has led to the development of a number of sets of operational definitions of key psychiatric disorders. The first of these were those produced by Feighner et al (1972) for each of the 16 psychiatric disorders in the second edition of the *Diagnostic and Statistical Manual* (American Psychiatric Association 1969). This was later revised to produce the Research Diagnostic Criteria (RDC) (Spitzer et al 1978) which contained operational definitions for 25 diagnostic categories. More recently, the development of the third edition of the *Diagnostic and Statistical Manual* (American Psychiatric Association 1980) provided an even more comprehensive operationally defined classificatory scheme. In parallel with these developments, research workers in both Britain and the United States were also addressing the need for standardized methods of eliciting from patients the information to which these operational criteria would be applied. This work led, in Britain, to the development of the Present State Examination or PSE (Wing et al 1974), and in the United States to the development of, amongst others, the Schedule of Affective Disorders and Schizophrenia or SADS (Endicott & Spitzer 1978). The use of such operational criteria and standardized interviews has resulted in greatly increased levels of inter-judge reliability for specific psychiatric diagnoses (Matarazzo 1983). For example, in an assessment of the reliability of diagnosis using RDC and the SADS, kappa coefficients of agreement for the major psychiatric disorders were between 0.80 and 0.89 (Spitzer et al 1978).

The achievement of acceptable levels of reliability in the diagnosis of psychological or psychiatric disorders suggests that there is nothing about these disorders which renders them unclassifiable in principle; nor does it appear to be the case that the traditional classificatory system was inherently inappropriate to the classification of these disorders. Technical improvement in the definition of the classificatory system and in the methods of eliciting information from patients has clearly demonstrated that the traditional system is indeed workable. However, although reliability is a prerequisite without which an acceptable level of validity cannot be achieved, as already noted, in itself it does not, of course, ensure validity.

Validity

Validity, as emphasized earlier, refers to the correlates of class membership, to the systematic import of classificatory concepts. As discussed at the beginning of this chapter, in the realm of the classification and diagnosis of psychiatric or psychological disorders there are two related aspects to the notion of validity. The first concerns the practical or functional usefulness of diagnosis; that is, whether assigning people to diagnostic categories has predictive validity in terms of important prognostic and therapeutic implications. The second aspect concerns the theoretical usefulness of the classificatory system; that is, whether the existing symptom-based system identifies disorders in such a way that it enables progress to be made towards the understanding and explanation of these disorders. A major problem of this way of assessing the validity of classificatory concepts is that whether a given concept is theoretically useful in this latter sense can only be firmly established once greater theoretical understanding of that particular disorder is achieved; but greater theoretical understanding of the disorder will only be achieved if it is first clearly recognized and distinguished from other disorders at a clinical level. As noted earlier, it is not clear that the existing system of classification could be said to be valid in either of these two respects. Very few attempts have been made directly to establish the predictive validity of psychiatric diagnoses. However, evidence of relevance to the issue is implicit in numerous therapeutic trials and outcome studies. In recent years it has been reasonably well established that lithium carbonate is an effective treatment for manic-depressive disorders (Coppen et al 1982); that phenothiazines are effective for acute schizophrenia (Hirsch 1983); that exposure and response prevention is the most effective treatment for obsessive–compulsive disorders (Rachman & Hodgson 1980); and that cognitive therapy is effective in the treatment of depression (Gelder 1986). The fact that each of the treatments mentioned is more effective with one category of disorder than with others, and that the use of such treatments is most likely to result in a certain known outcome, tends to establish the validity of these categories. These categories would be even more firmly established if there were treatments which were both specific to a single diagnostic category and invariably effective for members of that category. However, this is not the case in the treatment of these disorders. Many of the treatments mentioned are effective, to some extent, in other clinical conditions; and none is invariably effective even within one condition.

In the absence of knowledge about aetiology or underlying pathological processes on the basis of which to establish the theoretical validity of current classificatory concepts, various statistical methods have been employed in an attempt to establish discontinuities between categories of psychiatric disorder. A variety of multivariate techniques, such as factor analysis, cluster analysis and discriminant function analysis, have been used to measure either similarity (cluster analysis) or separation (discriminant function analysis) between groups, in an attempt to establish that such groups do indeed reflect independent categories. The use of these techniques as a means of validating classificatory systems has been discussed in detail by both Kendell (1975, 1982) and Paykel (1981). Both of these authors suggest that great caution needs to be exercised in interpreting the results obtained from studies using such statistical techniques, emphasizing that their limitations need to be clearly recognized. Kendell (1982) and Paykel (1981) both conclude that discriminant function analysis has largely failed to demonstrate obvious discontinuities between various diagnostic categories, such as between schizophrenia and affective disorder (e.g. Kendell & Gourlay 1970a, Brockington et al 1979), and between 'endogenous' and 'reactive' depression (e.g. Kendell & Gourlay 1970b). Factor analysis and cluster analysis have produced, particularly in the area of the classification of depression, evidence that various diagnostic categories do reflect distinct groups, although this has been less than definitive (Overall 1971, Paykel 1971).

Thus statistical techniques have tended to provide further support, albeit of a rather weak nature, for the validity of a number of existing categories. This evidence on validity is supplemented by evidence that the liability to develop some major disorders, such as schizophrenia and manic-depressive disorder, is genetically transmitted, that these disorders 'breed true', and that their symptom patterns remain stable over many years (Kendell 1982).

Taken together, the evidence on the validity of psychiatric diagnostic categories is far from conclusive. The fact that this evidence is weak certainly does not imply that the whole enterprise of classification is misconceived, but rather that the existing categories are in some cases not sufficiently well defined or sufficiently well distinguished from each other. This suggests that rather than abandoning classification and diagnosis, every attempt should be made to improve the existing system. It seems that this task can best be pursued by careful clinical observation rather than by the further application of sophisticated statistical techniques (Paykel 1981). An example of a recent improvement arising out of such clinical observation is Russell's (1979) account of bulimia nervosa (see Chapter 12) as a relatively distinct disorder.

CATEGORIES AND DIMENSIONS

Classification, as it has been discussed so far, is a categorical enterprise. A class is determined by some classificatory concept which represents its defining features, and a given object or member of a population either falls within this category or not, depending on whether it posseses the required defining characteristics. This system, used to great advantage in botany and zoology, appears to work well when the distribution of characteristics which form the basis of the classificatory system is discontinuous within the universe of discourse or population under study. However, objects within a universe of discourse or individuals within a population often resist categorization of this kind. This is because those characteristics which suggest themselves as a fruitful basis for classification are properties which are continuously distributed within that universe or population. Any given individual, therefore, does not either possess or lack this characteristic; rather, they exhibit this property to a greater or lesser extent. When this is the case, the relationship between individuals in the population is probably better expressed by assigning individuals to a position on one or more axes or dimensions. Assignment to such a position implies that the relationship between the individuals, as defined by their relative position on the dimension in question, is one of linear, or at least quasi-linear, ordering (Hempel 1961).

Although categorical classsificatory systems are much more widely used that dimensional ones, the latter do have a number of advantages. Dimensional systems obviously allow for much finer distinctions than categorical classification; and they are more flexible, particularly in dealing with cases which appear to fall on the borderline between two categories. Given these advantages, it has been argued that the existing categorical system of classification in psychiatry should be replaced with a dimensional one. Eysenck (1960, 1986) has been the foremost proponent of this view, arguing both against a categorical system of classification and for a dimensional approach. He has argued that the existing system of classification in psychiatry is based on a medical model of disease which is inappropriate because it assumes disease categories with separate and specific aetiologies, as is the case with physical illness. This assumption, he argues, leads to the development of arbitrary categories of disorder which totally fail to accord with reality. Eysenck notes that this arbitrariness is reflected in the system of multiple diagnosis whereby a patient may be diagnosed as an 'anxious hysteric with schizophrenic undertones'; or a 'depressive obsessive compulsive individual with psychopathic tendencies'. This state of affairs has arisen, Eysenck maintains, because 'slavish adherence' to the medical model has resulted in psychiatrists failing to recognize that mental disorder is not sharply discontinuous with normality. This conclusion, that the division between normality and abnormality is dimensional rather than categorical, is, he claims, supported by modern empirical research and the method of criterion analysis. In particular, he has suggested that a dimensional system consisting of the three major dimensions of psychoticism, neuroticism and extroversion–introversion replace the existing categorical system in psychiatry.

The argument Eysenck advances about the inappropriateness of the medical model has already been considered and will not be discussed further here. Eysenck's crucial claim of interest is that empirical research and the method of criterion analysis clearly support a dimensional rather than a categorical approach to psychiatric disorders. Eysenck (1986) has recently described the rationale of the procedure of criterion analysis. Briefly, it aims to elucidate the question of whether two groups, one of which is regarded as psychiatrically normal and the other of which is diagnosed as, for example, 'psychotic', are categorically distinct. It involves the selection of a number of objective psychological and physiological tests which clearly differentiate the two groups at a statistically significant level. These tests may then be said to be relevant to the distinction between the normal group and the psychotic group; but, obviously, they do not embody all possible distinctions between these two groups. The scores on these tests are then intercorrelated for each group. If the two groups are on a continuum from 'normal' to 'psychotic', it would be predicted that the pattern of intercorrelations would be similar for the two groups; while, if the groups were categorically distinct, there should be no such similarity of patterns of intercorrelations. Similarity of patterning is established by carrying out factor analyses separately for the two groups and testing whether the first factor extracted from the normal group could be formally identified with the first factor extracted from the psychotic group. Eysenck (1950, 1952) conducted a number of such analyses using data from both psychotic and neurotic groups, and concluded provisionally that both psychoticism and neuroticism are dimensionsal and not categorical variables. Eysenck (1986) has reviewed further work, using what he calls the 'proportionality method', which is a reduced form of criterion analysis, and has concluded that 'the proper model of psychiatric abnormality should be based on continuity rather than on categorical differences between diagnostic groups'.

The research evidence cited by Eysenck appears to establish that there is continuity between both psychotic and neurotic populations and normal populations. One limitation of these findings is that the continuity can only be said to exist between these populations in those respects measured by the test battery (Kendell 1975). Despite the fact that the tests were chosen in order to give maximum differences between the groups, they do not constitute tests of the usual aspects or attributes employed by clinicians to discriminate between clinical and non-clinical populations. Indeed, the meaning or theoretical rationale of the test battery employed in the early criterion analysis studies is obscure and it is unlikely that these measures illuminate the underlying condition responsible for psychotic or neurotic symptoms (Bishop 1977). Although this method of analysis may demonstrate that there is some underlying graded trait, in Eysenck's terms 'psychoticism' or 'neuroticism', on which those with psychological disorders may differ from normal people to varying degrees, this does not establish that, for example, schizophrenia or any other form of psychiatric disorder is, in fact, continuously distributed in this way.

Whilst Eysenck's argument, in particular the implication he draws for classification in psychiatry, is less than conclusive, it must also be conceded that the evidence supporting a categorical classificatory system is far from satisfactory. As discussed earlier, the search for discontinuities between one psychiatric disorder and another has yielded disappointing results. Discriminant function analyses which have been used in an attempt to establish that there are genuine 'points of rarity' between disorders have produced little convincing evidence that interforms between adjacent disorders are less common than the two disorders themselves (Kendell 1975). Cluster analysis has produced some evidence in support of categories, especially concerning the distinction between manic and depressive phases of manic-depressive disorder (Everitt et al 1971), and between 'psychotic' and 'non-psychotic' depression. It must be conceded that this evidence is not strong and neither is it extensive.

There is therefore some evidence to support both categorical and dimensional systems of classification in psychiatry and no clear evidence on which to base a definitive conclusion. In fact, the debate about dimensions and categories cannot ultimately be resolved by the application of statistical techniques which make prior assumptions about the underlying structure of the data (Maxwell 1971, Kendell 1975). Until knowledge advances about the aetiology and underlying processes involved in psychological disorders, it appears that which system is adopted is largely a matter of practicalities. As mentioned earlier, the main advantage of a dimensional system is that it is flexible and does not involve the loss of fine-grained information. Thus individuals on the borderline between two apparent disorders can be adequately characterized. Furthermore, dimensional information can always be converted into categories if the need arises. However, dimensional systems require representation in a somewhat inaccessible form. Any system involving more than one dimension can only be handled geometrically or algebraically, and with greater numbers of dimensions only algebraic representation is possible. This is not an intrinsic defect of such systems, but it does make them less accessible to clinicians without specialist mathematical knowledge. Also, in clinical practice, it is often the case that dimensions have to be converted to categories before the information they represent can be usefully applied. For example, any decision about treatment, such as whether cognitive therapy or electroconvulsive therapy (ECT) might be the most appropriate form of treatment, will require some way of grouping those who respond best to one or other of these treatments. As has been argued throughout this chapter, the great advantage of categorical systems is their ease of communication and their facilitation of aetiological research.

CONCLUSION

Throughout this chapter it has been emphasized that classification is necessary for both scientific and clinical purposes. There are clearly a number of problems with the existing Kraepelinian system in psychiatry. Although this system was originally based on a narrow and unacceptable interpretation of psychiatric disorders as disease entities, it is possible to retain the system without accepting this notion of disease entities. Problems of reliability have not turned out to be insuperable. This is of crucial significance, despite the fact that in ordinary clinical practice psychiatric diagnoses may often be unreliable. The major shortcoming of the system is that the validity of many of the diagnostic categories used is not firmly established. However, despite these problems, the system forms a framework, albeit flawed, on the basis of which further improvements can be made.

REFERENCES

American Psychiatric Association 1952 Diagnostic and statistical manual of mental disorders. 1st edn. APA, Washington, DC
American Psychiatric Association 1969 Diagnostic and statistical manual of mental disorders. 2nd edn. APA. Washington, DC
American Psychiatric Association (1980) Diagnostic and statistical manual of mental disorders. 3rd edn. APA, Washington, DC
Beck A T 1962 Reliability of psychiatric diagnoses: a critique of systematic studies. American Journal of Psychiatry 119: 210–216
Beck A T, Ward C, Mendelson M, Mock J, Erbaugh J 1962 Reliability of psychiatric diagnosis: a study of consistency of clinical judgements and ratings. American Journal of Psychiatry 119: 351–357
Bishop D V M 1977 The P scale and psychosis. Journal of Abnormal Psychology 86: 127–134
Bridgman P W 1927 The logic of modern physics. Macmillan, New York
Brockington I F, Kendell R E, Wainwright S, Hillier V F, Walker J 1979 The distinction between the affective psychoses and schizophrenia. British Journal of Psychiatry 135: 243–248
Cohen H, 1943 The nature method and purpose of diagnosis. Cambridge University Press, Cambridge
Cooper J E, Kendell R E, Gurland B J, Sharpe L, Copeland J R M, Simon R 1972 Psychiatric diagnosis in New York and London. Maudsley Monograph No. 20. Oxford University Press, London
Coppen A, Metcalfe M, Wood K 1982 Lithium. In: Paykel E (ed) Handbook of affective disorders. Churchill Livingstone, Edinburgh
Endicott J, Spitzer R L 1978 A diagnostic interview: the Schedule for Affective Disorders and Schizophrenia. Archives of General Psychiatry 35: 837–844
Everitt B J, Gourlay A J, Kendell R E 1971 An attempt at validation of traditional psychiatric syndromes by cluster analysis. British Journal of Psychiatry 119: 399–412
Eysenck H J 1950 Criterion analysis: an application of the hypotheticodeductive method to factor analysis. Psychological Review 57: 38–53
Eysenck H J 1952 Schizothymia–cyclothymia as a dimension of personality. Journal of Personality 20: 345–384
Eysenck H J 1960 Classification and the problem of diagnosis. In: Eysenck H J (ed) Handbook of Abnormal Psychology. 1st edn. Pitman, London
Eysenck H J 1986 A critique of contemporary classification and diagnosis. In: Millon T, Klerman G (eds) Contemporary directions in psychopathology: towards DSM IV. Guilford Press, New York
Eysenck H J, Rachman S 1965 Causes and Cures of Neuroses. Routledge & Kegan Paul, London

Feighner J P, Robins E, Guze S B, Woodruff R A, Winokur G, Munoz R 1972 Diagnostic criteria for use in psychiatric research. Archives of General Psychiatry 26: 57–63

Gelder M 1986 Cognitive therapy. In: Granville-Grossman K (ed) Recent advances in clinical psychiatry 5. Churchill Livingstone, Edinburgh

Hempel C G 1961 Introduction to problems of taxonomy. In: Zubin J (ed) Field studies in the mental disorders. Grune & Stratton, New York

Hirsch S R 1983 Medication and physical treatment of schizophrenia. In: Wing J K, Wing L (eds) Handbook of psychiatry 3: psychoses of uncertain aetiology. Cambridge University Press, Cambridge

Kanfer F H, Saslow G 1969 Behavioural analysis: an alternative to diagnostic classification. Archives of General Psychiatry 12: 529–538

Kendell R E 1975 The role of diagnosis in psychiatry. Blackwell, Oxford

Kendell R E 1982 The choice of diagnostic criteria for biological research. Archives of General Psychiatry 39: 1334–1339

Kendell R E 1983 The principles of classification in relation to mental disease. In: Shepherd M, Zangwill O L (eds) Handbook of psychiatry 1: general psychopathology. Cambridge University Press, Cambridge

Kendell R E, Gourlay J 1970a The clinical distinction between the affective psychoses and schizophrenia. British Journal of Psychiatry 117: 261–266

Kendell R E, Gourlay J 1970b The clinical distinction between psychotic and neurotic depression. British Journal of Psychiatry 117: 257–260

Kreitman N, Sainsbury P, Morrissey J, Towers J, Scrivener J 1961 The reliability of psychiatric assessment: an analysis. Journal of Mental Science 107: 887–980

Ledley R S, Lusted L B 1959 Reasoning foundations of medical diagnosis. Science 130: 9–21

Masserman J H, Carmichael H T 1938 Diagnosis and prognosis in psychiatry. Journal of Mental Science 84: 893–946

Matarazzo J D 1983 The reliability of psychiatric and psychological diagnosis. Clinical Psychology Review 3: 103–145

Maxwell A E 1971 Multivariate statistical methods and classification problems. British Journal of Psychiatry 119: 121–127

Menninger K 1948 Changing concepts of disease. Annals of Internal Medicine 29: 318–325

Menninger K 1963 The vital balance. Penguin, New York

Overall J E 1971 Major phenomenological sub-types in a general psychiatric population. Diseases of the Nervous System 32: 383–387

Passamanick B 1963 On the neglect of diagnosis. American Journal of Orthopsychiatry 33: 397–398

Paykel E S 1971 Classification of depressed patients: a cluster analysis derived grouping. British Journal of Psychiatry 118: 275–288

Paykel E S 1981 Have multivariate statistics contributed to classification? British Journal of Psychiatry 139: 357–362

Putnam H 1975 The meaning of meaning. In: Gunderson K (ed) Language, mind and knowledge. University of Minnesota Press, Minneapolis

Rachman, S J, Hodgson R J 1980 Obsessions and compulsions. Prentice-Hall, New Jersey

Rachman S J, Philips C 1978 Psychology and medicine. Penguin, New York

Rachman S J, Wilson G T 1980 The effects of psychological therapy. Pergamon Press, Oxford

Rosenhan D L 1973 On being sane in insane places. Science 179: 250–258

Russell G F M 1979 Bulimia nervosa: an ominous variant of anorexia nervosa. Psychological Medicine 9: 429–448

Scadding J G 1967 Diagnosis: the clinician and the computer. Lancet 2: 877–882

Schneider K 1959 Klinische Psychopathologie. Translation of 5th edn by Hamilton M W. Grune & Stratton , New York

Spitzer R L, Endicott J, Robins E 1978 Research diagnostic criteria. Archives of General Psychiatry 35: 773–782

Szasz T S 1960 The myth of mental illness. American Psychologist 15: 113–118

Watts F 1983 Mental illness In: Liddell A (ed) The practice of clinical psychology in Great Britain. Wiley, Chichester.

Wing J K, Cooper J E, Sartorius N 1974 The measurement and classification of psychiatric symptoms. Cambridge University Press, Cambridge

3   German E. Berrios

Historical background to abnormal psychology

INTRODUCTION

The development of abnormal psychology is treated with reticence by historians of psychology (Boring 1950, Watson 1978, Lowry 1971, Murphy 1967, Klein 1970, Reisman 1976, Schultz 1981, Maher & Maher 1979, etc.). This is not surprising as psychological historiography has mainly concentrated on the philosophical origins of its subject; on the historical mechanisms that led to its 'separation' from philosophy; and on the reliability and validity of competing psychological theories (Berrios 1975).

Things have not been different in the case of the history of psychiatry. Historians have mostly chronicled its social and political aspects and neglected the 'semiology' (study of signs) of insanity (Foucault 1972a, Castel 1977, Dörner 1969, Blasius 1980, Scull 1979, Donnelly 1983). Hence no effort has been made to understand why it was only towards the end of the nineteenth century that concepts of normal psychology began to be applied to the disorders of the mind. One answer to this latter question may be that psychological theorizing, as illustrated by the work of Rochoux (1842), Cabanis (Losserand 1967, Mora 1981, Staum 1980), Maine de Biran (Royer-Collard 1843, Drevet 1968), James Mill (Warren 1921), Royer-Collard (Swain 1978), Cousin (Ravaisson 1885), Herbart (Ribot 1885), Garnier (Ravaisson 1885) or Bain (Greenway 1973), was too abstract to be applied to disordered minds. Another is that the nineteenth century inherited what can be called a 'social' definition of madness and that it took the best part of the century to develop a medical and psychological account.

As a result of this endeavour two views on the symptoms of insanity can be found at the end of the nineteenth century. One, variously called psychological pathology, medical psychology, descriptive psychopathology or clinical semiology, included descriptions which originated in the asylum and was based upon the assumption that the behaviour of insanity was unrelated to normal behaviour (Berrios 1984a). Another, variously called abnormal psychology or pathological psychology, considered the symptoms of insanity to be exaggerations or quantitative deviations of normal behaviour (Dumas 1908). The 'discontinuous' view appeared earlier and it was not before the end of the century that the two converged in the work of Kraepelin, Ribot, Luys, Raymond, Janet and Freud. This convergence remains a source of tension in abnormal psychology.

DEFINITIONS AND HISTORIOGRAPHY

For the purposes of this chapter psychology is defined as a set of more or less technical languages that have as their main purpose the description of behaviour (both human and animal) and the explanation of its inner mechanisms and environmental contingencies. Psychopathology, *mutatis mutandis*, is defined as the description and/or explanation of deviancy or abnormality.

In the USA the terms psychopathology and psychiatry are used almost interchangeably. In Europe, since the late nineteenth century, the former term has had a narrower meaning and has been used to refer to the 'software' aspects of mental illness. Consequently a descriptive and a psychodynamic psychopathology are recognized. The former, in turn, is subdivided into phenomenological and experimental.

By 'language' is meant an array of terms, rules and models. Language is used here in a literal sense. It should be possible, therefore, to show that descriptive psychopathology is a system of 'signs' and is endowed with a grammar and a syntax. Consequently the existence of signs, signifieds and a community of interpreters can be postulated (Barthes 1972, Lantéri Laura 1966).

By 'behaviour' is meant overt, observable activity and also subjective experience, whether described by the individual himself or guessed by others; 'inner structures' include real or conceptual descriptions of the nervous system and various explanatory hypothetical constructs. 'Outer structures' include dyadic interactions, groups, crowds, Zeitgebers, pheromones and other real or conceptual cues considered as part of the contingency system.

The notion of 'sign' is not free from ambiguity in the context of abnormal psychology. A distinction must be made between cases where the sign relates to an underlying dysfunction in the same way in which smoke relates to fire (e.g. disorientation) and cases where the sign is unlikely to reflect a specific neurobiological disorder (e.g. 'approximate answers' or manipulative behaviour). In this latter case the sign only 'signifies' the fragment of abnormal behaviour in the same way that 'red sky means good weather'. Clearer agreements on meaning and related reliability issues may be more important in the second case.

An advantage of utilizing language as the 'guiding metaphor' is that it encourages the search for the mediational aspects of psychopathology. Thus the latter can be conceived of as an interphase (or mediational system) between clinical observer and patient; that is, as providing the purchase for social and political variables.

Operational definitions help the historian to organize historical reconstruction but also may foster overselective searching. Hence an effort must be made not to pass by expired psychological views as they are likely to have contributed, as much as those still extant, to the development of the discipline.

An additional difficulty in the case of abnormal psychology is the scanty information available on what actually went on behind closed doors between the nineteenth-century alienist or clinical psychologist and his patient. Hence the history of abnormal psychology will tend to be that of its written language rather than of its language in action.

Another source of bias must be mentioned. It is a historical fact that semiology was born out of the observation of the insane. The 'psychological' view of the neuroses, as entertained nowadays, did not exist before 1880 (López Piñero 1983, Drinka 1984). Hysteria, neurasthenia, hypochondria, peripheral vasomotor disorders, etc., did not yet fall within the purview of alienists and hence the rich variety of behavioural forms that characterized these states contributed little to the formation of psychiatric semiology. In other words the semiology of insanity and of the organic disorders was not only *the oldest* but also provided the conceptual matrix for the development of all subsequent psychiatric semiologies.

Finally it must be mentioned, although there will be no space to deal with it at any length, that two psychological theories, Faculty Psychology (Albrecht 1970, Brooks 1976) and Associationism (Warren 1921, Hoeldtke 1967, Oberg 1976), provide the ideological context in relation to which both normal and abnormal psychological descriptions took place. At the end of the nineteenth century both had reached an uneasy compromise.

THE DEVELOPMENT OF DESCRIPTIVE PSYCHOPATHOLOGY

Abnormal behaviour and mental experiences have been recognized and described in Western culture since antiquity. These descriptions combine verbal portraits of overt behaviour (e.g. mania) or theoretical accounts (e.g. melancholia) (Berrios 1987a).

At the beginning of the nineteenth century the view started in medicine (initially in France) that diseases were not situated in some conceptual inner space but occupied a real space in the body (Ackerknecht 1967, Lesch 1984). The definition of 'body' itself underwent gradual modification as it was successively based on the notions of organ, tissue and cell (Laín Entralgo 1978, Albarracin 1983). Three different conceptual realms were recognized: aetiology, site and manifestations of disease; the latter led to a 'semiology', i.e. to a science of the signs of disease (Barthes 1972).

The concept of 'sign' also changed during this period. A sign was no longer just a symbolic manifestation but became a real indicator or external representation of a localized inner pathology. The further development of medical manoeuvres such as palpation and auscultation (what Foucault called the refinement of the medical gaze) (Foucault 1972b) led to the identification of new signs and to operational definitions in terms of description, intensity and frequency. The complex realm of the 'pathological' yielded its mystery and, as Canguilhem (1966) has shown, became a source of signs. The gaze of the physician was directed away from the surface and towards the lesion sited deep in the body.

This momentous conceptual shift, called by historians the 'anatomo-clinical view' (López Piñero 1983), led to the establishment of a *correlational paradigm*. Signs led to organs, organs were examined pre- or postmortem and structural changes identified. The success of this approach (and also its limitations) depended upon the identification of a 'lesion' (Berrios 1985c). This was defined at the beginning of the nineteenth century (perhaps too optimistically) in anatomical terms. Repeated failure in the finding of specific anatomical lesions, technical limitations, and the progress of physiology, led after the 1850s to a redefinition of the concept of lesion in *physiological* terms. This made possible a third development towards the end of the century, namely its further redefinition in *psychological* terms. The neuroses went typically through these three stages (López Piñero & Morales Meseguer 1970).

A similar path was followed by the concept of disease in psychiatry. Madness had been a molar category until the early nineteenth century; mad behaviour was viewed 'in toto' and not as an array of individual 'signs'. The development of semiology during this period can thus be described as the gradual fractioning of the old categories (Berrios 1984a). The resulting fractions were called the 'elementary signs' (Griesinger 1867).

Hence there was little interest in how madness might relate to individual parts of the body. Once again the neuroses provide a good example. During the late eighteenth century this class included all affections of the nervous system, i.e. the 'nervous disorders' (Bowman 1975). But it would be wrong to equate it with any current concept of neurological disease (Berrios 1984b). In the case of the neuroses it was the most general properties of the nervous system, 'vibration' and 'motion' that were affected (Riese 1949, Jackson 1970).

According to the 'neuralpathology' medical theory the central nervous system was the supreme principle and controller of the body (Rath 1954). General and localized disorders of the nervous system could thus give rise to all manner of diseases. All these together went to constitute the class that Cullen in the late eighteenth century called 'neuroses'. It is not surprising therefore that it included conditions as wide apart as asthma, diabetes mellitus, apoplexy, hysteria and all the current neuroses and psychoses (Thompson 1827).

A movement away from this speculative holism was only possible in the wake of two major changes in medical thinking: one related to the reconceptualization of the body, i.e. the postulation of new units of analysis; the other to the development of a semantic or representational theory which could formalize the way in which symptoms related to disease (Lain Entralgo 1978).

The actors

The alienist cuts a reluctant figure during the early nineteenth century. A far cry from the greedy Scullian entrepreneur (Scull 1979), he was legislated into the asylums by the 1828 Amendment to Wynn's Act in Great Britain (Jones 1972) and by the 1838 Act in France (Petitjean et al 1982). Once caught in the medical, social and legal web that was the nineteenth-century mental asylum, the alienist had to confront the complexity of madness armed with almost no descriptive categories.

Analysis of clinical entries in earlier asylum logbooks (in most European countries) shows the traditional categories in operation; patients were described as globally manic, melancholic, phrenzied, demented or lethargic. Gross behavioural categories, added to simple putative causes, were about the only descriptions that the early asylum alienist could muster (Berrios 1984a).

Admission procedures and the remnants of the old 'wild beast test', i.e. the view that the insane person was no different from a beast (Platt & Diamond 1965, Walker 1968) determined the type of patient seen in the asylum before and during the early nineteenth century. All admissions were compulsory and hence clear evidence of marked behavioural disorganization was required. Severe delusional or hallucinatory states, aggression and agitation, acute delirium and suicidal behaviour, in addition to mental retardation, epilepsy and other paroxysmal organic states, qualified for admission. This meant that the underlying illness was either an acute or chronic brain syndrome or a severe psychosis. The mad behaviour seen in the asylum during this early period was, in general, so different from anything resembling 'the normal' that it would not often have occurred to alienists to resort to treatises of normal psychology to describe or understand it.

On the other hand, the authors of psychological books, mainly philosophers and naturalists, had little knowledge of asylum madness. Consequently there was little cross-fertilization. There are, of course, historical exceptions. Kant wrote with some interest on 'the diseases of the head' although there is little evidence that he did so out of personal acquaintance (Jalley et al 1977). In France, Cabanis (Mora 1981, Staum 1980), and the Royer-Collard brothers (one was a philosopher and the other an alienist) (Swain 1978) showed similar interest. But their impact was minimal at the time.

In spite of this Falret felt able to say, half a century later, 'all psychological doctrines have had some impact on the understanding of madness. We have seen, for example, how the ideas of Condillac o Laromiguière brought into psychiatry the concept of attention and soon various forms of madness were explained as resulting from increases or decreases of this function' (Falret 1864, Lantéri-Laura 1984).

Both components of the clinico-anatomical model presented the alienist with difficulties. On the one hand the subject matter of description — mad behaviour — was different from anything encountered in general medicine. On the other, the brain was less accessible to direct in vivo inspection than other parts of the body. This led to a real scarcity of in vivo anatomo-clinical correlations and encouraged much speculation which could not always be corrected by postmortem studies owing to observational distortions caused by cadaveric decay (Report 1883).

The alienist found that there was a crucial difference between medicine and alienism with regard to the use of 'signs'. In the case of the medical sign information was mostly carried in its physical attributes (e.g. heart murmurs, skin lesions, gait) and this facilitated public confirmation and encouraged the development of measuring or amplificatory instruments. Not so in the case of the psychopathological sign which did not occur in *a physical but a semantic space*. Operational definitions of signs could not be made on the basis of their physical attributes alone and without reference to the rest of the behaviour.

Assumptions and concepts

Since descriptive psychopathology has changed little since the nineteenth century, an analysis of the assumptions and conceptual innovations on which it was originally based may help explain the enduring quality of some of the current phenomenological categories (delusions, hallucinations, etc.).

The following will be discussed in this section: the 'form' and 'content' distinction, the origin of numerical descriptions, the use of iconographic representations, the relationship between mental disease and the time dimension, and the gradual incorporation of experiential information into the definition of mental illness.

The form and content of the symptom

The distinction between 'form' and 'content' of a symptom is one of the enduring contributions of nineteenth-century psychopathology. At the end of the century it was extended to provide a categorical dichotomy for the separation of phenomenological and psychodynamic psychopathology.

The concept of 'form' has a noble intellectual pedigree, starting with the Aristotelian 'eidos', essence or common character of objects. This meaning (with some modifications) lasted well into the seventeenth century, when Bacon proposed a less ontological definition and suggested that 'form' might be considered as a synonym of 'figure'. Kant redefined the antonyms 'content–form' and postulated that whilst the immediate 'datum' of perception (the raw sensation or Stoff) was to be considered as the 'content', the *sense modality* in which it took place, in conjunction with its attending cognitive relationships, should be called the 'form' (Abbagnano 1961, Leary 1982).

Nineteenth-century descriptive psychopathology, and indeed Jaspers at the beginning of the twentieth century, follow closely this definition of form:

> Form must be kept distinct from content which may change from time to time, e.g. the fact of a hallucination is to be distinguished from its content, whether this is a man or a tree . . . Perceptions, ideas, judgments, feelings, drives, self-awareness, are all *forms* of psychic phenomena; they denote the particular *mode of existence* in which content is presented to us. It is true, in describing concrete psychic events we take into account the particular content of the individual psyche, but from the phenomenological point of view it is only the form that interests us . . . (Jaspers 1963 pp. 58–59)

The 'form' of a psychopathological symptom refers to those aspects of the phenomenon that guarantee its stability in time and space; they provide its 'constancy'.

The 'form' of the sign is easier to conceive of in physical medicine. Colour, sound, surface, solidity, smell and temperature are the media in which it achieves expression and stability. The facility with which physical signs were defined in medicine might have inspired alienists in their quest to identify psychopathological signs. These were also expected to be stable, public and observable. Emphasizing 'form' helped to create this effect.

But they did do so at a cost. First of all they had to make a commitment to a metaphysics of 'natural kinds' (Mill 1898) according to which successful units of analysis (signs) were assumed to have ontological autonomy. Solutions of continuity were to be found 'in res' and hence were independent of the language of description. In the second place, emphasis on the 'form' led to a mechanical conception of the sign as a mere clue that indicated the way to some corner of the brain where the illness hid. This early neglect of the semantic aspects of insanity impeded the development of a workable model which reconciled the study of both form and content. As a result an exclusive model for the latter was to develop, with a vengeance, toward the end of the nineteenth century (Ellenberger 1970).

However, in clinical *practice* the 'contents' of the sign were not altogether neglected. They helped the alienist to establish aetiological connections between the subject's illness and his past; they told him why the subject was in his current state. By the second half of the century, and before Janet or Freud had come to the scene, associations between content and past history began to be taken as representing cause–effect chains. For example it was felt that the content of a delusion or a hallucination might tell something about the circumstances in which it was first acquired (e.g. trauma, financial loss, infection) (Bucknill & Tuke 1858).

The many cause–effect chains thus established created a second-order 'psychological' level of explanation (Billod 1861, Dagonet 1881, Despine

1876). This contradicts claims that psychiatric aetiology was totally 'somatic' during this period (Jacyna 1982). Not surprisingly these psychological accounts matched the beliefs of popular psychology. When the neuroses, particularly hysteria, became incorporated within the purview of the alienist (and this only occurred towards the end of the century) they provided him with the best evidence yet that the content of a sign could tell a great deal about the circumstances of its acquisition (e.g. Charcot's 'idea' expressing itself in the symptom) (Charcot 1971, Owen 1971).

The emphasis on 'form' led to important changes in the way in which some signs were conceived. For example, the 'form' of the hallucination drew attention towards the sense modality in which it occurred and suggested that it was but the manifestation of a localized dysfunction (Tamburini 1881); its content became irrelevant and the hallucination ceased to be considered, as it had been for centuries, a source of meaningful knowledge.

Numerical representation and measurement

The mathematization of the natural world started in Europe during the seventeenth century. However, the 'Newtonian paradigm' affected little psychological thinking during this period; both Cartesian and Lockean psychology coincided with the view that numerical descriptions did not apply to behaviour (Moravia 1983).

The suggestion that 'psychometry' (i.e. the measurement of experience) was possible and desirable is attributed to Christian von Wolff. Whilst describing ways of assessing the magnitude of pleasure and displeasure he stated, in a footnote of his *Psychologia Empirica* (1738): 'these theorems belong to "psychometry" which conveys a mathematical knowledge of the human mind and continues to remain a desideratum' (Ramul 1960). Ramsay, Baumgarten, Crusius, de Maupertuis, Buck, Mendelssohn and Ploucquet are mentioned amongst other eighteenth-century writers who prepared the conceptual terrain for the advent of measurement in psychology; no one, however, seems to have carried out experimental work (Ramul 1960).

The introduction of quantification to medicine follows a different path (Shryock 1961, Murphy 1981). Numerical management of data was already common to seventeenth-century epidemiology and demography (e.g. the bills of mortality) but inferential interpretations were scanty. The nineteenth century, however, began to utilize numerical analysis in a different way (Porter 1986). Inferential statistics based on probability theory help to produce educated guesses as to stability of certain symptom clusters. This is clear in the work of Louis and also in that of Esquirol, who made much use of inferential percentages.

Numerical descriptions extended only gradually to other areas of psychopathology and this occurred around the middle of the century (Parchappe

1856, Renaudin 1856). There is little historical evidence that during the first half of the nineteenth century efforts were made to measure individual signs or personality traits (Boring 1961, Zupan 1976, Bondy 1974). This is surprising as the ideas of Gall and Spurzheim made available to psychology a conception of individual differences that was perfectly susceptible to numerical description (Spoerl 1936, Lesky 1970). The brand of Faculty Psychology these great men developed (Bentley 1916), partially inspired by the views of the Scottish philosophers (Robinson 1986), contained a clear statement with regard to the view that human behaviour (or personality) was analysable into arrays of autonomous modules or traits that had brain representation. Indeed phrenology sought to establish correlations between anatomical and psychological magnitudes (Lantéri-Laura 1970).

The phrenological model stated that the magnitude of a personality trait (y) was a function of the size of an anatomical region (x), and that this correlation was governed by a rule of correspondence (r). Although Gall did not express the relationship quite like this (this looser form of mathematical function was formulated only by Lejeune Dirichlet in 1837) (Iyanaga & Kawada 1980) it helps to clarify his thought. In fact Gall, as a distinguished anatomist and psychologist, contributed handsomely to y and x but did little about r. This failure to provide a mediational theory made him vulnerable to being caricatured as a reader of head bumps. After the 1830s there developed an officially sponsored opposition to phrenology (Cantor 1975, Cooter 1976, Lantéri-Laura 1970). This might have discouraged alienists from espousing, at least publicly, Gall's interesting 'modular' view of the mind. As a consequence no attempt was made to measure personality traits.

To summarize so far, the long path of numerical description, originally suggested by Wolff (and opposed by Kant and Comte) had been continued by Herbart, who suggested the development of a 'statistics' of the soul (Ribot 1885, Leary 1978). This conceptual change made easier the work of Möller and Du Bois-Reymond (Rothschuh 1973) and the instruments (Sokal et al 1976) they designed facilitated, in turn, what Weber and Fechner were to do during the middle of the nineteenth century.

Thus when measurement of individual events developed in the 1850s, it did so in the most unexpected quarters for Fechner had no connection, at least of a professional nature, with psychopathology (Marshall 1982). Indeed his fervour might have resulted from the fact that he was a physicist who entertained quaint ideas about the relationship between mind and body. Nonetheless Fechnerian numerical description is important to later developments in descriptive psychopathology. As has been mentioned already, at the time Fechner started, neurophysiologists had already been able to measure tissular and tactile events (Rothschuh 1973). For example sensitive instruments were already available to measure nerve conduction. Fechner's preconception of the nature of the sense datum and of its relationship with the material world allowed him to posit a one-to-one correlation between stimulus intensity and its cognitive appraisal. So he proceeded to correlate the physical magnitude of the stimulus and its reported perception.

In the Fechnerian model there was a gap between stimulus and its cognitive acknowledgement. This gap he bridged with his metaphysical belief in the total connectedness of nature and in the existence of inner mechanisms. Fechner put it thus: 'Sensation depends on stimulation; a stronger sensation depends on a stronger stimulus; the stimulus however causes sensation only via the intermediate action of some internal process of the body. To the extent that lawful relationships between sensation and stimulus can be found they must include lawful relationships between the stimulus and this inner physical activity . . .' (Fechner 1966 p. 101).

Fechner does not seem to have carried out any measurements in the insane. Ribot, Janet, Ziehen, Wundt and, certainly, Kraepelin (1983) did. These numerical descriptions of symptoms included assessments of physiological variables such as pulse, usually considered as covariates of emotional states. The work of Galton (Bondy 1974, Buss 1976, Porter 1986) and Binet (Wolf 1973) should not be neglected in this regard, although it cannot be claimed that it was of direct relevance to the numerical analysis of the signs of insanity. Galton and Binet both suggested ways of describing personality traits and intellectual competence in numerical terms; the former also contributed to the development of correlational statistical techniques.

The psychopathology of non-verbal behaviour

The great diagnostic categories of the past (mania, melancholia, phrensy, lethargy) relied on the observation of what the individual did and looked like rather than on what he thought or felt. This is particularly so with regard to mania and melancholia. Much has been said (wrongly) about these being the forerunners of the current categories bearing the same name. There is little historical evidence, however, that elation or sadness (i.e. pathological mood) were part of their clinical definition before the nineteenth century. Mania was the generic name for any form of increased and disordered behavioural output; hence excited catatonia, organic delirium and presbyophrenia qualified for the title. Melancholia referred to states of reduced behavioural output; stuporous catatonia, organic or psychogenic akinesias and even obsessional hesitations would all be classed as melancholias (Berrios 1987a).

The use of overt behaviour as the basis of psychopathological description seems to have been started by the Greeks (Simon 1978, Roccatagliata 1973). Symptom mapping was influenced by their views on what constituted harmonious behaviour and gave rise to the Greek categories of madness. Whilst some of these views died out, the categories endured to become the archetypal forms of insanity that, with little change, lasted well into the eighteenth century.

Interest in the description of overt behaviour never disappeared completely and was renewed during the eighteenth century, particularly in the study of facial expression in normal and insane persons. Parsons (1747) for example made efforts to establish correlations between emotions and facial expressions. This iconography of madness determined to a large extent the modes in which the mentally ill were perceived up to the nineteenth century (Gilman 1982). Indeed, there is evidence that the icons were used as a diagnostic aid. Exaggerated or distorted facial expressions could even indicate the intensity of the underlying derangement.

During the nineteenth century a change occurred in the way in which the insane were represented. The old Hogarthian and Tardieuesque stereotypes gave way to attempts at capturing facial expression and behaviours as they 'really were'. After 1839 the availability of the daguerreotype technique made these efforts easier, although analysis of the results shows that, due perhaps to the need for the subjects to remain still, there was an emphasis on 'static' pathological conditions such as stupor.

Likewise correlations between inner states and the facies became less acceptable. Indeed, the view was developed that the two factors were dissociable and this in turn led, for the first time, to the idea that insanity could be on occasions either concealed or simulated. Morrison, Laurent and the great Pierret, for example, developed a complex theory of 'mimia' and 'paramimia' during the second half of the century (Régis 1906). Darwin's interest in this issue is also well known (Darwin 1904).

Disease and the time dimension

Asylum psychiatry allowed for the first time the longitudinal observation of groups of patients. Until this period the descriptions of insanity had, in a real sense, been atemporal. The presence, in the cross-sectional observation, of certain features and behaviours sufficed to make the diagnosis, which was based on the one-off clinical examination.

In a way this could not have been otherwise. Until this period the 'ontological definition' considered madness as an irreversible process; becoming mad meant emigrating to a land of no return. Periods of 'normal or lucid behaviour' did not necessarily mean that the illness had gone.

But in the 1850s a temporal dimension was gradually introduced (Lantéri-Laura 1972, 1986, Pistoia 1971). In practice this meant that the information obtained from longitudinal observations was used to correct or modify earlier diagnosis. Kahlbaum (1828–1899) used this with advantage in his new definition of mental disease, which included a distinction between acute and chronic insanity (Berrios 1987b). The time dimension, by the end of the century, had become all-important. For example in Kraepelin the evolution and outcome of a condition are crucial to confirm diagnosis (Berrios 1987b).

The incorporation of subjectivity

The main difference, with regard to source of signs, between early and late nineteenth-century descriptions of madness is the fact that the latter include more information on subjective states (Dagonet 1881). This shift towards subjectivity occurred gradually and led in the fullness of time to the development of the psychodynamic school. During the early stages, however, it was a modest enterprise encouraged, if not started, around 1859, by Moreau de Tours (1804–1884), the great French alienist (Bollote 1973, Ey & Mignot 1947).

In order for this shift to happen two conceptual changes were necessary: the development of a legitimate mechanism to collect subjective information, and the acceptance of the view that it was possible to establish an intelligible dialogue with the insane.

Introspection became an important information-gathering method during the middle of the nineteenth century (Boring 1953, Danzinger 1980). After its adoption by alienists it allowed for verbal pictures of inner experiences to be passed from the patient to the clinician. The subjectivity of the individual thus became another source of signs.

The effective incorporation of this information marks the change from the classical to the modern concept of mental illness. For example it led to the newer notions of melancholia and mania, based on information on the mood of the patient (Berrios 1987a), and to the modern notion of paranoia, based almost exclusively on delusional declarations (Lewis 1970). Likewise, the various forms of stupor, until then lumped together, were classified according to whether or not they included 'mental' content (Berrios 1981c). The classifications of religious, erotic and other forms of insanity and the description of the obsessional states (Berrios 1985a) were also accelerated by the simple step of incorporating subjective data.

THE HISTORY OF THE SIGNS OF MADNESS

The main contribution of the nineteenth century to psychopathology could be summed up in the claim that it established a new kind of relationship between sign and disease (Lantéri-Laura 1982). This was not an easy task. It meant first re-creating the concept of a sign and secondly suggesting new ways in which it would 'signify' or 'represent' disease. Until the eighteenth century, signs were 'symbols' of disease; after the 1840s they became proper signs, i.e they acquired a relation of significance (King 1968).

From then on, sign, disease and alienist formed a closed system and this allowed the alienist to embark on the long journey of professionalization. The old stereotypes of madness gradually died out and were replaced by subtle signs, by arcane indications, knowledge of which was no longer available to everyone. Signs became technical guidelines and hence the property of specialists.

It is an interesting clinical fact that the signs of madness are not very numerous. This was so even at the beginning. It has been suggested that during the first half of the nineteenth century the old insanity categories were subjected to 'parsing out (Daumezon 1957). A number of behavioural units of analysis resulted and only a few were retained. The criteria on which the choice was made are not always clear.

It can be suggested that nineteenth-century alienists selected symptoms with certain predictive value and they did so on the basis of longitudinal observation. A symptom can be said to predict when its presence suggests a certain expectation as to the future of the disease. The interesting question was then (as it is now) what makes this prediction possible.

All symptoms must have informational value. This information, one assumes, is generated by the fact that each symptom 'signifies' the existence of an inner disturbed state; so each will carry a hidden signal, often attenuated or enveloped in noise. Thus it can be further assumed that there is for each a different signal:noise ratio. The search for strategies that might identify this ratio has not yet started in descriptive psychopathology. It is suggested here that this strategy should have a historical, clinical and mathematical component.

Most of the important psychopathological symptoms were defined around the same period. Hence their histories should share some features in common. There is no space in this chapter to deal with all symptoms, so only a few examples will be included.

Symptoms were grouped during the nineteenth century according to the tripartite view of the mind enshrined in Kantian faculty psychology (Hilgard 1980, Leary 1978). The symptoms of *intellectual dysfunction* included perceptual, thought, attentional and memory disorders; those of *emotional or orectic function* included elation, depression, anhedonia and anxiety; those of *volitional function* included abulia and lethargy. To fit into their respective Procrustean beds the natural complexity of many symptoms had to be overlooked. Even then some resisted reduction (e.g. depersonalization). It is difficult to say to what extent excessive loyalty to this early classification has contributed to the current uncreative state of descriptive psychopathology.

Likewise, the history of any symptom can only be understood if it is placed against the backdrop of the history of nineteenth-century psychiatric and medical nosology. There is some evidence that even the choice of representative symptoms (such as thought disorder in schizophrenia or sadness in depression) might have been influenced by 'non-cognitive' variables. Thus it has recently been claimed that Kraepelin chose not to use delusions and hallucinations as the central symptoms of dementia praecox (schizophrenia) because he was at the time working in Dorpat and his patients only spoke Russian; hence it was easier to observe their behaviour than to assess their mental states (Hauser 1986).

The professionalization of psychiatry during the nineteenth century is another factor that cannot be overlooked. The order in which groups of diseases were taken on board by psychiatrists (and clinical psychologists such as Ribot or Dumas) is informative. There is little doubt that the organic disorders and the insanities were incorporated earliest and formed the very core of alienism practice. The neuroses arrived much later. Up to the 1890s cases thus affected were seen by general physicians and incipient neurologists (López Piñero & Morales Meseguer 1970, Drinka 1984). The so-called disorders of personality were an even later acquisition as they required an acceptable notion of personality before they could be described. The rest has come in much later and has no relevance to the history of abnormal psychology.

One crucial issue must be finally mentioned. It concerns the way in which the meaning of the neuroses and the psychoses changed so radically between 1845 and 1900. To start with the neuroses were conceived of as 'organic' and the psychoses, as defined by Von Feuchtersleben (1847), as subjective experiences. By the end of the century the former had become psychologized and the latter were considered as the organic diseases par excellence. There is no need here to account for this reversal in any detail but it must be kept in mind by anyone trying to understand the evolution of abnormal psychology.

Delusions

Of all symptoms of madness, delusions were recognized the earliest. For example the Greek descriptions of mania, phrensy or melancholia already include the bizarre claims made by subjects about themselves or the world. Indeed, this selective attention to delusions may have introduced a bias in the definition of insanity (Berrios 1985b). Delusion and obsession have a common genealogy in that they represent lay versions of 'possessio and obsessio' the theological dyad that referred to the two interactual modes between man and the devil. In the 'obsessio' state, man was under 'siege'; the devil remained external or 'dystonic' to the subject who fought against the intrusion. In the 'possessio' state the devil had gained entry and inhabited the subject's soul; he had become 'syntonic'; the subject no longer fought his presence. The structural features of these two modes were transcribed into clinical language and became the defining criteria for obsession and delusion, respectively (Berrios 1977).

John Locke also chose delusion as the essential feature for his redefinition of madness according to the new associationistic psychology (Locke 1959). He emphasized the irrational and unshifting nature of this symptom. Esquirol (1814) tidied up the defining criteria during the early nineteenth century and added insightlessness and cultural dislocation.

Faculty Psychology inspired the new classification of mental illness during the middle of the nineteenth century and delusions became the central feature of the intellectual insanities (Georget 1835). The concept of paranoia was resurrected during the 1860s, after an absence of centuries, to refer to forms of insanity where delusions were the only symptom (Lewis 1970).

A problem for the historian of European psychiatry is to differentiate the meanings of the supposedly equivalent terms delusion, *délire*, *Wahn* and *delirio*. Some have incautiously assumed their total correspondence, thus missing crucial differences (Arthur 1964). Indeed, one of the explanations for the lack of communication between French and Anglo-Saxon psychiatry must be found in the fact that delusion translates only part of the meaning of *délire*. By this term French psychiatrists mean unwarranted mental acts, whether reflected in ideas, speech, emotion, memory or motility. Thus the word *délire* encompasses a number of symptoms that cross the semantic boundaries of delusion (Ball & Chambard 1882). *Wahn* (the German term for delusion), on the other hand, has a wider referent than that of delusion but narrower than that of *délire*.

Another current difficulty in the understanding of the concept of delusion refers to its being considered as a 'pathological' belief. The historical origin of this miscategorization is interesting and takes one back to the period when there was an attempt to consider all symptoms as distorted forms of normal behaviour. Delusions may turn out to be just empty speech acts whose content has unfortunately been taken literally. If so their informational value will not reside in their content or social semantics but in their form (as is the case with tics).

Illusions and hallucinations

These two terms name subjective experiences ascribed to disordered perception. Illusions are defined as perceptual distortions and hallucinations as perceptual declarations, of varied degree of conviction, in the absence of a relevant external stimulus (Berrios 1982b, 1985d).

The current conceptual model of hallucination developed during the early nineteenth century out of the analysis of visions and other 'phantasmata'. 'Hallucinatio' was a term originally used to name visions and other disorders of visual function which, until this period, were considered as semantically pregnant; i.e. they were believed to be telling something about the visionary or about the world (Berrios 1982b).

Esquirol and others carried out what can be called the 'medicalization' of the symptoms of madness. One of the consequences of this was that hallucinations became emptied of content. Esquirol's crucial contribution, however, was his suggestion that the word hallucination, until then used only to name *visual experiences*, be generalized to refer to all forms of sensory deception. He wrote: 'if a man has the intimate conviction of actually perceiving a sensation for which there is no external object, he is in a hallucinated state: he is a visionary'. Then he went on to say that: 'vision is a term appropriate only for one perceptual modality. Who dares to talk about auditory visions, taste visions, olfactory visions? However, the brain alterations and clinical meaning related to these three disorders is probably *the same* as that of vision . . . Therefore a generic term is needed and I propose the word hallucination' (Esquirol 1838).

The importance of this suggestion for the subsequent history of hallucinations has not been sufficiently noted. In extending the term 'hallucinatio' from the visual to the other sense modalities, Esquirol forced upon the latter a common perceptual paradigm that since John Locke had assumed that a perception is the internal representation of an external stimulus. Whilst this worked well for vision, audition and olfaction, where, in general, the stimulus is in the public domain and hence is open to corroboration by fellow perceivers, it breaks down in relation to sense modalities such as touch: how to differentiate between a real itch and a hallucinated one (Berrios 1982b)?

But Esquirol also saddled hallucinations with another difficulty. They came to be accepted as being a *disturbance of perception* and this encouraged the search for the sense data themselves or their behavioural or neurophysiological concomitants. Do hallucinated subjects have images or do they simply believe that they do? Tamburini (1881) and the great Italian school of the late nineteenth century believed that they have the image. This encouraged the view that 'neurological' and 'psychiatric' hallucinations might be equivalent. The clinical limitations of this view started the chase for criteria that might differentiate the two types. The suggested criteria included presence or absence of insight, intensity and form of the sense perception, sense modality and repetitiveness (Berrios 1985d).

Economic as the 'continuity hypothesis' might be, it has limited heuristic value. None of these criteria has so far worked but this does not mean that they are the same phenomenon. To the clinician insane hallucinations appear as phenomenologically different from hallucinotic states such as those caused by epileptic auras, brain stimulation, drugs or tumours (Berrios 1985d). In this respect the French have suggested that psychiatric or psychotic hallucinations are only 'delusions of perception', i.e. the presence of a sense datum is irrelevant to their definition (Faure 1969).

Obsessions and compulsions

These terms name interloping fragments of behaviour characterized by inordinate repetition, anomalous content and resistance from the affected subject. Their iterative nature and offending content create uneasiness and cultural dissonance. Whether as thoughts, images or actions they often fracture and paralyse the flow of behaviour (Berrios 1985a).

Phenomena of the sort named by the words obsession and compulsion have been identified in most cultures and historical periods. Although the technical meaning of these terms only developed during the latter part of the nineteenth century, in ordinary language they had for long referred to acts and thoughts related directly or indirectly to the 'will'. Companion terms such as scruples, besetments, impulsions, contrary acts and imperative ideas once also in active currency have since fallen into desuetude (Berrios 1977, 1985a). A 'family resemblance', in Wittgenstein's sense, can also be found between the etymological stems from which the corresponding terms in the main European languages have derived. As has been said above, our current image of obsessional phenomena stems from a religious metaphor. On the other hand, the concept of compulsion, together with impulsion and other automatic and involuntary acts, has originated from a different source.

Obsessions and compulsions were brought together only towards the end of the nineteenth century. In the early Freudian model compulsions become subordinate to obsessions and the 'emotional hypothesis' led to the belief (probably unwarranted) that the meaning of the compulsion is parasitical upon that of the obsession and that, furthermore, the compulsion is mantained by its anxiety-reducing function. This might have had the effect of diverting attention away from the study of conpulsions in their own right. The obsessional disorders during the nineteenth century also included obsessional hallucinations, phobic states and a panoply of physical symptoms such as neurasthenia, blushing, etc. It was Freud who, in his classical paper of 1895, separated phobias from obsessions. This he did not on clinical but on theoretical grounds.

The bizarre nature of the obsessional disorders has always created classificatory difficulties. Earlier on they were grouped (perhaps rightly) with other forms of insanity. Then, in the 1860s, they were classified by Morel as 'neuroses' during the brief period when these conditions were considered as pathological disorders of the autonomic nervous system. When the neuroses were taken over by the developing psychodynamic doctrines (with Janet and Freud) the obsessional disorders found themselves trapped in an ideological interpretation that contributed nothing to their therapy. It has taken the best part of 50 years to realize that the class 'neuroses' is empty of useful meaning as it includes disparate behavioural phenomena. Once again the obsessional disorders have been set asunder (for an extended list of references see Berrios 1985b).

Disorders of consciousness

This group, one of the last to be incorporated into psychopathology, includes disorders that share common clinical features such as clouding of consciousness and disorientation. Their current clinical value resides in the fact that their presence identifies some of the 'organic disorders' in psychiatry (Berrios 1982a).

The history of the disorders of consciousness illustrates well how variations in the meaning of a concept (in this case that of consciousness) may reorganize observation. This 'noble' term had had up to the early nineteenth century a predominant philosophical meaning; the 'moral' meaning having been already separated off as early as the beginnings of Christianity (Abbagnano 1961, Eisler 1927). In languages such as German and English this is illustrated by the use of a separate word for the 'moral' dimension (i.e. conscience); in others such as French and Spanish the use of a single term for all the meanings is a reminder of the original complexity of the concept.

The psychological notion of consciousness, started by the Cartesian philosophy of mind (Cohen 1984), became fully operational only during the nineteenth century. In the work of (inter alia) William Hamilton (1859), Alexander Bain (1859) and Bastian (1870) the main issue concerned the nature of psychological consciousness, namely whether it was a higher level (independent) function developed to monitor all other mental functions or whether it was just a built-in attribute. The former view led to the search for the brain localization of consciousness and this, particularly in the work of Carpenter during the second half of nineteenth century, led to the conception of an 'automatic apparatus' (Walshe 1957).

A difficulty when dealing with the psychological role of consciousness is the need for an appropriate language. During the nineteenth century this was solved by resorting to the complementary metaphors of consciousness as the stage of a theatre or as a great eye; so the language of perception was employed throughout as illustrated by the use of adjectives such as clouded, blurred, narrow, sharp and acute (Berrios, unpublished).

A search for the clinical disturbances of conciousness (and for the illnesses they characterized) was started in the 1870s. By the 1890s, with the work of Chaslin (1895) on 'confusion' the analysis had been completed (Berrios 1981a). It was believed that consciousness could 'go wrong' in two dimensions: clarity and extension. It could be clouded (as in delirium and confusion) or 'narrowed' (as in hypnotic trances and other artificially induced pathological states). Sleep was, for a while, also considered to be a physiological modification of consciousness as were stupor (Berrios 1981b) and coma.

Much of this theorizing was abandoned as the early neurophysiology of consciousness developed in the 1920s and introspection and mental contents came under attack in the wake of Watsonian behaviourism (Burt 1962). The concepts of clouding and of disorientation, however, remained as central symptoms in psychiatric practice.

Disorientation was conceptualized as an instance of orientation failure; that is, a disorder in the subject's ability to monitor the relevant time, space and person reference systems (Berrios 1982a). Like the term hallucination, disorientation was supposed to refer to an ongoing mental state but, unlike it, it was defined as a negative state in which the subject failed to 'know that' (verbal disorientation) and to 'know how' (non-verbal disorientation).

The English word 'orientation' derives from the French *orienter* and was first used as a scientific term in astronomy. A psychological disturbance caused by cerebral atherosclerosis (consisting in the inability of the patient to find his way around) was called by Mott 'imperfect orientation'. Jaspers described four types: amnestic, delusional, apathetic and clouded. The latter was the central manifestation of a disordered consciousness.

Some readjustments in the conceptualization of the orientation failures have since taken place (Berrios 1983). For example, it has been suggested that verbal and non-verbal orientation can be found to be dissociated in clinical practice, i.e. patients can fail to reply to the usual questions but have no difficulty in finding their way in the ward. Likewise, at least three types of orientation failure can be recognized, depending on whether the subject chooses to use a public or a private (psychotic) reference system. If he oscillates between the two, as in the functional psychoses, 'double orientation' ensues; if he follows his private (delusional) reference system he shows 'false orientation'; if he cannot monitor at all any reference system, 'disorientation' proper appears (as in the organic states). It is further postulated that time, space and personal orientation break down in a hierarchical fashion in response to increases in disease 'severity', with time orientation being the most vulnerable. The sensitivity of the orientation failures is adequate, however they exhibit reduced specificity.

The disorders of affect, volition and motility

In addition to the disorders of intellecual function described above, nineteenth-century alienists also defined disorders of emotion, affect and mood, and disorders of will, volition and motility. There is insufficient space in this short historical introduction to deal with these at any length and only a few points will be made in relation to each.

The disorders of affect were recognized as primary only during the nineteenth century following the acceptance of Faculty Psychology as a taxonomic principle (Berrios 1985b). As has been said above, up to this period the concepts of melancholia and mania bore little resemblance to what nowadays goes under the same name. They were defined mainly in terms of overt behaviour and type and extension of delusional activity (Berrios 1987a).

This preference for intellectual symptoms continued late in the century. For example, efforts were made in the 1880s to reduce emotions to cognitive states (as in the case of the peripheralist theory of James and Lange) (Gardiner et al 1937) or to evolutionary programmes (as in the case of Darwin, Romanes, Spalding and Lloyd Morgan) (Kuper 1985, Mackenzie 1976, Richards 1977, 1982, Romanes 1888). This perpetuated the neglect of the psychopathology of affectivity. Recent efforts to reinterpret clinical depression in 'cognitive' terms are but a return to the old nineteenth-century view that people become depressed because they have a bad view of themselves.

The disorders of volition or of the 'will' (such as abulia) (Ribot 1904) suffered most from the change in philosophical fashion at the end of the nineteenth century (Daston 1982, Greenway 1973, Kimble & Perlmuter 1970). From being a very popular category during most of the century 'will' came under attack during the 1880s and eventually underwent eclipse. Thus the creative, self-help type of voluntarism that dominated the Victorian work ethos and education found little room in the philosophical anthropology that emerged from Darwinian evolutionism, Freudianism and the various historicisms that appeared towards the end of the century. These views had in common the assumption that conscious will-power was a mirage and that deeper forces, whether historical or unconscious, shaped the destiny of the individual.

Thus by the turn of the century the 'will' had ceased to be an explanatory category. Early twentieth-century psychiatry and psychology found themselves bereft of a shorthand term to name the link between intention and act. The concepts of drive and motivation were offered as a replacement. In the fashionable parlance of psychopathology, it no longer made sense to say that the alcoholic patient could not stop drinking because he had no will-power; the new way was to say that 'he had no motivation'.

The motility disorders refer to a gamut of motor symptoms that extend from the very complex stereotyped mannerisms of the catatonic patient to the simple tics of Gilles de la Tourette syndrome. Once again, during the nineteenth century these symptoms had been considered as reflecting cerebral pathology, particularly of the basal ganglia (Berrios 1981b).

The view that they reflected 'primary' brain pathology was championed by Karl Wernicke (Ajuriaguerra 1975). The early death of this great man made possible the triumph of the Kraepelinian and Bleulerian views of the motility disorders. According to the latter motility disorders had 'meaning' and hence were *secondary* to delusional ideas. A patient was 'akinetic' because he did not want to move; he did not want to do so because he had the delusion that if he did either himself or the world might be destroyed.

There never has been much evidence for this form of reductionism. Recent years have witnessed a healthy return of a 'primary view' of the motility disorders. Clinical states such as 'writer's cramp', spasmodic torticollis, Parkinsonian tremor and Gilles de la Tourette tics are no longer considered as the result of the subject not 'wanting' to write, or 'looking away' from a sexual fantasy, or 'trembling' in anger or substituting aggression, respectively. Instead, a heuristic view prevails that they reflect changes in the physiopathology of the basal ganglia (Lees 1985).

CONCLUSIONS

This chapter has touched upon aspects of the historical process that led to the formation of the descriptive language of abnormal psychology. Large regions of this process remain unresearched and hence the complete tale cannot yet be told. Sufficient is known, however, to believe that most of this language was compiled in the asylums for the insane between the 1830s and the end of the century. Hence symptom definition and the concept of mental disease itself were based upon the longitudinal observation of cohorts of subjects suffering from hard insanity and organic disorders.

The formation of this language can be considered as a conceptual vector resulting from the confluence of changes taking place in many intellectual provinces of the nineteenth century. These include the development of the anatomo-clinical view of disease in general medicine, the moulding influence of both Associationism and Faculty Psychology, the incorporation into medical description of areas of human experience occurring in spaces other than overt behaviour (subjective symptoms, particularly emotional experiences) which, until then, had been considered as beyond the reach of observational techniques, and the introduction of a time dimension in the definition and ascertainment of symptom and disease.

Symptoms thereby acquired the dual role of units of analysis and surface markers of disease. Insane behaviour was fractured or 'parsed out' and terms were adopted or coined to name fragments considered of clinical relevance. A distinction was made between the form and the content of the symptom: the form conveyed information on the bodily system involved; the content on aetiology, the patient's personality and on the circumstances in which the illness was acquired.

The descriptive language of abnormal psychology has changed little since the nineteenth century. This stability suggests that constancy factors, both external (i.e. social constructions) and internal (i.e. symptoms relate to real neurobiological phenomena), are in operation. The differential contribution of these factors must be calibrated by mathematical, clinical and historical techniques.

With respect to the latter, and as it is the case in other areas, the choice of historiographical method is important. Conceptual and contextual analyses are to be preferred to the more traditional biographical or presentistic approaches. The use of 'language' as a model (or metaphor) is particularly rewarding in this respect. Not only can psychopathological descriptions be analyzed in relation to their inner 'grammar' but also in relation to usage rules and social context. By the same token a distinction ought to be made between the history of psychiatric terms and of concepts. In this way the unhelpfulness can be shown of linear historical accounts, usually starting from Greek times, of terms such as mania, melancholia, hysteria and hypochondria. This chapter offers an alternative historical approach.

REFERENCES

Abbagnano N 1961 Dizionario di Filosofia. Unione Tipografico Torinese, Turin
Ackerknecht E H 1967 Medicine at the Paris Hospital 1794–1848. Johns Hopkins Press, Baltimore

Ajuriaguerra J de 1975 The concept of akinesia. Psychological Medicine 5: 129–137
Albarracin Teulon A 1983 La teoria celular. Historia de un paradigma. Alianza Editorial, Madrid
Albrecht F M 1970 A reappraisal of faculty psychology. Journal of the History of the Behavioural Sciences 6: 36–40
Arthur A Z 1964 Theories and explanations of delusions. American Journal of Psychiatry 121: 105–115
Bain A 1859 The Emotions and the Will. J W Parker, London, pp 599–646
Ball B, Chambard E 1882 Délire. In: Dechambre T (ed) Dictionnaire Encyclopédique des Sciences Médicales. Vol 26. Asselin et Masson, Paris, pp 315–434
Barthes R 1972 Sémiologie et Médécine. In Bastide R (ed) Les sciences de la folie. Mouton, Paris, pp 37–46
Bastian H C 1870 Consciousness. Journal of Mental Science 15: 501–523
Bentley M 1916 The psychological antecedents of phrenology. Psychological Review Monographs 21: 102–115
Berrios G E 1975 Nuevas tendencias en la historiografia de la psicologia. Revista de Occidente No 149, 154–169
Berrios G E 1977 Henri Ey, Jackson et les idées obsédantes. L'Evolution Psychiatrique 62: 685–699
Berrios G E 1981a Delirium and confusion in the 19th century: a conceptual history. British Journal of Psychiatry 139: 439–449
Berrios G E 1981b Stupor revisited. Comprehensive Psychiatry 22: 466–478
Berrios G E 1981c Stupor: a conceptual history. Psychological Medicine 11: 677–688
Berrios G E 1982a Disorientation states and psychiatry. Comprehensive Psychiatry 23: 479–490
Berrios G E 1982b Tactile hallucinations: conceptual and historical aspects. Journal of Neurology, Neurosurgery and Psychiatry 45: 285–293
Berrios G E 1983 Orientation failures in medicine and psychiatry: discussion paper. Journal of the Royal Society of Medicine 76: 379–385
Berrios G E 1984a Descriptive Psychopathology: conceptual and historical aspects. Psychological Medicine 14: 303–313
Berrios G E 1984b Epilepsy and insanity during the early 19th century. Archives of Neurology 41: 978–981
Berrios G E 1985a Obsessional disorders during the 19thC: terminological and classificatory issues. In: Bynum W F, Porter R, Shepherd M (eds) The Anatomy of Madness. Vol 1, People and Ideas. Tavistock, London, pp 166–187
Berrios G E 1985b The psychopathology of affectivity: conceptual and historical aspects. Psychological Medicine 15: 745–758
Berrios G E 1985c 'Depressive pseudodementia' or 'melancholic dementia': a 19th century review. Journal of Neurology, Neurosurgery, and Psychiatry 48: 393–400
Berrios G E 1985d Hallucinosis. In: Vinken P J, Bruyn G W, Klawans H L (eds) Handbook of clinical neurology. Vol 2: Neurobehavioural disorders. Elsevier Science Publishers, Amsterdam, pp 561–572
Berrios G E 1987a Depressive and manic states during the 19thC. In: Gorgotas T and Cancro J (eds) Handbook of Affective Disorders. New York (in press)
Berrios G E 1987b Historical aspects of the psychoses: 19thC issues. British Medical Bulletin 43: 484–498
Billod T 1861 De la lésion de l'association des idées. Annales Médico Psychologiques 18: 540–552
Blasius D 1980 Der verwaltete Wahnsinn. Eine Sozialgeschichte des Irrenhauses. Fischer, Frankfurt
Bollote G 1973 Moreau de Tours 1804–1884. Confrontations Psychiatriques 11: 9–26
Bondy M 1974 Psychiatric antecedents of psychological testing (before Binet). Journal of the History of the Behavioural Sciences 10: 180–194
Boring E G 1950 A history of experimental psychology. Appleton-Century-Crofts, New York
Boring E G 1953 A History of Introspection. Psychological Bulletin 50: 169–189
Boring E G 1961 The beginning and growth of measurement in psychology. Isis 52: 238–257

Bowman I A 1975 Classification of diseases: Sydenham and eighteenth-century attempts. In: Bowman I A 1975 William Cullen (1710–90) and the primacy of the nervous system. PhD Thesis, Indiana University, pp 153–225

Brooks G P 1976 The faculty psychology of Thomas Reid. Journal of the History of the Behavioural Sciences 12: 65–77

Bucknill J C, Tuke D H 1858 A manual of psychological medicine. Churchill, London

Burt C 1962 The concept of consciousness. British Journal of Psychology 53: 229–242

Buss A R 1976 Galton and the birth of differential psychology and eugenics: social, political and economic forces. Journal of the History of the Behavioural Sciences 12: 47–58

Canguilhem G 1966 Le normal et le pathologique. Presses Universitaires de France, Paris

Cantor G N 1975 The Edinburgh Phrenology Debate: 1803–1828. Annales Science 32: 195–218

Castel R 1977 L'ordre psychiatrique. L'âge d'or de l'aliénisme. Minuit, Paris

Charcot J M 1971 L'Hysterie. Textes choisis et préséntés par E Trillat. Privat, Paris

Chaslin P 1895 La confusion mentale primitive. Asselin et Houzeau, Paris

Cohen A 1984 Descartes, consciousness and depersonalization: viewing the history of philosophy from a strausian perspective. Journal of Medicine and Philosophy 9: 7–27

Cooter R J 1976 Phrenology and British alienists, c. 1825–1845. Medical History 20: 1–21, 135–151

Dagonet H 1881 Conscience et aliénation mentale. Annales Médico-psychologiques 5: 368–397; 6: 19–32

Danzinger K 1980 The history of introspection reconsidered. Journal of the History of the Behavioural Sciences 16: 241–262

Darwin C 1904 The expression of the emotions in man and animals. John Murray, London

Daston L J 1982 The theory of will versus the science of mind. In: Woodward W R, Ash M G (eds) The problematic science: psychology in 19thC thought. Praeger, New York, pp 88–115

Daumezon G 1957 Reflexions sur la sémiologie psychiatrique. L'Evolution Psychiatrique 22: 207–237

Despine P 1876 Du role de la psychologie dans la question de la folie. Annales Médico-Psychologiques 34: 161–175

Donnelly M 1983 Managing the mind. A study of medical psychology in early 19thC Britain. Tavistock, London

Dörner K 1969 Bürger und Irre. Zur Socialgeschichte und Wissenschaftssoziologie der Psychiatrie. Europäische Verlagsanstalt, Frankfurt

Drevet A 1968 Maine de Biran. Presses Universitaires de France, Paris

Drinka G F 1984 The birth of neurosis. Myth, Malady, and the Victorians. Simon & Schuster, New York

Dumas G 1908 Qu'est-ce que la psychologie pathologique? Journal de Psychologie Normale et Pathologique 5: 10–22

Eisler R 1927 Bewusstsein. In: Wörterbuch der philosophischen Begriffe, Vol 1. Ernst Siegfried Mittler, Berlin, pp 207–220

Ellenberger H F 1970 The discovery of the Unconscious. The history and evolution of dynamic psychiatry. Allen lane, London

Esquirol J E 1814 Délire. In: Dictionnaire des Sciences Médicales. Panckoucke, Paris, pp 251–259

Esquirol J E 1838 Des hallucinations. In: Des maladies mentales, Vol 1. Baillière, Paris pp 159–201

Ey H, Mignot H 1947 La psychologie de J Moréau de Tours. Annales Médico-Psychologiques 2: 225–241

Falret J P 1864 Des maladies mentales et des asiles d'aliénés. Baillière, Paris

Faure H 1969 Hallucinations et réalité perceptive. Presses Universitaires de France, Paris

Fechner G T 1966 Elements of psychophysics, Vol 1 (translated by Adler H E). Holt, New York

Foucault M 1972a Histoire de la folie à l'âge classique. Gallimard, Paris

Foucault M 1972b Naissance de la clinique. 2nd edn. Presses Universitaires de France, Paris

Freud S 1895 Obsessions et phobies. Revue Neurologique 3: 33–38

Gardiner H M, Metcalf R C, Beebe-Center J G 1937 Feeling and emotion. A history of theories. American Book, New York

Georget E 1835 Délire. In: Dictionnaire de Médicine, Vol 10. Béchet, Paris pp 19–29
Gilman S L 1982 Seeing the insane. Wiley, New York
Greenway A P 1973 The incorporation of action into associationism. The psychology of Alexander Bain. Journal of the History of the Behavioural Sciences 9: 42–52
Griesinger W 1867 Mental pathology and therapeutics (translated by Robertson C L, Rutherford J). New Sydenham Society, London
Hamilton W 1859 Lectures on Metaphysics and Logic, Vol 1. Blackwood, Edinburgh, pp 182–382
Hauser R 1986 The concept of dementia praecox in Kraepelin. M Phil thesis, University of Cambridge
Hilgard E R 1980 The trilogy of mind: cognition, affection and conation. Journal of the History of the Behavioural Sciences 16: 107–117
Hoeldtke R 1967 The history of associationism and British medical psychology. Medical History 11: 46–64
Iyanaga S, Kawada Y 1980 Encyclopedic dictionary of mathematics. 2 Vols. MIT Press, Massachusetts
Jackson S W 1970 Force and kindred notions in 18thC neurophysiology and medical psychology 64: 397–554
Jacyna L S 1982 Somatic theories of mind and the interests of medicine in Britain. Medical History 26: 233–258
Jalley M, Lefebvre J P, Feline, Kaufmann E et al 1977 Essai sur les maladies de la tête par E Kant. L'Evolution Psychiatrique 42: 203–230
Jaspers K 1963 General psychopathology (translated by Hoenig J, Hamilton M W). Manchester University Press, Manchester
Jones K 1972 A history of the mental health services. Routledge & Kegan Paul, London
Kimble G A, Perlmuter L C 1970 The Problem of volition. Psychological Review 77: 361–384
King L S 1968 Signs and symptoms. Journal of the American Medical Association 206: 1063–1065
Klein D B 1970 A history of scientific psychology. Routledge & Kegan Paul, London
Kraepelin F 1983 Lebenserinnerungen. Springer-Verlag, Berlin
Kuper A 1985 The development of Lewis Henry Morgan's evolutionism. Journal of the History of the Behavioural Sciences 21: 3–21
Laín Entralgo P 1978 Historia de la medicina. Salvat Editores, Barcelona
Lantéri-Laura G 1966 Les apports de la linquistique à la psychiatrie contemporaine. Masson, Paris
Lantéri-Laura G 1970 Histoire de la phrénologie. Presses Universitaires de France, Paris
Lantéri-Laura G 1972 La chronicité dans la psychiatrie française moderne. Annales 3: 547–568
Lantéri-Laura G 1982 La connaissance clinique: histoire et structure en médécine et en psychiatrie. L'Evolution Psychiatrique 47: 423–469
Lantéri-Laura G 1984 La sémiologie de J P Falret. Perspectives Psychiatriques 22: 104–110
Lantéri-Laura G 1986 Acuité et pathologie mentale. L'Evolution Psychiatrique 51: 403–418
Leary D E 1978 The philosophical development of the conception of psychology in Germany 1780–1850. Journal of the History of the Behavioural Sciences 14: 113–121
Leary D E 1982 Immanuel Kant and the development of modern psychology. In: Woodward W R, Ash M (eds) The problematic science: psychology in 19thC thought. Praeger, New York, pp 17–42
Lees A J 1985 Tics and related disorders. Churchill Livingstone, London.
Lesch J E 1984 Science and medicine in France. The emergence of experimental physiology 1790–1855. Harvard University Press, Massachusetts
Lesky E 1970 Structure and function in Gall. Bulletin of the History of Medicine 44: 297–314
Lewis A 1970 Paranoia and paranoid: a historical perspective. Psychological Medicine 1: 2–12
Locke J 1959 An essay concerning human understanding. 2 Vols. Dover, New York
López Piñero J M 1983 Historical origins of the concept of neurosis (translated by Berrios D.). Cambridge University Press, Cambridge
López Piñero J M, Morales Meseguer J M 1970 Neurosis y psicoterapia. Un estudio histórico. Espasa-Calpe, Madrid

Losserand J 1967 Les rapports du physique et du moral de L'homme de Cabanis à Auguste Comte. L'Evolution Psychiatrique 32: 573–601
Lowry R 1971 The evolution of psychological theory: 1650 to the present. Aldine & Atherton, Chicago
Mackenzie B 1976 Darwinism and positivism as methodological influences on the development of psychology. Journal of the History of the Behavioural Sciences 12: 330–337
Maher B A, Maher W B 1979 Psychopathology. In: Hearst E (ed) The first century of experimental psychology. Wiley, New York, pp 561–621
Marshall M E 1982 Physics, metaphysics and Fechner's psychophysics. In: Woodward W R, Ash M (eds) The problematic science: psychology in 19thC thought. Praeger, New York, pp 65–87
Mill J S 1898 A system of logic. Longmans Green, London, pp 76–86
Mora G 1981 Cabanis, neurology and psychiatry. In: Mora G (ed) On the relations between the physical and moral aspects of man by P J G Cabanis, Vol 1. Johns Hopkins Press, Baltimore pp 45–90
Moravia S 1983 The capture of the invisible for a (pre)history of psychology in eighteenth century France. Journal of the History of the Behavioural Sciences 19: 370–378
Murphy G 1967 Historical introduction to modern psychology. Routledge & Kegan Paul, London
Murphy T D 1981 Medical knowledge and statistical methods in early nineteenth-century France. Medical History 25: 301–319
Oberg B B 1976 David Hartley and the association of ideas. Journal of the History of Ideas 37: 441–454
Owen A R G 1971 Hysteria, hypnosis and healing. The work of J M Charcot. Dobson, London
Parchappe M J B 1856 Rapport sur la statistique de l'aliénation mentale. Annales Médico-Psychologiques 2: 1–6
Parsons J 1747 Human physiognomy explain'd. Cronian Lectures on muscular motion for the year 1746. Transactions Royal Society, pp 60–62
Petitjean F, Bonnefoy J P, Caroli F, Masse G 1982 Le secteur et la loi du 30 juin 1838. Annales Médico-Psychologiques 140: 301–319
Pistoia L D 1971 Le problème de la temporalité dans la psychiatrie française classique. L'Evolution Psychiatrique 36: 445–474
Platt A M, Diamond B L 1965 The origins and development of the 'wild beast test' concept of mental illness and its relation to theories of criminal responsibility. Journal of the History of the Behavioural Sciences 1: 355–367
Porter T M 1986 The rise of statistical thinking 1820–1900. Princeton University Press, Princeton
Ramul K 1960 The problem of measurement in the psychology of the eighteenth century. American Psychologist 15: 256–265
Rath G 1954 Neuralpathologische Anschauungen in 18. Jahrhundert. Deustche Medizinischen Journal 5: 125–127
Ravaisson F 1885 La philosophie en France au XIXe siècle. 2nd edn. Hachette, Paris
Régis E 1906 Précis de Psychiatrie. Doin, Paris, pp 116–118
Reisman J M 1976 A history of clinical psychology. Irvington, New York
Renaudin E 1856 Observations sur les recherches statistiques relatives a l'aliénation mentale. Annales Médico-Psychologiques 2: 339–360
Report 1883 Association of German physicians practising in lunacy. British Medical Journal 2: 1198–1199
Ribot Th 1885 La psychologie allemande contemporaine. 2nd edn. Alcan, Paris
Ribot Th 1904 Les maladies de la volonté. Alcan, Paris
Richards R J 1977 Lloyd Morgan's theory of instinct: from Darwinism to neo-Darwinism. Journal of the History of the Behavioural Sciences 13: 12–32
Richards R J 1982 The emergence of evolutionary biology of behaviour in the early nineteenth century. British Journal of History of Science 15: 241–280
Riese W 1949 An outline of a history of ideas in neurology. Bulletin of the History of Medicine 23: 111–136
Robinson D N 1986 The Scottish enlightenment and its mixed bequest. Journal of the History of Behavioural Sciences 22: 171–177

Roccatagliata G 1973 Storia della psichiatria antica. Hoepli, Milano
Rochoux, T 1842 Psychologie. In: Dictionnaire de Médécine ou Répertoire général des sciences médicales, Vol 26. Labé, Paris, pp 280–329
Romanes G J 1888 Mental evolution in man. Origin of human faculty. Kegan Paul, London
Rothschuh K E 1973 History of physiology (translated by Risse G B). Krieger, New York
Royer Collard A A 1843 Examen de la doctrine de Maine de Biran. Annales Médico-Psychologiques 2: 1–45
Schultz D 1981 A history of modern psychology. Academic Press, New York
Scull A 1979 Museums of madness. The social organization of insanity in 19thC England. Allen Lane, London
Shryock R H 1961 The history of quantification in medical science. Isis 52: 215–237
Simon B 1978 Mind and madness in ancient Greece. Cornell University Press, Ithaca
Sokal M M, Davis A B, Merzbach U C 1976 Laboratory instruments in the history of psychology. Journal of the History of the Behavioural Sciences 12: 59–64
Spoerl H D 1936 Faculties versus traits: Gall's solution. Character and Personality 4: 216–231
Staum M S 1980 Cabanis. Princeton University Press, Princeton
Swain G 1978 L'aliéné entre le medicin et le philosophe. Perspectives Psychiatriques 65: 90–99
Tamburini N 1881 Le théorie des hallucinations. Revue Scientifique Française et Etranger 27: 138–142
Thompson J D (ed) 1827 The works of William Cullen. 2 vols. Blackwood & Underwood, Edinburgh
Von Feuchtersleben E 1847 The principles of medical psychology (translated by Lloyd H E, Babington B G). Sydenham Society, London
Walker N 1968 Crime and Insanity in England. Vol 1. The historical perspective. Edinburgh University Press, Edinburgh
Walshe F M R 1957 The brain-stem conceived as the 'highest level' of function in the nervous system; with particular reference to the 'automatic apparatus' of Carpenter (1850) and to the 'centrencephalic integrating system' of Penfield. Brain 80: 510–539
Warren H C 1921 History of the association psychology. Scribners, New York
Watson R I (Sr) 1978 The great psychologists. J.B. Lippincott, New York
Wolf T H 1973 Alfred Binet. University of Chicago Press, Chicago
Zupan M L 1976 The conceptual development of quantification in experimental psychology. Journal of the History of the Behavioural Sciences 12: 145–158

4
Edgar Miller

Methodological issues in abnormal psychology

INTRODUCTION

In general the methodological issues that arise in abnormal psychology are much the same as those encountered in other aspects of psychology. To this extent the inclusion of a special chapter on methodology in a book like this might appear superfluous. Nevertheless there are certain methodological problems that are particularly prone to arise in abnormal psychology and which have attracted solutions that are not so frequently exploited in other branches of psychology. It is with these more limited aspects of methodology that the present chapter is concerned.

One immediate problem that arises in abnormal psychology is that many phenomena of particular interest are quite rare, thus making it difficult to collect sizeable groups of subjects. Although well described in psychiatric textbooks, examples of schizophrenics with florid thought disorder rarely arise in clinical practice, and a great many other infrequent phenomena could also be listed. Even in the case of relatively common disorders, such as phobias or psychoses with paranoid delusions, it may still be difficult to collect substantial groups that are reasonably homogeneous and not contaminated by other factors. Two responses to this situation have been devised. One is the use of small N or even single-case experimental designs. The other is the use of analogue subjects.

Another limitation is that research is often carried out on clinical samples. Because the subjects are hospital patients being investigated or treated for their problems this means that certain arrangements or procedures may not be possible for ethical or practical reasons. The most desirable and elegant experimental design may then have to be sacrificed because of other considerations. The investigator may be forced back onto quasi-experimental designs (see p. 60). Even if what might be regarded as conventional research methodology is possible certain problems still remain. Essentially these revolve around the question of experimental control and the consequences of having to design experiments where an entirely adequate control group or condition is just not possible.

Within the relatively small space available, the aim of this chapter is to outline these problems of experimental design and to examine some of the solutions that have been offered. No attempt can be made to describe specific experimental designs within each class but such details can be obtained from other sources and a number of these will be cited at appropriate points. It is also not possible to deal with a number of other issues that arise in designing experiments and especially that of ensuring adequate measurement. Measurement problems are just too varied and alter with the particular experimental situation. Where measurement is a particularly pressing issue it will be taken up in the various chapters on specific topics. In general the approach taken is informed by the views on experimentation put forward by writers like Cook & Campbell (1979). This book is particularly recommended for those not otherwise familiar with the general thrust of the arguments offered in this chapter.

As a final preliminary it is always useful to have an agreed terminology when discussing complex issues. This chapter will use three particular terms very much in the sense used by Cook & Campbell (1979) when dealing with different aspects of the validity of an experimental design. In brief, *internal validity* refers to the degree to which it is possible to assume that changes in the dependent variable really are produced by the relevant experimental manipulations. Thus if an alteration in a subject's environment is made and a change appears in some measured symptom, then how confident is it possible to be that the environmental manipulation really did produce the symptomatic change, as opposed to some other factor that may coincidentally have changed at about the crucial time? *External validity* concerns the degree to which the results of the experiment can be generalized to other similar populations, as opposed to just indicating something that is applicable only to that particular experimental situation. Finally, *statistical conclusion validity* is rather like the concept of power in inferential statistics. In other words it is concerned with the ability of the experiment to detect the looked for effect assuming that the effect is there to be detected. Despite the use of the adjective 'statistical' in the phrase 'statistical conclusion validity' it is important to remember that the sensitivity of an experiment to show up the effect being sought is still an important issue, even for experiments where no formal statistical procedures are used in the analysis of data.

SMALL N AND SINGLE-CASE DESIGNS

These are particularly applicable where the problem being investigated is not encountered frequently and substantial groups of subjects cannot be collected, or where the investigator's circumstances do not otherwise allow the collection of such groups. This is not to imply that single-case or small N designs are always just used as something to fall back upon when the more typical group designs are not possible. In fact advocates of single-case research have claimed positive advantages for the use of these designs, which could make them preferable to group designs even when group designs are possible (Kazdin 1982). These alleged advantages will be considered later. Moreover, as Peck (1985) has pointed out, a number of eminent and influential figures in the history of psychology have based their work on the intensive study of single cases or small groups of cases. These include Pavlov, Freud, Skinner and Piaget. Small N and single-case research therefore has a respectable pedigree although its particular advocacy is a relatively recent phenomenon.

Shapiro (1961) was probably the first to draw attention to the potential value of systematic single-case experiments in the field of abnormal and clinical psychology. Since then a number of extensive descriptions of single-case methodology have appeared, with Hersen & Barlow (1976) and Kazdin (1982) being amongst the most detailed. A surprisingly large number of single-case or small N designs are available but the two most commonly used are undoubtedly the ABAB reversal design and the multiple baseline design. Good descriptions of these, as well as some other single-case or small N designs, can be found in Kazdin (1982).

A major concern with all single-case or small N research is its external validity (Cook & Campbell 1979). (For ease of exposition the discussion of this point, as well as some others, will concentrate on single-case designs. This is possible because the single-case design can be seen as the extreme instance of small N research and what applies to the one applies to a greater or lesser degree to the other.) The subject used in a single-case experiment is usually selected either because he is the only one available with the key characteristic, or because he represents an especially good example of that characteristic in a pure form. No selection procedure will have been gone through to ensure that this subject is in some way representative of those who have, say, checking rituals or early infantile autism. In fact the subject may be rather atypical in being a relatively 'pure' case. The researcher will want to say something about the phenomenon in general rather than about this one example in particular. If such generalization is not possible then the value of single-case research is very limited indeed.

If it is assumed that, say, compulsive checking is mediated by the same mechanisms in all compulsive checkers then a single-case experiment that throws some light on this mechanism should have some validity for all such subjects. It should be noted that this same assumption about homogeneity of mechanism also underlies group experiments designed to investigate the same processes. If subjects in a group of checkers perform their rituals for a number of different reasons then the whole basis of averaging data across subjects from manipulations designed to elucidate the causal mechanism is undermined. This means that as far as research into processes is concerned, and this is the main issue for abnormal psychology, the problem of generalization from single-case experiments, whilst present, is not as great as it might seem at first. In addition replication of single-case experiments is just as important as the replication of research findings from other types of investigation. Replication of findings over a small series of single cases also adds confidence to any generalizations from the results.

Here lies one of the strengths that has been claimed for single-case research. Averaging data across subjects can lead to a misleading picture, where the average is not typical of any individual in the group. For example, Zeaman & House (1963) found that plotting average learning curves in the ordinary way for severely handicapped children yielded a picture of their discrimination learning which was completely erroneous. Single-case research helps to get round the problem of averaging across individuals. In theory the same problem could occur from averaging data within subjects, but this is less likely. Researchers using group studies can get round the problem of misleading averages by carefully inspecting the raw data before averaging, but it is sometimes all too easy to fail to do this. Advocates of single-case methodology also suggest that focusing on the one subject makes the experimenter pay closer attention to what is going on in order to demonstrate effects and this leads to a more penetrating level of analysis (e.g. Kazdin 1982).

Even if these arguments are accepted single-case designs do have real limitations. They may help to illuminate processes but they can say very little about the likely size of an effect (including the size of a treatment effect) in other subjects. If the investigator wants to answer a question concerning the extent to which compulsive checking is also associated with ruminations in obsessionals in general, this is something that can only be answered by a group design.

Another important aspect of single-case (and small N) designs lies in their statistical conclusion validity or their ability to show up the sought for effect if it really is there. Given that some supporters of single-case research deplore the use of statistics, preferring to make judgements on the basis of 'eyeballing' graphs, this is a situation where the use of the term 'statistical conclusion validity' is a little unfortunate. Nevertheless, as already indicated, the question of the sensitivity of an experiment in detecting the sought after effect still remains even if the findings are not analysed statistically. Whether the experiment could show the effect looked for is a particularly important consideration when the results appear to be negative, because a good hypothesis might then be rejected on the basis of an inadequate experimental test.

As Kazdin (1978a) has argued, the common single-case designs (multiple baseline and ABAB designs) work by establishing a baseline level of functioning and then showing that this level alters after intervention such that it becomes clearly different from what would have been expected had baseline conditions continued to operate. This is illustrated by the two hypothetical examples in Figure 4.1. In each case the solid line offers a summary of the actual baseline and its subsequent change, and the interrupted line a continuation of the baseline.

Such designs depend on two conditions that are not always easy to

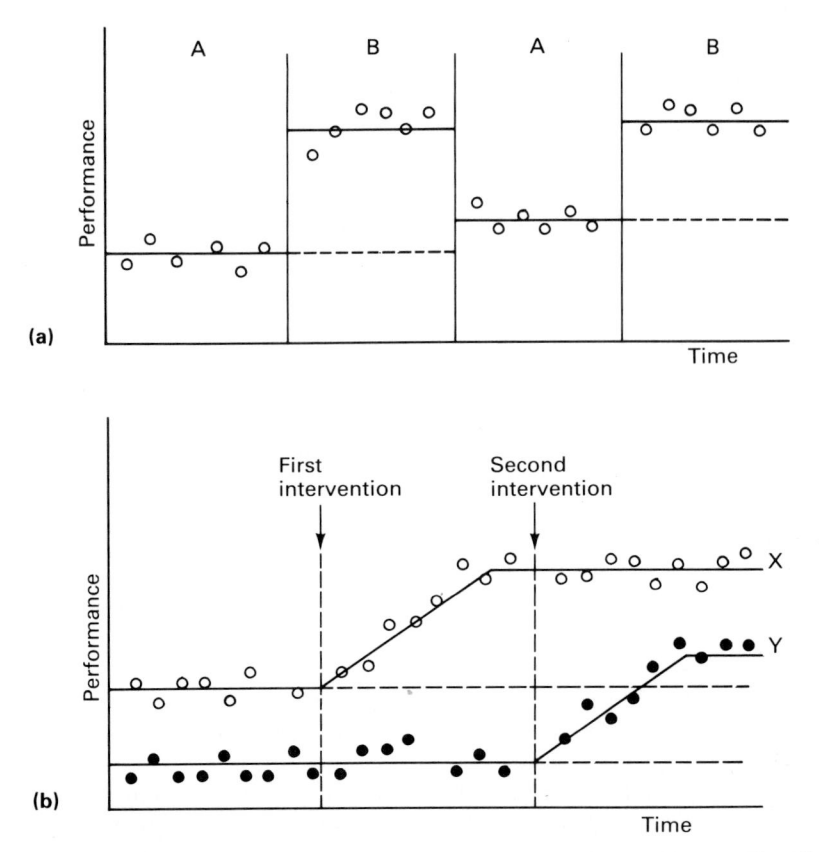

Fig. 4.1 Hypothetical illustrations of two common types of single-case design. (a) The ABAB or reversal design with A = baseline and B = intervention. (b) Multiple baseline design using two measures (X and Y).

achieve in practice. One is the ability to study individuals over relatively long periods of time and free from unprogrammed variations in circumstances that might affect the dependent variable. The second is the ability to obtain or devise measures that can be used repeatedly over time without marked fluctuations from occasion to occasion or being subject to appreciable practice effects. In theory these designs should be able to detect effects against the background of a steady change in the dependent variable. In reality such trends will act so as to blur the sought after effect. Frequent use of a measure can also give problems. For example, practice effects may produce a ceiling against which it becomes impossible to detect any change.

The need to study subjects intensively over long periods of time can also lead to threats against 'internal validity' or the confidence with which the experimenter can claim that a change in the independent variable is really due to the effects of the experimental manipulation. In the multiple baseline experiment shown in Figure 4.1(b) it appears that the two aspects of behaviour being measured really are selectively sensitive to the two manipulations. It is possible that some other influence on the subject's behaviour might be slowly changing and that this change might push both measures in an upward direction. If the variable expected to respond to the first intervention is also more sensitive to these unplanned background changes it might respond earlier than the other and thus produce a picture like that shown in Figure 4.1(b). An alternative explanation of this kind does not seem very convincing on the basis of the rather idealized data shown in Figure 4.1(b) but in practice the picture is often nothing like as clear as this. Thus effects of the kind just described can be difficult to discriminate from a true response to the independent variables.

The lengthy period over which many single-case experiments need to run therefore offers an appreciable opportunity for various uncontrolled events to operate and thus obscure the results. Of course, not all single-case and small N designs need to run over protracted periods and this particularly applies to such designs based on analysis of variance models (e.g. Maxwell 1958). The point is that many single-case experiments do run over relatively long periods of time.

A final issue is the role of statistical analyses in single-case designs. This is controversial, with some rejecting statistical inference and arguing that unless the effects of manipulations are clear-cut enough to be detected without statistical help they are not large enough to be of any consequence. As Peck (1985) indicates, data can be confused and ambiguous, thus requiring some more sophisticated level of analysis than just inspecting graphs. Even though an effect is difficult to detect, this does not mean that the underlying phenomenon is of no real significance or lacks reliability. For example, it could be difficult to detect because the available measures are inadequate. Appropriate statistical procedures are discussed by Kazdin (1976) and these are briefly outlined, together with the most immediate pitfalls, by Peck (1985).

In summary, single-case and small N designs are of considerable value in some situations and are not as limited with regard to making generalizations as might at first be thought. There are, however, some questions that just cannot be answered with single-case designs, or even satisfactorily with small N designs. This is where it is necessary to establish the average size of an effect or to look at the relationship between variables across subjects.

ANALOGUE RESEARCH

Analogue research offers another way of dealing with an inadequate flow of suitable subjects. It also offers a possible way of coping when research with clinical samples does not permit the desired experimental manipulations, whether for ethical or practical reasons. In this context 'analogue research' involves the use of subjects who are not taken from the key population of interest but who show some feature in common with that population. For example, much work on certain models of depression has been carried out on subjects (often students) who are not depressed patients but who score relatively highly on some scale of depression known to discriminate depressed patients from normal samples. It assumed here that the purpose of analogue studies is to throw light on the clinical disorder. This point is made because it occasionally seems to be the case that analogue research generates a momentum of its own, with little concern for truly abnormal populations. As a final preliminary point Kazdin (1978b) has argued that the term 'analogue' in this context is misleading since almost all experiments deal with what is in some way an analogue of the 'real' situation. This point is conceded but this discussion will stick with the commonly used term in its usual meaning.

It is obvious that the crucial issue in analogue research is one of external validity or generalization. Analogue research is useful in so far as the results will generalize to the key population with which the researcher is ultimately concerned. Miller & Morley (1986) have attempted to set out the logical basis for a consideration of this. Analogue subjects can be considered in terms of three sets of characteristics:

A. Features they share with the key population.
B. Features they clearly do not share with the key population.
C. Features they may or may not share with the key population.

Typically the features that fall into category A are such things as a high score on a scale of depression or a fear of some potentially phobic stimulus like a spider. These show that the analogue subject shares to some degree a characteristic that helps to define the abnormal population of interest. There must be some features in category B which distinguish the analogue subject from the key subject, e.g. not having presented as a psychiatric patient. If this were not so the analogue subject would be regarded as being the same, or potentially the same, as the key subject.

The features of interest in analogue experiments will belong to category C. This is necessarily so since the analogue experiment is being carried out because the answer is not known for the key population. If the status of this feature, the factors influencing it, etc. are not known for the key population then it cannot be assigned to category A or B with any certainty. The key question is then the extent to which it is reasonable to assign the findings of any experiment to category A.

In taking the discussion further it should be noted that some of the examples to be considered come from treatment research which is certainly not the main focus of this volume. This is because analogue research has roused the greatest interest in treatment research and most major considerations of its value have been from this standpoint (e.g. Kazdin 1978b, Borkovec & Rachman 1979). Since the real concern at present is with the logic of analogue research which remains much the same regardless of its context, the use of examples from treatment studies is far from inappropriate.

As both Kazdin (1978b) and Miller & Morley (1986) indicate, analogue subjects can differ from clinical samples along a number of dimensions. A particularly important dimension is that of symptom intensity, with the analogue subjects usually being less severe. For example, in one of the earlier studies of the learned helplessness model of depression (Miller & Seligman 1975) students were asked to complete the Beck Depression Inventory. The 'depressed' group was selected from those scoring above the mean on this scale for a general student sample. In this experiment a 'depressed' subject could have a score on the scale well below that associated with clinically significant levels of depression.

In studies of fear it has been found that subjects with lesser degrees of fear are more open to influence by the demand characteristics of the experiment than those with greater levels of fear (Bernstein & Neitzel 1977, Trudel 1979). Trudel (1979) used female students with varying levels of fear for harmless snakes. Moderately and highly afraid subjects were compared on a behavioural avoidance test to see how close subjects would approach a harmless snake, whether they could touch it, pick it up, etc. Half the subjects in each group were given fairly neutral instructions whilst the rest had high demand instructions stressing that subjects had to complete all tasks for the experiment to be successful. As expected, the degree of fear was related to performance on the test but there was a strong interaction between fear level and instructions. High demand instructions did have an effect for both groups but this was much more powerful in the case of the moderately afraid group.

This is only one of many ways in which analogue subjects may differ from clinical populations. In addition they are often students, who will generally be younger, of higher intelligence and come from a more homogeneous social background. They will be recruited by the experimenter in different ways and the investigation may be carried out in a laboratory rather than a hospital. These differences are also likely to induce variations in the level of motivation which are difficult to predict, in that it is easy to think of reasons why clinical subjects might be better motivated and also reasons why the reverse might be the case. In a field like psychology where fairly minor variations in experimental circumstances can sometimes exert quite a marked effect on the results, the potential dangers of analogue research are very real.

Although there is a strong threat to external validity, analogue research has many potential advantages if this threat can be overcome. It is often not possible to use the optimal experimental design with clinical subjects. Analogue experiments can be devised which are better able to neutralize threats to other types of validity, especially internal validity and statistical conclusion validity (i.e. more sensitive in detecting any effects that might be there as well as enabling the relationship between independent and dependent variables to be specified with greater confidence). Probably the best way of overcoming the threat to external validity is to integrate analogue studies into an overall programme of research which includes testing out major findings from analogue subjects on clinical samples as well. Ley (1977) reviews work on doctor–patient communication, which illustrates this very well. Detailed experiments to look at the influence of potentially important variables that could not be readily manipulated in the clinical setting were carried out with analogue subjects. Having drawn conclusions from these as to how doctors might better communicate with their patients, these lessons were put into practice and tested out in the 'real life' setting. Of course it is always possible to argue that what emerged as optimal for analogue subjects might not be optimal in reality, and it was only the suggested optimal solution that was tested out with clinical samples. Nevertheless, this final clinical test does give a much greater confidence in the overall outcome than would otherwise have been possible. It is unfortunate that those carrying out analogue research in other areas, e.g. depression, have generally not tried to integrate analogue and non-analogue research in this close way.

A final limitation of analogue research is that it is not a universally applicable strategy. Analogues of such phenomena as depression and fear or anxiety are easy to find. It is difficult to conceive of convincing analogues for things like paranoid delusions or hypomania.

QUASI-EXPERIMENTAL DESIGNS

These offer another way of coping with situations where an ideal experimental design is not possible. A large number of different quasi-experimental designs exist and these have been explored in some detail by Cook & Campbell (1979). Again all that can be offered here are a few general comments relating to the principles that have to be considered when using these designs.

A fairly typical situation leading to the use of quasi-experimentation is where an investigator is interested in the effect of the social environment on the negative symptoms of chronic schizophrenia. Manipulating a social environment is usually not something that can be done for an individual patient alone, and the investigator will introduce the manipulation to a residential unit such as a ward and note its effect. Just looking at the change in measures before and after the intervention would offer the simplest investigation. However, measures may change over time for a number of reasons unconnected with the effects of any intervention. The investigator may then decide to introduce a control ward with a similar population of chronic schizophrenics. An ideal control may not be possible because the subjects on the control ward may not be matched with those on the experimental ward on variables that might influence outcome, including what are the dependent measures for the experiment. Reassignment of the total pool of patients to achieve matching or a random allocation of subjects to wards is often not possible (for practical and/or ethical reasons). The investigator may use the available control ward to create a more sophisticated quasi-experiment but still one with a much less than perfect degree of experimental control. Even if after the intervention the level of negative symptomatology appears to have decreased more in the experimental group than the control group, it is still quite possible that this differential change is due to factors other than the effects of the experimental manipulation. One possibility is simply that reassessment with the measures has itself produced a change in score and the degree of this 'practice effect' is strongly related to the initial starting level.

As this example illustrates, the main difficulty with quasi-experimentation arises from the fact that the degree of experimental control is far from perfect, leading to threats to internal validity; in other words to problems in assigning any change in dependent variable to the effects of the experimental manipulation. In consequence a wide range of alternative hypotheses may have to be entertained as potential explanations of the findings. Just how serious a limitation this is in practice depends on the context in which the experiment is carried out. If there is other evidence indicating that the most likely alternative explanation of any findings does not in fact operate under similar experimental conditions, then greater confidence can be placed in the results. In some circumstances it is also the case that obtaining some evidence consistent with a hypothesis can be useful even if it still leaves certain other explanations open.

Generally speaking the quasi-experiment is not more open than other forms of experimentation to threats to other forms of validity. Since the restrictions that force the experimenter to use quasi-experimentation arise most commonly out of doing research in applied settings (i.e. in the 'real-life' situation) the external validity of such investigations is usually quite high, assuming that the limitations in internal validity can be overcome.

EXPERIMENTS IN GENERAL: THE PROBLEM OF COMPARISON

Essentially, experiments are concerned with comparison. Subjects are compared under two or more conditions, or two or more groups of subjects are compared under the same conditions. This means that a central concern of any investigation is what is being compared with what, and whether the particular comparison involved is the right one, given the hypothesis that the experiment is designed to test. In the terms of Cook & Campbell (1979) this is a question that is fundamentally tied up with 'internal validity'. This is also an issue that arises in all experimentation and even that which does not involve the special forms of experimental design, such as single-case or quasi-experimental designs, that were discussed earlier in this chapter.

In many group experiments the selection of a control group is not as simple a matter as it might seem. It is always easier to discuss the issues with a specific example in mind, and the present account will consider that of the investigator who is interested in the possible role of attentional impairments in explaining performance decrements, or even the presence of certain symptoms, in schizophrenic subjects. Nevertheless the same basic problems of methodology arise in a wide range of contexts.

It might be hypothesized more specifically that hallucinations in schizophrenics are a consequence of attentional deficits. Assuming that hallucinating schizophrenics can be identified with a reasonable degree of reliability and that a suitable measure of attention can be obtained (and these goals may not themselves be achieved all that easily), one strategy is to compare hallucinating schizophrenics with normal controls. This is obviously inadequate since poor attention may be a characteristic of schizophrenics in general and not just those who hallucinate.

Ideally the control group should be identical in every possible way to the experimental group but for the key feature, which is the presence of hallucinations. In practice this may be difficult or even impossible to achieve. The perfect control group for this experiment would be schizophrenics of similar age, length of hospitalization, length of illness, etc., but who are not hallucinating. Given that schizophrenics who do and do not hallucinate generally differ in other ways (e.g. age and presence of other schizophrenic symptoms), the ideal control group may not be possible. The investigator may have to settle for controls that match the experimental group in some ways but not others. In this case the matching should relate, as far as possible, to those factors that might offer the most plausible alternative explanation of any positive findings. Thus if older schizophrenics are known or suspected to be more prone to hallucinate and older subjects are also more likely to do badly on the measure of attention, then it might be particularly important to match for age. Similarly if chronicity was known to be unrelated to hallucinating and to attentional performance (other than through age) then controlling for the level of chronicity in the subjects would be of much less importance.

A common kind of prediction in abnormal psychology involves comparing two groups in their response to a particular intervention in relation to some baseline performance. Again with the example of attention and schizophrenia in mind it might be hypothesized that schizophrenics do badly on certain tasks (e.g. tasks demanding continuous performance of some type) because their selective attention is poor and they are more readily distracted by background stimuli. A prediction from this might be that lowering the level of background stimulation (e.g. by doing the task in an anechoic chamber) would enhance performance in the schizophrenics but have little effect on normal controls because their selective attention can cope with a moderate degree of background noise. The expectation is that the experiment may give results like those in Figure 4.2, which are at least consistent with the hypothesis.

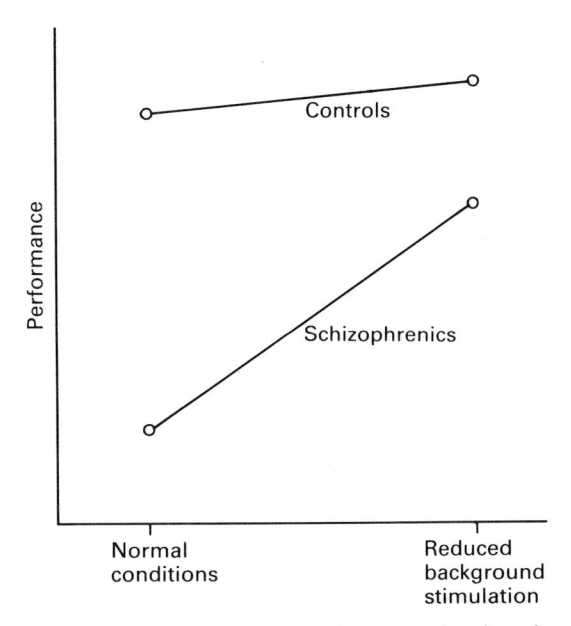

Fig. 4.2 Results of hypothetical experiment comparing schizophrenic and control groups under different levels of background noise.

In this case explanations of the results other than the hypothesized mechanism are possible. It could be, for example, that the control group is experiencing a ceiling effect on the measure and is just not capable of showing much further improvement from the level at which the control group starts. Even if there is no ceiling effect it may be that the measure is not equally sensitive to factors that might produce change over the whole of its range. Finally, it is often quite arbitrary with measures used in psychological experiments whether one uses, say, the number of correct responses, the proportion of correct responses, or some transformation of one of these scores (e.g. the logarithm or square root). Such transformations of the data can sometimes make interactions of the kind shown in Figure 4.2 appear and disappear. Which then offers the correct interpretation of the results? In general such threats to the internal validity of the experiment can only be obviated in situations where the experimental and control groups start off at the same level and then one shows a bigger change in score with the manipulation or, alternatively, where there is a crossover effect where one group benefits from the manipulation and the other has its performance depressed by the same intervention. Such situations occur quite rarely.

Problems like this frequently arise in abnormal psychology. They indicate the value of an alternative kind of strategy for research in abnormal psychology (Miller 1979, Zeaman 1965). The traditional research design for investigating problems in abnormal psychology is to compare an abnormal group on some task of interest with the way in which normal controls (or sometimes some other abnormal group) perform on the same task. The alternative approach, which avoids the difficulty of comparison with often less than ideal control groups, is to use only groups of subjects with the abnormal feature of concern. Thus instead of comparing schizophrenics with normal controls or schizophrenics of a different type, the experimenter looking at attentional mechanisms in schizophrenics may compare matched groups of schizophrenics of the same type in carrying out the attentional task under different conditions or on different types of attentional task. This can be taken even further in some circumstances by using the same group as its own control, i.e. by carrying out the task under different conditions. There are some strong advocates of designs which use subjects as their own controls (i.e. within-subject designs) but it should be noted that these designs can have their own problems and threats to internal validity (Poulton 1982). Essentially these concern possible order effects, such that doing the one version of a task before the other may affect the way the subject performs on the second occasion in a manner or degree different from that if the two versions were administered in the reverse order.

As Zeaman (1965) has indicated, a lot depends here upon what interests the investigator. If the investigator is interested in the *unique* laws that govern the behaviour of the abnormal group of interest, then comparison with normal control groups or other groups of abnormal subjects becomes essential, with all the problems that this may raise. However, if the investigator is interested in the laws that govern, say, the behaviour of schizophrenics or elderly people with dementia, regardless of whether these are different from those applying to any other group, then this can be done without reference to subjects not belonging to the population of interest. In practice the problem of carrying out experiments comparing different kinds of subjects only becomes really acute when dealing with situations where there is a substantial difference in performance between the abnormal group of interest and the control subjects. This is especially the case in comparing severely mentally handicapped or elderly demented subjects with normal controls, but the problem can arise in many other contexts. For example, where speed of performance is important, groups such as institutionalized chronic psychiatric patients or those with severe obsessional states may turn out to be extremely slow.

CONCLUDING COMMENT

This chapter has attempted to outline some major methodological problems that arise in research in abnormal psychology. It has also attempted to discuss and evaluate some of the more commonly adopted solutions to these problems. A proper consideration of methodology would require a substantial text in its own right. All this chapter can try to do is to highlight some of the major issues.

An important general point is that the perfect experiment does not exist. Whatever solution is adopted to any particular problem in experimental design it will always be possible for some critic to argue that there is a factor that has not been adequately controlled and which could therefore furnish an alternative explanation for the data. The skill of the experimenter therefore lies in designing experiments which most closely meet the needs of the hypothesis under investigation, and which have the best chance of demonstrating what has to be demonstrated, given the circumstances involved. In doing this experiments should control for, or rule out, the most likely alternative explanations for the results that the experiment is hoped to produce. Sometimes all the likely alternative explanations cannot be ruled out in one experiment and further investigations may need to be carried out, simply to test the possible impact of these alternative explanations.

Different experimental designs are applicable in different contexts and each type of design carries its own problems of interpretation. Single-case designs have many legitimate uses and are of inestimable value in certain areas of work. They also have important limitations. There are potential problems in relation to external validity and they cannot of themselves answer questions which relate to the likely size of an effect across subjects or which concern the extent to which two or more variables co-vary across subjects. Group designs, and sometimes large group designs, are then essential. Analogue research and quasi-experimental designs similarly have their own advantages and limitations.

Since the perfect experiment does not exist it is no use the experimenter looking for some ideal form of experiment that will answer all problems of experimental design. The investigator has to think out the logic of what is intended and then plan the study to take into account the factors that are most likely to confound the interpretation of the results. Similarly, the consumer of the final report of that work cannot reasonably expect to encounter an investigation that is flawless and not open to any possible criticism or alternative explanation. Acceptance of the results as valid and as having certain implications for the future means accepting that, on balance, the investigation appears to have suggested that something is the case, with alternative explanations being inherently less plausible than the interpretation that is being accepted.

Another implication that follows from this is that issues are not generally decided, either for or against, on the basis of a single experiment. Ideas or theories in any branch of psychology become accepted or rejected on the basis of an accumulation of evidence that converges so as to point towards one particular model as an explanation of the observed phenomena, and where there is a general consensus amongst psychologists and other relevant scientists that the likely confounding effects have been excluded. Good methodology in individual experiments makes this convergence of findings easier to achieve and gives the user of that research greater confidence in any decisions based upon the results.

REFERENCES

Bernstein D A, Neitzel M T 1977 Demand characteristics in behaviour modification: the natural history of a nuisance. Progress in Behavior Modification 4: 119–162

Borkovec T D, Rachman S 1979 The utility of analogue research. Behaviour Research and Therapy 17: 119–126

Cook T D, Campbell D T 1979 Quasi-experimentation: design and analysis issues for field settings. Rand McNally, Chicago

Hersen M, Barlow D H 1976 Single case experimental designs: strategies for studying behavior change. Pergamon Press, Oxford

Kazdin A E 1976 Statistical analyses for single-case experimental designs. In: Hersen M, Barlow D H (eds) Single case experimental designs: strategies for studying behavior change. Pergamon, New York

Kazdin A E 1978a Methodological and interpretive problems of single-case experimental designs. Journal of Consulting and Clinical Psychology 46: 629–642

Kazdin A E 1978b Evaluating the generality of findings in analogue therapy research. Journal of Consulting and Clinical Psychology 46: 673–686

Kazdin A E 1982 Single case research designs: methods for clinical and applied settings. Oxford University Press, New York

Ley P 1977 Psychological studies of doctor–patient communication. In: Rachman S (ed) Contributions to medical psychology, Vol. 1. Pergamon Press, Oxford

Maxwell A E 1958 Experimental design in psychology and the medical sciences. Methuen, London

Miller E 1979 Memory and ageing. In: Gruneberg M M, Morris P E (eds) Applied problems in memory. Academic Press, London

Miller E, Morley S 1986 Investigating abnormal behaviour. Weidenfeld & Nicolson, London

Miller W R, Seligman M E P 1975 Depression and learned helplessness in man. Journal of Abnormal Psychology 84: 228–238

Peck D F 1985 Small N experimental designs in clinical practice. In: Watts F N (ed) New developments in clinical psychology. British Psychological Society/Wiley, Chichester

Poulton E C 1982 Influential companions: effects of one strategy on another in the within-subjects design of cognitive psychology. Psychological Bulletin 91: 673–690

Shapiro M B 1961 The single case in clinical psychological research. British Journal of Medical Psychology 34: 255–262

Trudel G 1979 The effects of instructions and level of fear. Behaviour Research and Therapy 17: 113–118

Zeaman D 1965 Learning processes of the mentally retarded. In: Osler S F, Cook R E (eds) The biological basis of retardation. Johns Hopkins University Press, Baltimore

Zeaman D, House B J 1963 The role of attention in retardate discrimination learning. In: Ellis N R (ed) Handbook of Mental Deficiency. McGraw Hill, New York

Social perspectives on depression and schizophrenia

INTRODUCTION

Social aspects of psychiatric disorder have generated considerable interest, particularly since the 1950s. There is substantial disagreement about how much weight should be given to the role of social factors in such disorders. Research has focused on the influence of social factors on onset, course and treatment. In this chapter two major psychiatric disorders, depression and schizophrenia, will be examined in the light of the research evidence. In depression, attention has been directed chiefly to onset and risk factors such as gender, class, race, unemployment and social supports and stressors. Less attention has been given to the role of such factors on course and outcome. In contrast, research into the social aspects of schizophrenia has moved away from the examination of precipitating factors and concentrated on the course of the disorder. The social factors that have been implicated in this condition are familial, societal, social networks and cultural. For both depression and schizophrenia, there has been recent interest in the idea of preventing or ameliorating the adverse impact of social stressors.

There are important methodological difficulties in investigating the role of social factors in both depression and schizophrenia. In depression there has been a fundamental issue of defining a 'case' (Wing et al 1981); when does one person's sadness and loss of interest become a depressive disorder? The definition of depression employed has varied widely between research studies. However, a broad distinction can be drawn between those studies which use some measure of depressive symptoms, most commonly a self-report questionnaire such as the Beck Depression Inventory (BDI, Beck et al 1961), and those which employ a clinically based categorical definition of a depressive disorder, e.g. the DSM III definitions or those diagnoses derived from the PSE CATEGO ID system (Wing et al 1974). For present purposes, only those studies which have investigated non-psychotic depression will be considered, since the role of social factors is most closely implicated and widely studied in relation to this type of depression.

In schizophrenia, where self-report may be the sole method of gaining information about symptoms, in the past diagnostic practices have been liable to error and misinterpretation. However, the use of standardized and reliable interviews, like the Present State Examination (Wing et al 1974), has become the norm in the more recent studies reviewed below. A further methodological problem is how to assess social factors reliably and with high validity. Thus, the question of how to measure life events has generated much debate (Brown 1974). There still remains some controversy in this area, concerning such issues as what is to be measured, biases in recall, and whether events can be assessed independently of psychiatric state.

In respect of the outcome and treatment of depression and schizophrenia, there has been a move towards investigation of the possibility of protecting against life stresses. In depression the emphasis has been on the interactions between social supports and social stressors and how these might alleviate the severity or duration of the disorder. In schizophrenia there have been some recent intervention studies arising from research into social factors in families. While it is not clear whether such interventions can do more than delay relapse in schizophrenia, they are an interesting example of the application of social research via a novel treatment approach.

Overall the research into social factors in these disorders is still at an early stage. While some progress has been made in methodology, the results have reflected the complexities of the areas being investigated, and the necessarily interactive nature of social factors. Many gaps and many questions remain. This chapter attempts to review and consolidate the most recent research in these areas, to illustrate how the methodological problems have been tackled, and to highlight how different social factors have been emphasized in depression and schizophrenia.

DEPRESSION

A great number of social factors have been implicated in the onset and maintenance of depression. In the following section five main categories will be examined: gender; social class; race and migration; unemployment; and social supports and stressors.

Onset and risk

Gender

Women have been found to have a greater risk of both clinical depression and depressive symptoms than have men. Overall, women are about twice as likely as men to be depressed. However, most of the studies that have looked at sex differences in depression have been conducted in Western countries and it is unclear whether such a sex difference would be observed in other countries. In two comprehensive reviews of sex differences in depression, Weissman & Klerman (1977, 1985) assessed the available evidence from a variety of sources. They concluded that a consistently greater number of women than men were treated for depression and were identified as depressed in epidemiological studies. They also report that suicide attempters are more likely to be women. The ratio of women to men in all these cases is roughly 2 : 1.

Boyd & Weissman (1981) compared depression rates by sex among bipolar and unipolar depressions separately. They found that it was only rates of unipolar depression that were higher for women than for men, there being no differences in rates of bipolar depression. Results from the New Haven site of the NIMH Epidemiological Catchment Area study have been reported by Weissman et al (1984). The NIMH Diagnostic Interview Schedule was used to collect information about symptoms, and diagnoses were made using DSM III. The diagnosis of major depression was found to be significantly more common in women than in men (2.4 : 1). However, there was no difference by sex in rates of bipolar depression.

In a longitudinal study, Hagnell et al (1982) compared the rates of depression in a Swedish population over many years and suggested that, although there may have been an overall increase in the rate of major depression recently, the difference in rates between men and women may be decreasing. In Weissman & Klerman's (1985) review of recent epidemiological studies in the USA, they note an increase in rates of major depression in women. However, for bipolar disorders the sex ratios are equal.

The above studies have examined rates of the clinical syndrome of depression; and results from studies looking at depressive symptoms have largely confirmed these findings. For example, Amenson & Lewinsohn (1981) in a community study in the USA used both the Research Diagnostic Criteria (RDC, Spitzer et al 1978) and the CES-D measure of depressive symptoms (Radloff 1977). They found that roughly twice as many women as men met the RDC criteria for unipolar depression and that this greater risk was accounted for by the fact that women with previous episodes of depression were more likely to have subsequent episodes than were men. In a community study of a black Southern community in the United States, Dressler & Badger (1985) found that women reported a substantially greater number of depressive symptoms than men.

A number of explanations have been offered to account for women's increased risk of depression. Some of the main ones are:
1. Artefactual explanations suggest that women are more likely to recall and report psychological symptoms than are men. However, there is little direct support for this explanation, and some contrary evidence. For example, a study by Byrne (1981) confirmed that the observed sex difference in depression was not an artefact of women's style of reporting distress. He found that the sex differences held for the somatic symptoms of depression as well as the affective and emotional symptoms. Similarly Amenson & Lewinsohn (1981) did not find that women were more likely to label themselves 'depressed' than men with the same severity of symptoms.

2. Social status explanations have located women's greater risk of depression in their social conditions. Such explanations would include reference to the role restrictions (Gove 1972, Radloff 1975) suffered by women, which limit their experiences of success and mastery, as well as material restrictions which lead to legal and economic dependence. Kessler (1979a), using data from an earlier community survey (Myers et al 1975), found that, relative to men, women were both more exposed to stressful life events and more vulnerable to the impact of such stressors. Women were found to use less effective coping strategies and to be less helped by the family's financial resources.
3. Cognitive or personality explanations suggest that women have acquired, through their socialization and later life experiences, a bias against independence and self-assertion which makes them more at risk of depression. Some studies have found evidence of a 'learned helplessness' style in females (Deaux et al 1975) but personality studies have not found evidence for a specific depressive personality type in women when compared with men (Hirschfeld et al 1983).

It is worthwhile bearing in mind, as Weissman & Klerman (1985) point out, that it is unlikely that any single explanation will adequately account for the increased risk of depression in women.

Social class

One of the earliest studies to highlight the differential risk of psychiatric disorder by social class was carried out by Hollingshead & Redlich (1958) in New Haven. All patients receiving psychiatric care were assessed and it was found that there was an excess of patients from the lower socio-economic groups. In a follow-up study of Hollingshead & Redlich's original sample, Myers & Bean (1968) reported that social class position in 1950 was predictive of psychological adjustment in 1960.

In a community survey, Brown & Harris (1978) found a greater prevalence of psychiatric disorder among working-class women than among middle-class women in London. This class difference held only for women with children at home. Since single women and married women without children at home are more likely to be in paid employment, this class difference may have been accounted for, in part, by differences in actual or disposable income. Brown & Harris (1978) also found that the class difference could be explained in terms of certain 'vulnerability' factors being more likely among the working-class women. These were loss of mother before the age of 11, lack of an intimate confiding relationship, lack of paid employment and having three or more children under the age of 14 living at home. It seems likely that these vulnerability factors are themselves markers of deficits in social and material resources (Campbell 1983). Additional support for this interpretation comes from a study of poverty in Britain by Layard et al (1978). They found that about half of those families in which there were three or more children and the woman was not in paid employment had incomes below the official poverty line. It is clear that it might be expected that some of Brown & Harris's most vulnerable women would be expected also to be among the poorest families.

The relationship between social class and depression may be mediated by some particular correlate of class membership such as income, an interpretation supported by Hagnell's (1966) Swedish study. No relationship was found between social class and psychological disorder once poverty had been taken into account. Pearlin & Johnson (1977) have reported that level of depression varied directly with level of economic strain. Similarly, in a community sample in the USA, Dean et al (1981) found that the best predictors of depressive symptoms were family income and reported monetary problems. Together these accounted for almost 34% of the variance in depressive symptoms.

Two recent British community studies have produced conflicting findings. Surtees et al (1983), using the same definitions of social class and psychiatric disorder as Brown & Harris (1978), found a significantly higher prevalence of psychiatric disorder among working-class than middle-class women. However, Bebbington et al (1981a) failed to find any statistically significant class differences in prevalence in a male and female sample. Nevertheless, in the latter study, there was a trend for a higher prevalence of depression in the working-class group.

One of the first large-scale surveys of psychological disorder in the community was the Midtown study, which was carried out in a random sample in Manhattan (Srole et al 1962, Langner & Michael 1962). This and many later studies have consistently reported that the highest prevalence of depressive symptoms is found among lower socio-economic groups (Berkman 1971, Warheit et al 1973). In a large community study in the USA, Comstock & Helsing (1976) found that low-income groups had the highest frequency of individuals with depressive symptoms. This finding is consistent with those of a similar community study conducted by Ilfeld (1978), in which associations between symptom measures and a number of socio-demographic factors were examined. He found a significant association between higher levels of symptoms and lower levels of education, income and occupational status.

There has been, therefore, a consistent finding that lower social classes are at greater risk of the depressive syndrome and depressive symptoms. Most writers have invoked some version of a social causation hypothesis to explain these findings. This hypothesis suggests that a lower social class position is associated with a number of stressful factors. In addition, working class membership is thought to reduce the individual's resources for coping with stress (Kessler & Cleary 1980, Brown & Harris 1978, Liem & Liem 1978). Such a social causation model suggests that both cultural (beliefs and values) and material (financial support, access to professional help) aspects of class membership must be taken into account in explaining the greater prevalence of depression among lower class groups. It seems difficult to avoid the conclusion (Liem & Liem 1978) that 'social class is a principal aspect of social structure relevant to the psychological well-being of the individual'.

Race and migration

The results of studies examining the association between ethnic origin and risk of depression have been inconsistent. However, recent studies have found that once age, sex and social class are taken into account, there are few if any racial risk factors for depression. There have been relatively few British studies conducted in this area. In these studies it has often not been possible to study increased risk associated with membership of a particular ethnic group independently of any increased risk that may be a function of the migratory process itself.

There have been two early general practice studies in Britain comparing the psychological health of different ethnic groups (Pinsent 1963, Hashmi 1968). Both of these studies suggested that West Indians had a greater risk of psychiatric disorder. Unfortunately, neither used standardized methods of assessing psychiatric disorder. A more recent community study was conducted by Bebbington and his colleagues (Bebbington et al 1981b). They compared rates of psychiatric disorder, using the Present State Examination, in West Indian-born and native-born residents of London. Among West Indian men there tended to be lower rates of disorder than among native-born men, but there was no such difference among women. In a Swedish study, Halldin (1985) found no difference in the prevalence of disorder between Swedish-born and foreign-born individuals.

There have only been two community studies of symptom rates in different ethnic groups in Britain. In their first study, Cochrane & Stopes-Roe (1979) compared the mental health of immigrant Irish, native Irish and native English. The immigrants were found to have fewer symptoms than the native Irish, but the native English had a greater number of symptoms than either of the Irish groups. In their second study (Cochrane & Stopes-Roe 1980) comparisons were made between samples born in England, India and Pakistan. The Indians had fewest psychiatric symptoms, with the English and Pakistanis having similar levels of symptoms.

Many more studies have been conducted in the United States. Dohrenwend & Dohrenwend (1969), in an early review, discussed the findings from eight studies. Of these, half reported higher rates for blacks and half reported higher rates for whites. Later studies have found that blacks score significantly higher than whites on symptom scales; but, when the results were controlled for age, sex and socio-economic status, this difference disapeared (e.g. Warheit et al 1975, Steele 1978, Ilfeld 1978). Therefore, these more recent studies have concluded that race is not in itself an important predictor of level of psychiatric symptoms.

Unemployment

In general the benefits of paid employment have been suggested to include psychological, social and material aspects. The psychological benefits include a sense of confidence and self-esteem and the affording of social identity and status. However, women's relationship to paid employment has been different from that of men's for a number of reasons. Most women of working age will have the primary responsibility in their families for the tasks of child care and housekeeping. Women are therefore often simply not available for work outside the home because of their commitments within it. This family-based work can provide women with a socially legitimated and potentially gratifying alternative to paid employment with the result that many women who are 'unemployed' are not actively seeking paid employment and do not consider themselves to be without a work role. It is perhaps not surprising therefore that while unemployment has been found to be a clear risk factor for depression in men, the picture is a more complicated one for women.

It has consistently been found that unemployment among men is associated with an increased risk of psychiatric disorder (Finlay-Jones & Eckhardt 1981, Dooley & Catalano 1980, Warr 1982). Both cross-sectional and longitudinal studies have been carried out to investigate the association between unemployment and depression. Between 20 and 30% of men report an increase in psychological symptoms or a deterioration in psychological health following job loss (Warr & Jackson 1985, Payne et al 1984). Warr (1984) concluded from his review of previous studies that it was not the case that the chronically psychologically distressed were more likely to become unemployed, but rather that it was the fact of unemployment that led to psychological disorder.

The results from studies of women and unemployment have been mixed. In their London study, Brown & Harris (1978) found that lack of employment acted as a 'vulnerability' factor (a risk factor only when in combination with some severe life stress), but only among women without a confiding relationship. However, the role of unemployment as such a vulnerability factor was not confirmed in a similar study of women in the Outer Hebrides (Brown & Prudo 1981) or in studies in other localities (Solomon & Bromet 1982, Costello 1982, Campbell et al 1983).

In another London community study, Bebbington et al (1981a) found that women in part-time or full-time employment were significantly less likely than women without paid employment to be diagnosed as having a psychiatric disorder. Similarly, in Edinburgh, Surtees et al (1983) found that significantly more unemployed working-class women (11.5%) were cases of depression than were employed working-class women (2.5%).

Certain factors appear to mediate between employment status and psychiatric disorder in women. Warr & Parry (1982a) re-examined data from the surveys conducted by Bebbington et al (1981a) and Brown &

Harris (1978). In both studies the association between lack of employment and psychiatric case status held only for working-class women.

In a large American community survey, Roberts et al (1982) found that women who were not employed had significantly more psychological symptoms than women who were employed. However, when amount of social contact was taken into account, the relationship between employment status and levels of symptoms was non-significant.

Most British studies have found that women in paid employment are less likely to have psychiatric symptoms. In a study of working-class women with children, Warr & Parry (1982b) found that women in full-time employment had significantly lower scores on a measure of depressed mood than women in part-time work or non-employed women. Cochrane & Stopes-Roe (1981) also found that women in paid employment had fewer symptoms than women at home. Warr & Parry (1982a) have produced a comprehensive review of the association between paid employment and psychological well-being in women, in which they caution against the search for a simple association between work and psychological health. They reassessed previous studies of women's employment and psychiatric disorder by subdividing the samples according to lifestyle, marital status and the presence of children. They concluded that in the case of single women there does appear to be a strong positive association between psychological well-being and paid employment. However, no simple association, between employment and psychiatric symptoms, was found among married women. Results from studies conducted in North America and Australia largely confirm the above findings. A recent review of these studies can be found in O'Brien (1986).

Social supports and social stressors

The degree and quality of social contact has been considered to be an important factor in determining the risk of developing a psychiatric disorder and the risk of having a chronic rather than a short-lived episode. The social network that is available to an individual has been thought to provide a variety of different resources, from emotional support to practical advice and assistance (Caplan 1981).

Some researchers have emphasized almost exclusively the emotional and psychological provisions of the social network, while others have given primary emphasis to its practical and instrumental aspects. As well as diversity in conceptualization of the role of social contact, there has been a considerable diversity in its measurement. It is therefore difficult to compare results from different studies and to draw any unequivocal conclusions about the role of friends and kin in relation to the risk of psychiatric disorder.

A common distinction that has been made is between 'close' contacts and support and 'diffuse' contacts and support. Individuals providing 'close' support would include spouses and confidants, or the 'principal attachment figures' as Henderson et al (1978) have termed them. 'Diffuse' social contacts would include friends, kin and the social contacts and supports provided by neighbourhood or community affiliations such as belonging to a social club or attending a church.

In Brown & Harris's (1978) study in London, it was found that divorced, separated and widowed women had a higher prevalence of psychiatric disorder than married women. However, in another British community survey women who had never been married were found to have the lowest prevalence of psychiatric disorder (Surtees et al 1983); and women who were divorced, widowed, separated or cohabiting had the highest rates, almost one in five having a disorder of case severity. Married women had intermediate rates. These findings were very similar to those of Bebbington et al (1981a) in their London study. They found that the divorced, widowed and separated had the highest prevalence of psychiatric disorder; but women who had never been married had a lower rate of disorder than married women.

Some studies have examined the relationship between the simple presence of a spouse or confidant and level of psychiatric symptoms. In a large American community study, Pearlin & Johnson (1977) found that married people had fewer depressive symptoms than unmarried. Those formerly married, whether widowed, divorced or separated, had the highest scores on depression symptom scales. Those who had never been married had symptom scores which were intermediate between those of the formerly married and the currently married. These results were true both for men and for women. Pearlin & Johnson (1977) also found that being unmarried was associated with having fewer social contacts. The unmarried were more likely to experience social isolation, to have fewer local friends and were less likely to belong to voluntary associations. Further American community studies found that the absence of a spouse was associated with greater psychiatric symptom scores. Warheit (1979) found that married people had lower symptom scores than non-married people, as did Comstock & Helsing (1976). Dean et al (1981) also found that unmarried people reported more depressive symptoms, while in Ilfeld's (1978) survey married individuals had considerably less symptoms than others, even after controlling for age and sex.

Roberts et al (1982) distinguished between the never-married and those who were single because of separation, divorce or widowhood. In their large community survey of American women, they found that those individuals who had never married reported less symptoms than married individuals, who in turn had fewer symptoms than those who had been divorced, separated or widowed. They then calculated the equivalent proportions from Finlay-Jones and Burvill's (1979) study of Australian women and found a very similar distribution of psychiatric disorder by marital status. These last results suggest that the mere absence of a spouse is not necessarily associated with a greater risk of having psychiatric symptoms, but the fact of having had a spouse and then lost that person is associated with an increased risk.

In conclusion, the simple absence of a spouse does not in itself seem to be a risk factor for psychiatric disorder. Although not all studies have broken down their results to allow a comparison between those single individuals who have never married and other unmarried people, on the whole it appears that it is worse to have had and lost a spouse than not to have had one at all. This may be because they are still suffering some bereavement reaction or because divorced, separated or widowed people have greater life stresses to cope with, such as financial hardship.

Some investigators have not been content with examining the effect of the mere presence of a spouse but have attempted to relate the risk of psychiatric disorder to the quality of any such relationship. In a British sample drawn from general practitioner attenders, Miller & Ingham (1976) found that having a confidant was associated with lower levels of tiredness, anxiety and depression. However, these findings were true only for women and not for men. Similarly, the quality of communication with their husband was found to be associated with depressive symptoms in British women six weeks after childbirth (Paykel et al 1980). In a British sample of depressed patients, Surtees (1980) found that patients with a close, confiding relationship had less severe symptoms at follow-up than those patients without such a relationship.

In contrast, Henderson's Australian community study (Henderson et al 1981) did not find that the availability of close relationships was consistently related to levels of psychiatric symptoms. However, he did find that the perceived adequacy of close relationships was significantly associated with both concurrent and subsequent symptoms.

The role of diffuse support has been examined by a number of researchers. A number of British studies have found that having many friends is associated with having few psychological symptoms (Cooke 1981, Miller & Ingham 1976). However, there have been conflicting results from two Australian studies. A community study by Andrews et al (1978) did not find a significant association between diffuse support, as measured by neighbourhood interaction and community participation, and psychological impairment. They did find that perception of the support that would be available in a crisis was related to symptom score. In Henderson et al's (1981) community study, both the availability of diffuse relationships and their perceived adequacy were significantly positively correlated with concurrent and subsequent symptoms.

There have been a number of studies which have examined the role of life stress in the onset of clinical depression in community samples. The most methodologically sound have been those studies which have employed the method of assessment of life events developed by Brown and his colleagues (Brown et al 1975, Brown & Harris 1978).

Brown & Harris (1978) in a sample of London women found that 89% of women with an onset of depression had had a severe life event or difficulty prior to the onset of their depression. This was a significantly greater proportion than amongst those who were not cases, of whom 30% had had a similar stress in a comparable time period. In a study in the Outer Hebrides, Brown & Prudo (1981) found that severe life events and difficulties played the same aetiological role as they had in the London sample. These findings have been confirmed in a number of studies which used the same measures of life stress and psychiatric disorder as the two studies mentioned above (Tennant et al 1981a, Costello 1982, Campbell et al 1983).

There has been a considerable debate about the inter-relationships between life stress, social support and psychiatric symptoms. There have been several studies which have confirmed Brown & Harris's (1978) original finding that having an intimate, confiding relationship is protective in the face of severe life stress (Solomon & Bromet 1982, Costello 1982, Campbell et al 1983). These studies have been reviewed by Tennant (1985).

In Surtees' (1980) study of depressed psychiatric patients it was found that those individuals who had close and reciprocal confiding relationships were protected against psychological distress when faced with severe life stress. Surtees (1980) then examined the data to see if the variation in depression scores could be accounted for by the independent and separate effects of life stress and social support or if there was some interaction effect of these two variables over and above their separate and joint effects. He found different results depending on the different statistical analyses used, and the issue remains undecided. Warheit (1979) found that close social contact had a protective effect at all levels of life stress. In a community study in Los Angeles County, Aneshensel and Stone (1982) found that no interaction term was needed to explain the effects of support and life stress on symptoms.

Evidence for diffuse social contact buffering the effects of life stress has been found by several researchers (Frydman 1981, Henderson et al 1981, Warheit 1979, Miller & Ingham 1976). However, some others have found that level of diffuse social support does not relate to the development of psychiatric symptoms in the face of life stress (Brown & Harris 1978, Andrews et al 1978, Surtees 1980). There is therefore less consensus about the stress-buffering role of diffuse social contact than there is about the protective effect of close social contact. Those individuals who experience some life stress but have close social contacts, particularly confiding relationships, appear to be relatively protected from developing psychiatric symptoms. However, the majority of studies have relied upon retrospective accounts and have employed correlational statistics. It is very difficult therefore to rule out the alternative explanation that psychiatric disorder itself is responsible for low levels of support or the lack of an intimate relationship. Certain depressive symptoms (e.g. social withdrawal, loss of interest, self-depreciation) could bring about the diminution of social contacts. The direction of causality is therefore unclear.

Maintenance and remission

The influence of each of the above social factors will be examined briefly in the following section in relation to the course and outcome of depression. There has been considerably less research in this area than in the area of risk factors in relation to depression.

There are very few studies which have specifically addressed the issue of sex differences in outcome of depression. Amenson & Lewinsohn (1981) did not find that women had longer-lasting episodes of depression than men but did observe that women who had previously been depressed were more likely than men to have a further episode. In a five-year follow up of a community sample, Beiser (1976) found that men were less likely to recover from psychiatric disorder than women. There were no significant sex differences in outcome in the follow-up studies conducted by Billings & Moos (1985) and by Mann et al (1981).

In two studies of the outcome of neurotic disorders in British psychiatric outpatients, Huxley & Goldberg (1975) and Huxley et al (1979) found that one of the best predictors of clinical outcome at one year was material circumstances, including quality of housing, number of consumer durables and adequacy of income. Beiser (1976) concluded that such circumstances afforded a wider range of resources which might contribute to recovery from psychological disorder. He found that the chronically ill were more likely to be in the lowest of his socio-economic categories. A number of other studies have found that improvement in neurotic symptoms is associated with higher social class (Gift et al 1986, Rance 1976, Wheaton 1978).

There have been virtually no longitudinal studies of the association between race and maintenance of depression and only a few such studies examining the role of unemployment. Warr & Jackson (1985) found that men who were continuously unemployed over a nine-month period showed a deterioration in psychological health across time. Re-employment has been found to be associated with a decrease in symptoms in this and other studies (Banks & Jackson, 1982). Feather & Davenport (1981) failed to find any association between duration of unemployment and affective reactions; however, they did not attempt to measure chronic depression as such.

The roles of stressors and supports has also been examined in relatively few studies. Billings & Moos (1985), in their follow-up study of patients with unipolar depressive disorders, found that stressors were predictive of outcome. However, post-treatment stressors and resources were found to be more important than those that occurred pre-treatment (Billings & Moos, 1985). In addition, in relation to outcome, the quality of social support available was more important than its quantity. Mann et al (1981) also found that the perceived quality of social and family life was associated with outcome at 12 months follow-up. In another follow-up study of depressed patients, Surtees & Ingham (1980) found that patients with a moderate level of depressive symptomatology at follow-up had had significantly more life events and difficulties than patients with none or fewer symptoms. Other studies examining the role of life events in relapse include Monroe et al (1983) and Paykel & Tanner (1976). As well as examining the role of stressful negative events in relation to outcome, some researchers have looked at the effects of 'positive' events (Cohen & Hoberman 1983). Billings & Moos (1985) found that post-treatment positive events were associated with fewer depressive symptoms and greater levels of self-esteem. Tennant et al (1981b) found that remission of symptoms was related to 'neutralizing' life events which counteracted the impact of previously occurring negative events.

Conclusion

Many different social characteristics have been found to be implicated in the onset, prevalence and maintenance of depression. For the purposes of this review, each of these factors has been examined separately. However, there are complex inter-relationships between them which are just beginning to be explored in relation to depression. As Liem & Liem (1978) observe, the social processes which are investigated by researchers are artificially abstracted from the wider social context.

The broad conclusion that can be drawn is that certain social positions probably carry with them a disproportionate exposure to stress as well as increasing the vulnerability of the individual to those stresses. The processes by which social risk is translated into the psychological reality of depression for any given individual are still only poorly understood. The elucidation of these processes is a vital research task.

SCHIZOPHRENIA

Schizophrenia has been defined as

> a group of psychoses in which there is a fundamental disturbance of personality, a characteristic distortion of thinking, often a sense of being controlled by alien forces, delusions which may be bizarre, disturbed perception, abnormal affect out of keeping with the real situation and autism. Nevertheless, clear consciousness and intellectual capacity are usually maintained. The disturbance of personality involves its most basic functions which gives the person his/her feeling of individuality, uniqueness and self direction.
> (WHO, International Classification of Diseases)

The lifetime risk of developing schizophrenia is 1 in 100, and its prevalence is 0.5 in 100. It is not confined to any particular society or culture and has been found to exist to a similar extent in various countries (WHO, International Pilot Study of Schizophrenia 1973). It ranks as a major disorder, of the same magnitude as diabetes in the general population. It is more likely to affect men than women, and has a typical onset in early adulthood, although sometimes onset is in middle age, often associated with a paranoid illness. It is not confined initially to a particular social class, although after onset more people cluster in the lower social classes due to its disabling effects on factors such as employment status and social relationships.

Onset and risk

Family factors

Early studies of the families of schizophrenic patients concentrated on causes: how did this family produce this 'sick' individual? A variety of suggestions were proposed to answer this question. For instance, Bateson et al (1956) proposed that schizophrenia was the result of a family's 'double bind' communication. Wynne & Singer (1963, 1965) also focused on communication difficulties and found that parents of schizophrenic patients had a 'fragmented' or 'amorphous' communication style. Lidz (1975) identified parents with schizophrenic offspring as having 'schism' or 'skew' in the marriage and narcissistic egocentricity. Alternatively, Laing & Esterson (1964) considered schizophrenia in terms of a valid and understandable response to particular family and societal pressures.

Hirsch & Leff (1975), in an extensive review of the role of parents in the aetiology of schizophrenia, looked closely at the experimental evidence on which these ideas were based. As a result they concluded, very parsimoniously:

> In our view the following statements are *reasonably* supported by the experimental evidence [page 104].
> (1) More parents of schizophrenics are psychiatrically disturbed than parents of normal children, and more of the mothers are 'schizoid'.
> (2) There is a link between allusive thinking in schizophrenics and their parents but this is also true in normal people in whom it occurs less frequently.
> (3) The parents of schizophrenics show more conflict and disharmony than parents of other psychiatric patients.
> (4) The pre-schizophrenic child more frequently manifests physical ill health or mild disability early in life than the normal child.
> (5) Mothers of schizophrenics show more concern and protectiveness than mothers of normals both in their current situation and in their attitude to children before they fell ill.
> (6) The work of Wynne and Singer strongly suggests that parents of schizophrenics communicate abnormally, but their most definite findings have not been replicated.

There is little definitive evidence up to 1975 of family factors accounting for the onset of schizophrenia. This has not changed in the last decade. Theories have often been vague and, as a consequence, difficult to test. The studies rely on retrospective data so that even if differences are found it is not clear whether they are causal factors or constitute a reaction to the problem. Family theories fail to explain why one particular sibling becomes schizophrenic. If, on the other hand, there are several cases in the same family, one cannot ignore the possibility of a genetic explanation. There are also methodological problems in choosing 'normal' families for comparison purposes (Haley 1972). One possible way of elucidating causal family factors is to carry out a longitudinal study of families with children who may be at 'high risk' of developing schizophrenia (e.g. Venables 1977, Goldstein 1985). These, however, have their own problems (Shakow 1973), such as the length of time required to complete the study, the ethics of non-intervention, and high drop-out rates.

Societal factors

There was some early interest in labelling theory interpretations of the origins of schizophrenia. Scheff (1966) hypothesized that society's reaction to odd or eccentric behaviour in individuals caused them to be labelled as 'deviant' and that this label was self-fulfilling. An individual called 'schizophrenic' and placed in a mental hospital would then behave even more oddly and be reinforced by the institution for 'sick' behaviour rather than normal behaviour (Goffman 1961). This hypothesis called into question the wide range of odd behaviour that could at that time be used as a basis for the diagnosis of schizophrenia, particularly in the USA, and the problems of using self-report data as the only indicator of a schizophrenic illness.

There is little real evidence that labelling by itself has a causal role. In contrast to labelling theory predictions, follow-up studies of children attending child guidance clinics do not suggest that they go on to become severely mentally ill (Waring & Ricks 1965). Wing (1978a) has argued strongly that labelling theory fails to account for most of the known facts concerning schizophrenia.

Life events

Although it is received opinion that acute environmental stresses can act as causal factors in schizophrenia the empirical evidence is rather unsatisfactory. George Brown and colleagues developed an interview whereby a major change or crisis, involving either positive or negative factors, could be precisely dated and classified as to whether it was independent of a subject's mental state. Brown & Birley (1968) and Birley & Brown (1970) showed that in the three-week period before onset of schizophrenia there was a significantly higher frequency of life events than for normal controls: 60% of the patients had had an independent or possibly independent life event in the three weeks preceding onset, compared to about 15% of the controls. Events were as likely to precede first as subsequent admissions. They concluded that this was reasonably sound evidence that environmental factors can precipitate a schizophrenic episode and that such events tend to cluster in the few weeks before onset (Brown & Birley 1968). However, they added a note of caution by saying that life events were likely to interact with other factors. They did not suggest that a life event would by itself be sufficient cause of a schizophrenic episode, even though many of the patients were experiencing a first episode.

In a subsequent investigation, Jacobs & Myers (1976) examined subjects with well-dated first episodes of schizophrenia and compared them with a well-matched sample of normal controls. Unfortunately they examined the frequency of life events throughout the whole period of six months before onset. Once they had eliminated events that could have been caused by the illness, there were no significant differences. However, because of the long period examined, any important influence of life events within a much shorter antecedent period, as suggested by Brown & Birley (1968), may have been swamped.

Canton & Fraccon (1985) reviewed the methodological pitfalls of such research, but it is clear that they did not avoid them in their own study, which adds little to the argument. Alkhani and his colleagues (1986) showed suggestive evidence for an effect of life events, but only in some subgroups of their patients, and the Saudi Arabian location of their study adds to the difficulty of interpretation. The published results of the cross-national studies of the WHO are awaited, and it is to be hoped that they will clarify this issue.

Brown and his colleagues (1973) suggested that there was some specificity to the effect of life events in schizophrenia, by comparing it with that in depression. First, the effect is smaller in schizophrenia, and Brown et al (1973) argue that events have more of a 'triggering' role. Secondly, the period within which events seem to operate appears to be shorter in schizophrenia than in depression. However, any real resolution of the mechanisms by which events produce their effects must await firmer establishment of the effects themselves. There seems little doubt that any role of life events is minor in the face of the other potential contributions to the cause of the disorder (Zubin et al 1983, Liberman 1986).

Social networks

Deficiences in the social network have also been suggested as aetiologically relevant to schizophrenia. One of the functions of social networks is the provision of social support, and it has been proposed that defective social support may be a causal factor (Hammer et al 1978). It has certainly been documented that people with schizophrenia tend to have small, family-centred networks (Beels 1981). Pattison et al (1975) report that whereas the normal population has a primary group of 20 to 30 people, neurotic patients average 10 to 12 people and psychotic patients only 4 or 5. However, again the evidence for causality 'is unsatisfactory and likely to remain so' (Henderson 1980).

Cultural factors

Although a certain amount is known about the clinical picture and course of schizophrenia in non-western cultures (WHO 1973, 1979, Leff 1981), very little is known about the possible influences of culture on onset. Culture determines the nature of the hazards that people have to face and also the coping strategies and social resources that they might use to deal with them, so it would not be surprising if there were such effects. On the face of it, however, there do not appear to be major differences in the prevalence of schizophrenia in different cultures, although even here authorities do not agree on the interpretation of the evidence (Leff 1981, Torrey 1980). There are many interesting questions that could be asked about the influence of specific aspects of culture, but until there is some consensus on what the important cultural dimensions might be, it seems premature to speculate from scanty and unreliable evidence.

Maintenance and remission

While theories for social factors having causal effects in schizophrenia have been plentiful, evidence has not. Moreover, it is almost always possible to suggest an alternative explanation for the findings: for instance, that they represent consequences, not causes. The evidence overall suggests that social factors are important because of their effect on the course or outcome of the illness. In this sense, they have implication for social treatments and prevention programmes. This shift away from causality towards the course of schizophrenia has been more productive. The influence of some of the factors discussed above on the course and outcome of schizophrenia will be examined in the following section.

Family factors

Studies of how schizophrenic patients fared when they went out of hospitals and started living in the community began to emerge in the late 1950s and have been previously reviewed (Kuipers 1979, Hooley 1985, Leff & Vaughn 1985). Brown et al (1958, Brown 1959) were interested in the social influences that such patients would encounter, and looked specifically at the relapse rates of schizophrenic patients returning to different types of living group on discharge from hospital. Their study provided some evidence that discharged long-stay male patients tended to relapse if they returned to parents or wives, rather than if they lived in hostels alone. Attempts to measure possible mediating social factors led to the development of a semi-structured interview in which the emotional atmosphere in the home could be assessed (Brown et al 1962). This interview was refined and validated and called the Camberwell Family Interview (CFI) (Brown & Rutter 1966,

Rutter & Brown 1966). Affective ratings were made of the number of critical comments and positive remarks plus overall warmth, hostility, emotional over-involvement and dissatisfaction expressed in the interview. These measures were found to predict relapse rates in a follow-up study of 101 schizophrenic patients returning to their relatives (Brown et al 1972). A cut-off point of seven critical comments, marked over-emotional involvement or hostility defined high 'Expressed Emotion' (EE) relatives. Of patients returning to high-EE homes, 58% relapsed, compared to 16% of those living with low-EE relatives. The difference persisted when the groups were controlled for the patients' previous work impairment and behavioural disturbance. Drug therapy was unrelated to relapse in low-EE homes, and showed only a trend for a relationship in high-EE homes. On the other hand, mutual family contact of more than 35 hours per week in the same room was associated with relapse for patients living with high-EE relatives.

These findings were almost exactly replicated by Vaughn & Leff (1976a). Using a shortened version of the CFI (Vaughn & Leff 1976b) they compared a group of depressed neurotics with schizophrenic patients. Again they found that returning to live with high-EE relatives was associated with a high risk of relapse in schizophrenic patients in the nine months following discharge from hospital. This finding was independent of all other social and clinical factors investigated. As their methods were so similar to the 1972 study they were able to combine the data and look more closely at the relapse rates in a total sample of 128 schizophrenics.

It was possible to see that not only was high EE associated with relapse (51% of patients with high-EE relatives relapsed compared to 13% of patients with low EE), but that there were other protective factors operating. The schizophrenic patients in high-EE homes were less likely to relapse if they were on regular maintenance drug therapy and if they were in reduced face-to-face contact with their relatives (less than 35 hours per week). Those in high-EE homes with neither of these factors operating had very high relapse rates. There were several implications of these findings. First, relapse rates in schizophrenia were associated with social factors. Second, it was possible to identify those schizophrenic patients with a high risk of relapse. Finally, since some of the factors associated with relapse had been pinpointed, the targets of a possible intervention programme had been elucidated; namely, the effective provision of medication, a reduction of face-to-face contact and a lowering of expressed emotion in the family.

These early findings have not been fully supported by some recent research, which suggests that following a first admission for schizophrenia EE may have less predictive power. In a sample of 82 first-episode patients MacMillan and her colleagues (1986) failed to demonstrate that critical comments or social contact were significant determinants of relapse. They found similar rates of relapse over two years to those presented in earlier studies by Leff & Vaughn (1981), but pointed out that many patients lived alone or were not in high contact with their families, suggesting that these social factors were less important than the effects of neuroleptic medication. As they mention, their results are not decisive and their different methods of analysis make direct comparisons with the earlier data difficult. Other methodological problems have been pointed out by Leff & Vaughn (1986). Nevertheless, these findings inject a 'note of caution' for the significance of these factors with first-admission schizophrenics.

A similar lack of enthusiasm for the EE measure and findings based on it is apparent in the work of Birchwood et al (1987). They completed a retrospective follow-up of 153 first-admission patients over two years and investigated the relationship between relatives, coping characteristics and the outcome of the disorder in terms of relapse, social adjustment and psychopathology. Their objections to EE appear to be theoretical in that they see EE as a trait on which the traditional cut-off points are imposed arbitrarily. They present instead a feedback or adjustment model whereby families' coping efficacy and coping style, along with other predictors such as the quality of family relationships, will develop over time. They also see concentration on 'high-EE' families as too narrow and liable to exclude other families with problems from effective help. Interestingly, what Birchwood and colleagues appear to have done is to approach the question of family factors in schizophrenia from a different perspective, and with an interest in describing and quantifying families' coping behaviour and coping styles. This means that the work overlaps with the previous EE research, but provides new data on family behaviour in this situation.

Birchwood et al identify eight categories of coping behaviour, ranging from coercive to reassuring. They found that their family outcome scale was significantly related to relapse in the patients, independent of patient disturbance. A subscale 'signs of rejection' contributed most to this effect. Their tolerance (coping) index was strongly correlated with all the family outcome scales. They also replicated a social contact effect, with poor outcome associated with high contact with a relative, although they add that much poorer social adjustment was evident in high-contact patient groups. Finally, coercive coping strategies were associated with relapse, particularly in relation to patients' 'negative' impairments.

This study does go some way towards providing evidence for the idea that EE develops over time, and may be due to exposure to difficult behaviour and coping failure. There is certainly a lower relapse rate in first admissions (35%) when compared to subsequently admitted patients (69%) (Leff & Brown 1977), although other explanations of this are possible. Both the descriptions of the coping behaviours of these families and their development of a role-play video of families' problems as an assessment device are valuable. It is a pity, however, that these studies (Birchwood et al 1987, Birchwood & Smith 1987) have been developed independently of any EE assessment, as the ability to link family coping styles and EE now remains descriptive rather than substantive. Hogarty (1985) has recently reviewed the EE studies and argues that EE is only predictive of relapse in men, not women. This point has not been made before and seems to have some support from the available evidence.

Finally, there has also been some disquiet that EE is an attitudinal rather than a behavioural measure and that there has been relatively little evidence for its construct validity (Kuipers 1979). This is beginning to be rectified, however. Miklowitz et al (1984) suggested that measures of EE were related to ongoing family interactions in that high-EE parents exhibited more negatively charged emotional verbal behaviour in direct transaction with their children than did low-EE parents. Kuipers et al (1983) also found it possible to distinguish between high- and low-EE relatives (spouses and parents) on the basis of the amount of speech. During interviews including the patient high-EE relatives talked for longer and were poor listeners compared to low-EE relatives. Greenley (1986) provides some data for EE as a theory of social control used by families. Thus there is some reason to think that EE is of value as a predictor because it is associated with aspects of ongoing family interactions.

Societal factors

Ever since the classic three-hospital study of Wing & Brown (1970), when it became clear that the category 'doing nothing' in hospital was associated with increased symptomatology, it has been evident that some environments are not conducive to a good outcome in schizophrenia, particularly because of the risk of exacerbating negative symptoms. Poor environments are not of course confined to hospitals, and there has been recent concern that moving patients out into the community, whether to families, hostels or bedsits, may provide another sort of institutionalization in a different setting (Carle 1984). Conversely over-enthusiastic attempts at making changes in hospital or in other settings have also been associated with relapses in schizophrenia, especially the re-emergence of florid symptoms (Wing et al 1964, Hemsley 1978).

Life events

Brown & Birley (1968) reported that in their group of 31 schizophrenic patients with relapses, the excess of antecedent life events was as apparent as in their first onset cases. Alkhani et al (1986), in contrast, found the influence of life events less remarkable in those experiencing a relapse. Leff et al (1983) have reported a simple additive model whereby relapse in schizophrenia is determined by the total number of 'risk' factors, such as an adverse social environment, refusing medication, or life events. This fits in with Zubin et al's (1983) vulnerability model of relapse in schizophrenia, which suggest that a variety of factors, genetic, physiological and social, can combine to trigger or moderate a schizophrenic attack in an individual. However, neither model has been tested empirically.

Cultural factors

The two-year follow-up of the International Pilot Study of Schizophrenia (WHO 1979) found that developing countries reported a better course and outcome for schizophrenia than developed ones. Possible reasons for this are only now being investigated. Suggestions have been made that the larger network of the extended family and the lower expectations and fatalistic attitudes more common in developing countries may be beneficial in schizophrenia, rather than the competitive, individual oriented culture, and small, isolated family units of industralized countries.

Expressed Emotion has now been studied in the USA, where the principal British findings have been replicated (Vaughn et al 1984), as well as in Denmark where a similar pattern exists (Menon et al 1987). It is now possible to compare these findings in the West with others in India. EE ratings were completed in 93 relatives of both rural and city dwellers near Chandigarh. Despite the low relapse rates in these samples, particularly in the rural areas, there was still an association between hostility expressed by relatives and subsequent relapse a year later. This suggests that familial factors might also be implicated in the outcome of schizophrenia in this culture (Leff et al 1987).

Most of the evidence for the effects of social factors on the course of the illness comes from the research into family influences in schizophrenia. This has led to guidelines for intervention studies, which are discussed in the next section. It is now clear that the wider environment, such as a hospital or hostel, may also affect the course of the illness. Changes in social circumstances in the form of life events are probably implicated also. These operate in association with other factors, and are not specific to the onset or relapse of a schizophrenic illness. Although research has shown impoverished social networks in schizophrenic patients, these are likely to be a result of the illness. They may, however, be associated with its impact on the individual. Cultural factors may be responsible for a better outcome in some developing countries.

Implications for social treatment

Family interventions

Family-based social treatments of schizophrenia have recently been reviewed by Barrowclough & Tarrier (1984). The first such study was reported by Goldstein et al (1978), who compared family therapy with six weeks of medication after patients were discharged from hospital. They found that no patient relapsed when they had received family therapy and a standard drug dosage, while 24% of patients relapsed in the group provided with low-dosage drug therapy alone. This study had a very brief exposure to treatment and family members were not rated for EE.

Leff et al (1982) specifically investigated 'high-risk' families; that is, those who were in high contact and had high levels of EE towards the patient. Neuroleptics were prescribed for all patients; but, while the control group ($N=12$) had standard hospital care, the experimental group ($N=12$) were given education sessions at home, a relatives group consisting of low- and high-EE families, and sessions at home with the patient and family. The aim of these interventions was twofold: to reduce EE in the relatives and to reduce the social contact below 35 hours a week. Either one of these objectives was achieved in 75% of the experimental families (9/12) and there were no relapses over the nine months after discharge from hospital in these families. Overall, the experimental group had an 8% relapse rate (1/12), whereas the control group had the predicted 50% relapse rate (6/12). Critical comments, a main component of EE, were significantly reduced only in the experimental group, but emotional over-involvement showed only a trend towards reduction. A two-year follow-up (Leff et al 1985) suggests that for those patients who remained on medication there was a 20% (2/10) relapse rate in the experimental group compared with 78% (7/9) rate in the control group. However, if all the study patients are included and a broader definition of outcome is used, two subsequent suicides in the experimental group mean that only half the patients (6/12) remain well in contrast to 75% (9/12) in the control group, a non-significant difference. The suicides appeared to be due to intervening circumstances: there was no evidence to connect them with treatment given during the study.

Falloon et al (1982) reported an intervention study of 36 parental families. Most of these were rated as high EE, but some families were included because they showed high levels of 'tension'. Again, all patients were medicated. The control group ($n=18$) had the best 'standard care' available, which consisted of individual treatment taking up a total amount of time comparable to that received by the experimental group. Thus this study controlled for the 'attention only' effects of treatment. The experimental group ($n=18$) received education sessions and family intervention at home. The latter was based on a problem-solving approach and consisted of a structured attempt to delineate problems and enable the family to come to some consensus. The results were similar to the previous study in that 44% of the control group relapsed over the next nine months but only 6% of the experimental group did so. The authors do not state whether EE was changed significantly. A two-year follow-up (Falloon et al 1985) again suggests a lasting effect of this type of intervention. By this time 83% of their control patients had had a major episode of schizophrenia compared with only 17% of the family-treated patients. There are also indications of less subjective burden in the experimental families (Falloon & Pederson 1985) and a reduction in negative affective style (Doane et al 1986). The experimental patients complied more with medication and this could have confounded the long-term effects of family treatment. However, the overall levels of medication were lower in the experimental group than in controls, so this is unlikely.

The latest study of this type has been reported by Hogarty et al (1986). This comprised a large trial of social treatment and medication in the prevention of schizophrenic relapse. They had a sample of 134 parental high-EE families, of whom 90 accepted all the treatments. They divided them into four groups; family treatment and medication ($N=21$); social skills and medication ($N=20$); family treatment, social skills and medication ($N=20$); and medication alone ($N=29$). Family treatment consisted of a multi-family educational workshop, followed by sessions at home. The latter aimed to increase information about the illness, to reduce isolation by augmenting social networks, and to help the families cope with problems and reduce long-standing difficulties. Social skills training was aimed at helping patients improve their social perception and be more assertive with their families but was conducted individually. They reported no relapses over the next year for those receiving the combination of family treatment, social skills and medication; a 19% relapse rate for those receiving the family treatment and medication; a 20% relapse rate for those receiving social skills and medication; and a 41% relapse rate for those receiving medication only. Mini episodes which responded to treatment in two to three weeks were not counted as relapses, which makes the study harder to compare with the other studies. Interestingly, as this study did not specifically aim to lower EE in the families, they also found no significant relationship between change in EE and outcome; even in the family treatment conditions the majority of the families remained high EE.

Social skills training appeared to have a significant additional effect when combined with the family treatment. Hogarty et al (1986) also address the problem of whether social treatments merely delay relapse. In a thoughtful critique, they suggest this might be all that the results so far can show. Their own study with its impressive combination of treatments has not yet completed the follow-up of patients.

There have been two other intervention studies with schizophrenic samples. Vaughan (1986) replicated an association between EE and relapse in 91 schizophrenic patients in an Australian study but reports that a family counselling approach with high-EE relatives in the absence of the patient was not successful. Kottgen et al (1984), using a much more psychodynamic approach, have published a nine-month trial of family group therapy. Their relapse rate of 33% in the treatment group was not appreciably less than the 50% in their control group.

Finally, a brief education intervention with 23 families has recently been completed (Smith & Birchwood 1987). This suggests that education is useful both in its own right and in facilitating possible engagement in later family treatment.

Other intervention studies are in progress. Leff and colleagues are comparing education and a relatives group with education and family therapy. Kuipers and colleagues are evaluating the addition of education plus a relatives group to the standard clinical care of an extremely long-term group of patients. Birchwood and colleagues are looking at interventions with first-episode schizophrenic patients and their families. There is also some evidence of an emerging interest in applying some of these ideas to routine clinical practice, as argued by Kuipers & Bebbington (1985).

Effects of environment

Environmental factors associated with a good outcome have now been fairly clearly delineated. These are not just a matter of resources or large numbers of staff, but of practices oriented towards residents rather than towards staff (King et al 1971, Raynes et al 1979), which encourage higher levels of positive staff-patient interaction (Shepherd & Richardson 1979). Other relevant factors are the provision of structure, individualized programmes for patients, and patient involvement in deciding their own treatment goals (Shepherd 1983). The importance of staff involvement and morale (Raynes et al 1979) has also become apparent. In order to avoid adverse institutional practices, the long-term care of patients should involve a team of professionals rather than isolated staff who may become 'burned out'. It is also important to ensure that junior staff are part of the decision-making process about patients. Such practices form the basis of good rehabilitative care and are discussed in detail elsewhere (Watts & Bennett 1983). There is also evidence that it is possible to 'institutionalize' resident-oriented practice even in long-term settings (Garety & Morris 1984).

It is possible to think of treatments directed at the other social factors already identified, for instance the effect of increasing the size of a psychotic patient's social network. No controlled trials have been reported as yet.

The main social treatments so far evaluated have fallen into two groups. On the one hand there are the recent family studies; and, on the other, changes in institutional practices towards resident-oriented management styles. Both these developments have implications for the move into the community currently in process, particularly for many long-term schizophrenic patients; institutions do not just consist of hospitals. When schizophrenic patients live in the family home the relatives are likely to become or remain the primary source of care. The limitations of the family interventions are that the benefit apparent from these early studies may not be substantiated and more certainly that many patients do not have families to return to. In long-term patient samples, about 50% of patients may live with or be in contact with a family member or live with another patient (Creer et al 1982). However, that leaves the other 50% living alone in hostels or other settings. It is not yet clear whether the EE results also apply to hostel environments, although preliminary studies are under way.

Despite the interest in social factors in schizophrenia, and the recent treatment advances suggested and implemented by the research, there is a distinct paucity of explanatory models to provide a framework for the processes involved. The most usual one is that propounded by Wing (1978b), which suggests that schizophrenic patients are particularly sensitive to the social environment, either to a lack of appropriate structure or stimulation, leading to an increase of negative symptoms, or to too much stimulation, leading to an increase in positive symptoms or relapse. The Zubin et al (1983) vulnerability model also accords broadly with these ideas. However, there is little evidence to illuminate the exact pathways and there are many gaps. The situation is not helped by our general lack of information about the causes and processes involved in schizophrenic illnesses. At a psychological level one of the best potential bridges between experimental research and clinical phenomena is the evidence on cognitive deficits in schizophrenia put forward by Hemsley (1977, 1984, 1985); see also Chapter 6. He postulates that too much information might 'overload' schizophrenic patients because of their inefficient 'pigeon-holing' and cause increased symptomatology as a kind of adaptation to the environment. This suggests that a structured and predictable environment would be helpful for patients with these cognitive impairments. In support of this idea MacCarthy et al (1986) have recently found that highly critical relatives appear to provide an unpredictable home environment for schizophrenic patients.

'Arousal' has been implicated as a possible mediating factor that might be measured in schizophrenic patients in these stressful situations. Despite the obvious problems of invoking such an imprecise concept (Andrew 1974) and deciding how to measure it, there have been some studies using psychophysiological measures in schizophrenia, reviewed by Turpin (1984). These can be linked with the EE studies. For example, Tarrier et al (1979) examined the skin conductance (SC) recordings of schizophrenic patients in the presence and absence of their relatives. They showed that patients had high levels of arousal when high-EE relatives entered the room, but not if the relative was low EE. The effect was apparent only on the first occasion of testing. Sturgeon et al (1984) also showed significantly higher levels of skin conductance response frequencies in patients interviewed with high-EE relatives, compared to those with low-EE relatives. However, despite changes in EE due to a successful social intervention programme, there were no concomitant changes in the SC recordings of patients, which were independently related to relapse. It is not therefore clear whether this modality is an inaccurate reflection of this attribute of the social environment, or if changes in EE are not mediated via an arousal system. As Turpin (1984) notes, there are all sorts of methodological problems in this research, ranging from the relevance of the testing situation for psychotic patients to their levels of medication and institutionalized behaviour; and the imprecision of psychophysiological measures themselves. This area of research has so far not produced conclusive results and the processes involved in mediating social circumstances in schizophrenic illnesses have not been clarified.

Conclusions

Over the last thirty years the research into social factors in schizophrenia has diversified, and while it now seems clear that social events have an impact on schizophrenic illnesses, the range of factors involved and the mechanics of the effect are still being elucidated. There is currently less interest in social factors as a distant cause of the onset, although the evidence suggests that they may mediate the timing and affect the severity of an acute attack. More usefully, social factors have emerged as important in determining the course and extent of recovery of the illness. This has resulted in considerable recent research which has substantiated social interventions as useful treatments for those schizophrenic patients still living with relatives, over and above the effects of neuroleptic medication. This research, while founded on a variety of theoretical approaches and using ostensibly different treatment packages, has common features of a positive approach to families, the provision of education and information about schizophrenia to participants, and structured and specific treatment aims. The whole family is involved at home and treatments last for at least a year. These elements appear to constitute the common features of the current interventions, and to distinguish them from some of the previous and less successful attempts in this field.

The research into Expressed Emotion, while not universally accepted, has nevertheless fuelled these interventions. There is considerable evidence to suggest that a better outcome in schizophrenia is linked to a calm home atmosphere where people can cope with difficulties that arise, whether this is labelled as EE or not (Birchwood et al 1986). This has been reinforced by the success of the recent intervention studies (Leff et al 1985, Doane et al 1986). By providing a precise and replicable measure of family attitudes to the patient that appears predictive of relapse, EE has provoked renewed interest in the problems of families living with a schizophrenic patient. It has also generated social treatments whose effects can be evaluated. This research suggests it is possible at least to delay relapse and to reduce the burden on families who are becoming increasingly involved in caring for patients in the community. Even if EE itself does not become the preferred method of assessing family attitudes, this will not detract from its usefulness in formulating these early and promising social interventions.

The other social factors discussed, such as life events and social networks, are usually seen as additive in their effects on schizophrenia. A large number of life events, or an unstimulating environment, appear to increase the risk of developing in the former case an acute illness, or in the latter of worsening negative symptoms. The small social network, typical of those with psychotic illness, while not causal, will affect the resources available to a patient recovering from an attack. Cultural factors suggest that the course of the illness may be worse in the more competitive, encapsulating and perhaps less tolerant, cities of the developed world.

The models invoked to explain how these social factors have an effect on a schizophrenic illness are so far merely descriptive. The most common one, the 'arousal' hypothesis which states that too little or too much stimulation in the environment can lead to increases in negative or positive symptoms in a patient, fits quite well with the observed social data. However, evidence on the underlying psychophysiological pathways is not conclusive and, even if it were, would still not explain how relapse occurs. The cognitive deficits model also fits with some of the symptomatic behaviour of schizophrenic patients, and at present provides useful hypotheses in terms of information-processing difficulties in schizophrenia. Vulnerability, the proposal that a genetic loading for schizophrenia may be added to or moderated by social factors, is another version of the arousal idea, but again only describes the phenomena. However, given our limited understanding of schizophrenia itself it may not be surprising that these models are not more useful.

The study of social factors in schizophrenia has led to new ideas on its course and on possible methods of treatment. They have emphasized the universality of schizophrenia by plotting its occurrence in diverse cultures. The research is still at a very early stage, however, and future studies on social factors will continue to clarify and hopefully alleviate the effects of this extremely disabling condition.

REFERENCES

Alkhani M, Bebbington P, Watson J, House F 1986 Life-events and schizophrenia: a Saudi-Arabian study. British Journal of Psychiatry 148: 12–22
Amenson C S, Lewinsohn P M 1981 An investigation into the observed sex difference in prevalence of unipolar depression. Journal of Abnormal Psychology 90: 1–13
Andrew R J 1974 Arousal and the causation of behaviour. Behaviour 51: 135–165
Andrews G, Tennant C, Hewson D, Vaillant G E 1978 Life event stress, social support, coping style and risk of psychological impairment. Journal of Nervous and Mental Disease 166: 307–316
Aneshensel C S, Stone J D 1982 Stress and depression; a study of the buffering model of social support. Archives of General Psychiatry 39: 1392
Banks M H, and Jackson P R 1982 Unemployment and risk of minor psychiatric disorder in young people: cross-sectional and longitudinal evidence. Psychological Medicine 12: 789–798
Barrowclough C, Tarrier N 1984 'Psychosocial' interventions with families and their effects on the course of schizophrenia: a review Psychological Medicine 14: 629–42
Bateson G, Jackson D, Haley J, Weakland J 1956 Towards a theory of schizophrenia. Behavioural Science 1: 251–264
Bebbington P, Hurry J, Tennant C, Sturt E, Wing J K 1981a The epidemiology of mental disorders in Camberwell. Psychological Medicine 11: 561–579
Bebbington P E, Hurry J, Tennant C 1981b Psychiatric disorders in selected immigrant groups in Camberwell. Social Psychiatry 16: 43–51
Beck A T, Ward C H, Mendelson M, Mock J, Erbaugh J 1961 An inventory for measuring depression. Archives of General Psychiatry 4: 561–571

Beels C C 1981 Social support and schizophrenia. Schizophrenia Bulletin 7: 58–72
Beiser M 1976 Personal and social factors associated with the remission of psychiatric symptoms. Archives of General Psychiatry 33: 941–945
Berkman P L 1971 Measurement of mental health in a general population survey. American Journal of Epidemiology 94: 105–111
Billings A G, Moos R H 1985 Life stressors and social resources affect posttreatment outcomes among depressed patients. Journal of Abnormal Psychology 94: 140–153
Birchwood M, Smith J 1987 Schizophrenia. In: J. Orford (ed) Coping with disorder in the family. Croom Helm, London
Birchwood M, Cochrane R, Moore B 1987 Family coping behaviour and the course of schizophrenia: a follow up study. Psychological Medicine (in press)
Birley J L T, Brown G W 1970 Crises and life changes preceding the onset or relapse of acute schizophrenia: clinical aspects. British Journal of Psychiatry 116: 327–333
Boyd J H, Weissman M M 1981 Epidemiology of affective disorders — a re-examination and future directions. Archives of General Psychiatry 38: 1039–1046
Brown G W 1959 Experiences of discharged chronic schizophrenic mental hospital patients in various types of living group. Millbank Memorial Fund Quarterly 37: 105–131
Brown G W 1974 Meaning, measurement and stress of life events. In: Dohrenwend B S, Dohrenwend B P (eds) Stressful life events: their nature and effects. Wiley, New York
Brown G W, Birley J L T 1968 Crises and life changes and the onset of schizophrenia. Journal of Health and Social Behaviour 9: 203–214
Brown G W, Harris T 1978 Social origins of depression. Tavistock Publications, London
Brown G W, Prudo R 1981 Psychiatric disorder in a rural and an urban population: 1. Aetiology of depression. Psychological Medicine 11: 581–599
Brown G W, Rutter M L 1966 The measurement of family activities and relationships. Human Relations 19: 241–63
Brown G W, Carstairs G M, Topping G C 1958 The post hospital adjustment of chronic mental patients. Lancet 2: 685–689
Brown G W, Monck E M, Carstairs G M, Wing J K 1962 Influence of family life on the course of schizophrenic illness. British Journal of Preventive and Social Medicine 16: 55–68
Brown G W, Birley J L T, Wing J K 1972 Influence of family life on the course of schizophrenic disorders: a replication. British Journal of Psychiatry 121: 241–258
Brown G W, Harris T O, Peto J 1973 Life events and psychiatric disorders, part II: nature and causal link. Psychological Medicine 3: 159–176
Brown G W, Ni Bhrolchain M, Harris T P 1975 Social class and psychiatric disturbance among women in an urban population. Sociology 9: 225–254
Byrne D G 1981 Sex differences in the reporting of symptoms of depression in the general population. British Journal of Clinical Psychology 20: 83–92
Campbell E A 1983 Depression in women: the role of life events, social factors and psychological vulnerability. Unpublished DPhil thesis, University of Oxford
Campbell E A, Cope S, Teasdale J D 1983 Social factors and affective disorders: an investigation of Brown and Harris' model. British Journal of Psychiatry 143: 548–553
Canton G, Fraccon I G 1985 Life events and schizophrenia: a replication. Acta Psychiatrica Scandinavica 71: 211–216
Caplan G 1981 Mastery of stress: psychosocial aspects. American Journal of Psychiatry 138: 413–420
Carle N 1984 Common experiences of people with handicapping conditions. In: Simpson S, Higston P, Holland R, McBryan J, Williams J, Henneman, L (eds) Facing the challenge: common issues in work with people who are handicapped, elderly or chronically mentally ill. British Association for Behavioural Psychotherapy, Rossendale, Lancs
Cochrane R, Stopes-Roe M 1979 Psychological disturbance in Ireland, in England and in Irish emigrants to England: a comparative study. Economic and Social Review 10: 301–320
Cochrane R, Stopes-Roe M 1980 Social class and psychological disorder in natives and immigrants to Britain. International Journal of Social Psychiatry 27: 173–183
Cochrane R, Stopes-Roe M 1981 Women, marriage, employment and mental health. British Journal of Psychiatry 139: 373–381
Cohen S, Hoberman H M, 1983 Positive events and social supports as buffers of life

change stress. Journal of Applied Social Psychology 13: 99–125
Comstock G W, Helsing K J, 1976 Symptoms of depression in two communities. Psychological Medicine 6: 551–563
Cooke D J 1981 Life events, depression and vulnerability factors: a theoretical and empirical evaluation. Paper presented at British Psychological Society Annual Conference 1981
Costello C G 1982 Social factors associated with depression: a retrospective community study. Psychological Medicine 12: 329–339
Creer C, Sturt E, Wykes T 1982 The role of relatives In: Wing J K (ed) Long term community care: experience in a London borough. Psychological Medicine Monograph Supplement 2.
Dean A, Lin N, Ensel W M 1981 The epidemiological significance of social support systems in depression. Research in Community and Mental Health 2: 77–109
Deaux K, White L, Farris E 1975 Skill versus luck: field and laboratory studies of male and female preferences. Journal of Personality and Social Psychology 32: 629–636
Doane J A, Goldstein M J, Miklowitz D J, Falloon I R H 1986 The impact of individual and family treatment on the affective climate of families of schizophrenics. British Journal of Psychiatry 148: 279–287
Dohrenwend B P, Dohrenwend B S 1969 Social status and psychological disorder. Wiley, New York
Dooley D, Catalano R 1980 Economic change as a cause of behavioural disorder. Psychological Bulletin 87: 450–468
Dressler W W, Badger L W 1985 Epidemiology of depressive symptoms in black communities: a comparative analysis. Journal of Nervous and Mental Disease 172: 212–220
Falloon I R H, Pederson J 1985 Family management in the prevention of morbidity of schizophrenia: adjustment of the family unit. British Journal of Psychiatry 147: 156–163
Falloon I R H, Boyd J L, McGill C W, Razani J, Moss H B, Gilderman A M 1982 Family management in the prevention of exacerbations of schizophrenia: a controlled study. New England Journal of Medicine 306: 1437–1440
Falloon I R H, Boyd J L, McGill C W et al 1985 Family management in the prevention of morbidity of schizophrenia: clinical outcome of a two year longitudinal study. Archives of General Psychiatry 42: 887–896
Feather N T, Davenport P R 1981 Unemployment and depressive affect: a motivational analysis. Journal of Personality and Social Psychology 41: 422–436
Finlay-Jones R A, Burvill P W 1979 Women, work and minor psychiatric morbidity. Social Psychiatry 14: 53–57
Finlay-Jones R, Eckhardt B 1981 Psychiatric disorder among the young unemployed. Australian and New Zealand Journal of Psychiatry 15: 265–270
Frydman M D 1981 Social support, life events and psychiatric symptoms: a study of direct, conditional and interaction effects. Social Psychiatry 16: 69–78
Garety P, Morris I 1984 A new unit for long stay psychiatric patients: organisation attitudes and quality of care. Psychological Medicine 14: 183–192
Gift T E, Strauss J S, Ritzler B A, Kokes R F, Harder D W 1986 Social class and psychiatric outcome. American Journal of Psychiatry 143: 222–225
Goffman E 1961 Asylums: essays on the social situation of mental patients and other inmates. Doubleday, New York
Goldstein M 1985 Family factors that antedate the onset of schizophrenia and related disorders: the results of a 15 year prospective longitudinal study. Acta Psychiatrica Scandinavica 71 (suppl. 319): 7–18
Goldstein M, Rodnick E H, Evans J R, May P R, Steinberg M 1978 Drug and family therapy in the aftercare of acute schizophrenia. Archives of General Psychiatry 35: 1169–1177
Gove W R 1972 The relationship between sex roles, marital status and mental illness. Social Forces 51: 34–44
Greenley J R 1986 Social control and Expressed Emotion. Journal of Nervous and Mental Disease 174: 24–30
Hagnell O 1966 A prospective study of the incidence of mental disorder. Svenska Bokförlaget, Lund

Hagnell O, Lanke J, Rorsman B, Ojesjö L 1982 Are we entering an age of melancholy? Depressive illnesses in a prospective epidemiological study over 25 years: the Lundby study, Sweden. Psychological Medicine 12: 279–289

Haley J 1972 Critical overview of present status of family interaction research. In: Framo J L (ed) Family interaction: a dialogue between family researchers and family therapists. Springer, New York

Halldin J 1985 Prevalence of mental disorder in an urban population in central Sweden in relation to social class, marital status and immigration. Acta Psychiatrica Scandinavica 71: 117–127

Hammer M, Makiesky-Barrow S, Gutwirth L 1978 Social networks and schizophrenia. Schizophrenia Bulletin 4: 522–544

Hashmi F 1968 Community psychiatric problems among Birmingham immigrants. British Journal of Social Psychiatry 2: 196–201

Hemsley D R 1977 What have cognitive deficits to do with schizophrenic symptoms? British Journal of Psychiatry 130: 167–173

Hemsley D R 1978 Limitations of operant procedures in the modification of schizophrenic functioning: the possible relevance of studies of cognitive disturbance. Behavioural Analysis and Modification 2: 165–173

Hemsley D R 1984 Cognitive impairment in schizophrenia. In: Burton A (ed) The pathology and psychology of cognition. Methuen, London

Hemsley D 1985 Information processing and schizophrenia. Paper presented at EABY Munich. To appear in: Straube E, Hahlweg K (eds) Schizophrenia: models and intervention

Henderson S 1980 Personal networks and the schizophrenias. Australian and New Zealand Journal of Psychiatry 14: 255–259

Henderson S, Byrne D, Duncan-Jones P, Scott R, Adcock S 1978 Social bonds in the epidemiology of neurosis: a preliminary communication. British Journal of Psychiatry 132: 463–466

Henderson A S, Byrne D C, Duncan-Jones P 1981 Neurosis and the social environment. Academic Press, Sydney

Hirsch S R, Leff J P 1975 Abnormalities in the parents of schizophrenics. Maudsley Monograph No. 22. Oxford University Press, Oxford

Hirschfeld R M A, Klerman G L, Clayton P J, Keller M B, McDonald-Scott P, Larkin B H 1983 Assessing personality: effects of the depressive state on trait measurement. American Journal of Psychiatry 140: 695–699

Hogarty G E 1985 Expressed Emotion and schizophrenic relapse. Implications from the Pittsburgh study. In: Apert M (ed) Controversies in schizophrenia. Guilford Press, New York

Hogarty G E, Anderson C M, Reiss D J et al 1986 Family psycho-education social skills training and maintenance chemotherapy in the aftercare treatment of schizophrenia. I one year effects of a controlled study on relapse and Expressed Emotion. Archives of General Psychiatry 43: 633

Hollingshead A B, Redlich F C 1958 Social class and mental illness: a community study. Wiley, New York

Hooley J M 1985 Expressed emotion: a review of the critical literature. Clinical Psychology Review 5: 119–139

Huxley P J, Goldberg D P 1975 Social versus clinical prediction in minor psychiatric disorder. Psychological Medicine 5: 96–100

Huxley P J, Goldberg D P, Maquire P, Kincey V 1979 The prediction of the course of minor psychiatric disorders. British Journal of Psychiatry 135: 535–543

Ilfeld F W 1978 Psychologic status of community residents along major demographic dimensions. Archives of General Psychiatry 35: 716–724

Jacobs S, Myers J 1976 Recent life events and acute schizophrenic psychosis: a controlled study. Journal of Nervous Disease 162: 79–87

Kessler R C 1979a Stress, social status and psychological distress. Journal of Health and Social Behaviour 20: 259–272

Kessler R, Cleary R 1980 Social class and psychological distress. American Sociological Review 45: 463–478

King R D, Raynes N V, Tizard J 1971 Patterns of residential care. Routledge & Kegan Paul, London

Kottgen C, Sonnichsen I, Mollenhauer K, Jurth R 1984 Group therapy with the families of schizophrenic patients: results of the Hamburg Camberwell family interview study III. International Journal of Family Psychiatry 5: 84–94

Kuipers L 1979 Expressed Emotion: a review. British Journal of Social and Clinical Psychology 18: 237–243

Kuipers L, Bebbington P E 1985 Relatives as a resource in the management of functional illness. British Journal of Psychiatry 147: 465–471

Kuipers L, Sturgeon D, Berkowitz R, Leff J P 1983 Characteristics of Expressed Emotion: its relationship to speech and looking in schizophrenic patients and their relatives. British Journal of Clinical Psychology 22: 257–264

Laing R D, Esterson A 1964 Sanity, madness and the family. Penguin, London

Langner T S, Michael S T 1962 Life stresses and mental health: the Midtown study. Free Press, Glencoe, Ill.

Layard R, Piachaud D, Stewart M 1978 The causes of poverty. HMSO, London

Leff J P 1981 Psychiatry around the globe: a transcultural view. Marcel Dekker, New York

Leff J P, Brown G W 1977 Family and social factors in the course of schizophrenia. British Journal of Psychiatry 130: 417–420

Leff J P, Vaughn C E 1981 The role of maintenance therapy and relatives' Expressed Emotion in relapse of schizophrenia: a two year follow up. British Journal of Psychiatry 139: 102–104

Leff J P, Vaughn C E 1985 Expressed Emotion in Families. Guilford Press, New York

Leff J P, Vaughn C 1986 First episodes of schizophrenia. British Journal of Psychiatry 148: 215

Leff J P, Kuipers L, Berkowitz R, Eberlein-Fries R, Sturgeon D 1982 A controlled trial of social intervention in schizophrenic families. British Journal of Psychiatry 141: 121–134

Leff J P, Kuipers L, Berkowitz R, Vaughn C E, Sturgeon D 1983 Life events relatives' Expressed Emotion and maintenance neuroleptics in schizophrenic relapse. Psychological Medicine 13: 799–806

Leff J P, Kuipers L, Berkowitz R, Sturgeon D 1985 A controlled trial of social intervention in the families of schizophrenic patients: two year follow up. British Journal of Psychiatry 146: 594–600

Leff J P, Wig N, Ghosh A et al 1987 Influence of relatives' Expressed Emotion on the course of schizophrenia in Chandigarh. British Journal of Psychiatry 151: 166–173

Liberman R P 1986 Coping and competence as protective factors in the vulnerability–stress model of schizophrenia. In: Goldstein M J, Hand I, Hahlweg K (eds) Treatment of schizophrenia. Springer-Verlag, Berlin

Lidz T 1975 The origins and treatments of schizophrenic disorders. Basic Books, New York

Liem R, Liem J 1978 Social class and mental illness reconsidered: the role of economic stress and social support. Journal of Health and Social Behaviour 19: 139–156

MacCarthy B, Hemsley D, Shrank-Fernandez C, Kuipers L, Katz R 1986 Unpredictability as a correlate of Expressed Emotion in the relatives of schizophrenics. British Journal of Psychiatry 148: 727–730

MacMillan J F, Gold A, Crow T J, Johnson A L, Johnstone E C 1986 The Northwick Park study of first episodes of schizophrenia IV Expressed Emotion and relapse. British Journal of Psychiatry 148: 133–143

Mann A H, Jenkins R, Belsey E 1981 The twelve-month outcome of patients with neurotic illness in general practice. Psychological Medicine 11: 535–550

Menon D K, Leff J P, Kuipers L et al 1987 The distribution of Expressed Emotion among relatives of schizophrenic patients in Aarhus and Chandigarh. British Journal of Psychiatry 151: 160–166

Miklowitz D J, Goldstein M J, Falloon R H, Doane J A 1984 Interactional correlates of Expressed Emotion in the families of schizophrenics. British Journal of Psychiatry 144: 482–487

Miller P M, Ingham J G 1976 Friends, confidants and symptoms. Social Psychiatry 11: 51–58

Monroe S M, Bellack A S, Hersen M, Himmelhock H M 1983 Life events, symptom course and treatment outcome in unipolar depressed women. Journal of Consulting and Clinical Psychology 51: 604–615

Myers J K, Bean L L 1968 A decade later: a follow-up study of social class and mental illness. Wiley, New York

Myers J K, Lindenthal J J, Pepper M P 1975 Life events, social integration and psychiatric symptomatology. Journal of Health and Social Behaviour, 16: 421–427

O'Brien G E 1986 Psychology of work and unemployment. Wiley, Chichester

Pattison E M, De Francisco D, Wood P, Frazier H 1975 A psychosocial kinship model for family therapy. American Journal of Psychiatry 132: 1246–1251

Paykel E S, Tanner J 1976 Life events, depressive relapse and maintenance treatment. Psychological Medicine 6: 481–485

Paykel E S, Emms E M, Fletcher J, Rassaby E S 1980 Life events and social supports in puerperal depression. British Journal of Psychiatry 136: 339–346

Payne R, Warr P, Hartley J 1984 Social class and psychological ill health during unemployment. Sociology of Health and Illness 6: 152–174

Pearlin L I, Johnson J S 1977 Marital status, life-strains and depression. American Sociological Review 42: 704–715

Pinsent R J P H 1963 Morbidity in an immigrant population. Lancet 1: 437–438

Radloff L 1975 Sex differences in depression: the effects of occupation and marital status. Sex Roles 1: 249–265

Radloff L S 1977 The CES-D scale: a self report depression scale for research in the general population. Applied Psychological Measurement 1: 385–401

Rance L 1976 The causal priority between socioeconomic status and psychiatric disorder: a prospective study. International Journal of Social Psychiatry 22: 1–8

Raynes N V, Pratt M, Roses S 1979 Organizational structure and the care of the mentally retarded. Croom Helm, London

Roberts C R, Roberts R E, Stevenson J M 1982 Women, work, social support and psychiatric morbidity. Social Psychiatry 17: 167–173

Rutter M L, Brown G W 1966 The reliability and validity of measures of family life and relationships in families containing a psychiatric patient. Social Psychiatry 1: 38–53

Scheff T J 1966 Being mentally ill. Aldine, Chicago

Shakow D 1973 Some thoughts about schizophrenic research in the context of high risk studies. Psychiatry 36: 353–365

Shepherd G 1983 Planning the rehabilitation of the individual. In: Watts F N, Bennett D (eds) Principles of psychiatric rehabilitation. Wiley, Chichester

Shepherd G, Richardson A 1979 Organization and interaction in psychiatric day centres. Psychological Medicine 9: 573–579

Smith J, Birchwood M J 1987 Specific and nonspecific effects of educational intervention with families living with a schizophrenic relative. British Journal of Psychiatry 150: 649

Solomon Z, Bromet E 1982 The role of social factors in affective disorders: an assessment of the vulnerability model of Brown and his colleagues. Psychological Medicine 12: 123–130

Spitzer R L, Endicott J, Robins E 1978 Research Diagnostic Criteria: rationale and reliability. Archives of General Psychiatry 35: 773–782

Srole L, Langner T, Michael S, Opler M, Rennie T 1962 Mental health in the metropolis. McGraw-Hill, New York

Steele R E 1978 Relationship of race, sex, social class and social mobility to depression in normal adults. Journal of Social Psychology 104: 37–47

Sturgeon D, Turpin D, Kuipers L, Berkowitz R, Leff J 1984 Psychophysiological responses of schizophrenic patients to high and low expressed emotion relatives: a follow-up study. British Journal of Psychiatry 145: 62–69

Surtees P G 1980 Social support, residual adversity and depressive outcome. Social Psychiatry 15: 71–80

Surtees P G, Ingham J G 1980 Life stress and depressive outcome: application of a dissipation model to life events. Social Psychiatry 15: 21–31

Surtees P G, Dean C, Ingham J G, Kreitman N B, Miller P McC, Sashidharan S P 1983 Psychiatric disorder in women from an Edinburgh community: associations with demographic factors. British Journal of Psychiatry 142: 238–246

Tarrier N, Vaughn C E, Lader M H, Leff J P 1979 Bodily reactions to people and events in schizophrenics. Archives of General Psychiatry 36: 311–315

Tennant C 1985 Female vulnerability to depression. Psychological Medicine 15: 733–737

Tennant C, Bebbington P, Hurry J 1981a The role of life-events in depressive illness: is there a substantial causal role? Psychological Medicine 11: 379–389

Tennant C, Bebbington P, Hurry J 1981b The short-term outcome of neurotic disorders in the community: the relation of remission to clinical factors and to 'neutralizing' life events. British Journal of Psychiatry 139: 213

Torrey E F 1980 Schizophrenia and civilisation. Aronson, New York

Turpin G 1984 Psychophysiology, psychopathology and the social environment. In: Gale A, Edwards J (eds) Physiological correlates of human behaviour. Academic Press, London

Vaughan K 1986 Personal communication

Vaughn C, Leff J P 1976a The influence of family and social factors on the course of psychiatric illness: a comparison of schizophrenic and depressed neurotic patients. British Journal of Psychiatry 129: 125–137

Vaughn C E, Leff J P 1976b The measurement of Expressed Emotion in the families of psychiatric patients. British Journal of Clinical and Social Psychology 15: 157–165

Vaughn C E, Snyder K S, Jones S, Freeman W B, Falloon I R H 1984 Family factors in schizophrenic relapse: replication in California of British research in Expressed Emotion. Archives of General Psychiatry 41: 1169–1177

Venables P 1977 Psychophysiological high risk strategy with Mauritian children: methodological issues. Paper read at Psychophysiological Conference, London

Warheit G J 1979 Life events, coping, stress and depressive symptomatology. American Journal of Psychiatry 136: 502–507

Warheit G J, Holzer C E, Schwatz J J 1973 An analysis of social class and racial differences in depressive symptomatology. Journal of Health and Social Behaviour 14: 291–299

Warheit G J, Holzer C E, Arey S A 1975 Race and mental illness: an epidemiologic update. Journal of Health and Social Behaviour 16: 243–256

Waring M, Ricks D M 1965 Family patterns of children who became adult schizophrenics. Journal of Nervous and Mental Disorders 140: 351–364

Warr P 1982 Psychological aspects of employment and unemployment. Psychological Medicine 12: 7–11

Warr P 1984 Job loss, unemployment and psychological well-being. In: Allen V L, van de Vliert E (eds) Role transitions. Plenum, New York

Warr P, Jackson P 1985 Factors influencing the psychological impact of prolonged unemployment and of re-employment. Psychological Medicine 15: 795–807

Warr P, Parry G 1982a Paid employment and women's psychological well-being. Psychological Bulletin 91: 498–516

Warr P, Parry G 1982b Depressed mood in working-class mothers with and without paid employment. Social Psychiatry 17: 161–165

Watts F N, Bennett D (eds) 1983 Principles of Psychiatric Rehabilitation. Wiley, Chichester

Weissman M M, Klerman G L 1977 Sex differences and the epidemiology of depression. Archives of General Psychiatry 34: 98–111

Weissman M M, Klerman G L 1985 Gender and depression. Trends in Neurosciences 8: 416–419

Weissman M M, Leaf P J, Holzer C E, Myers J K, Tischler G L 1984 The epidemiology of depression: an update on sex differences in rates. Journal of Affective Disorders 7: 179–188

Wheaton B 1978 The sociogenesis of psychological disorder: re-examining the causal issues with longitudinal data. American Sociological Review 43: 383–403

Wing J K 1978a Reasoning about madness. Oxford University Press, London

Wing J K 1978b Schizophrenia: towards a new synthesis. Oxford University Press, London

Wing J K, Brown G W 1970 Institutionalism and schizophrenia. Cambridge University Press, Cambridge

Wing J K, Monck E, Brown G W, Carstairs G M 1964 Morbidity in the community of schizophrenic patients discharged from London mental hospitals in 1959. British Journal of Psychiatry 110: 10–21

Wing J K, Cooper J E, Sartorius N 1974 The measurement and classification of psychiatric symptoms: an instruction manual for the Present State Examination and CATEGO program. Cambridge University Press, London

Wing J K, Bebbington P, Robins L N (eds) 1981 What is a case? Grant McIntyre, London

World Health Organization 1973 The international pilot study of schizophrenia. Vol 1. Geneva
World Health Organization 1979 Schizophrenia: an international follow-up study. Wiley, Chichester
Wynne L C, Singer M, 1963 Thought disorder and family relations of schizophrenics I. Archives of General Psychiatry 9: 191–206
Wynne L C, Singer M, 1965 Thought disorder and family relations of schizophrenics II. Archives of General Psychiatry 12: 187–212
Zubin J, Magaziner J, Steinhauer J R 1983 The metamorphosis of schizophrenia: from chronicity to vulnerability. Psychological Medicine 13:551–571

6
Psychological models of schizophrenia

David R. Hemsley

INTRODUCTION

It is first necessary to present briefly the phenomena upon which a diagnosis of schizophrenia is based. However, this should not be taken to imply acceptance of the view that these behavioural and experiential abnormalities represent a single disorder. Although the reliability of the diagnosis of schizophrenia has been subject to considerable criticism, satisfactory levels of inter-rater agreement as to the presence of specific symptoms can now be achieved by the use of systematic and structured interviews. However, the important question is whether the resultant classification schemes possess utility at either the practical or theoretical level. The present chapter will adopt Neale & Oltmanns' (1980) position that schizophrenia is best viewed as an open scientific construct, capable of being partially defined via a series of measurement operations. Further definition and validation of the construct then involves specifying the network of lawful relationships into which it enters. The importance of specific symptoms is thus dependent on their relationship to other factors, and they may be seen as mediated by a range of biological and psychological processes.

The selection of an optimal set of criteria for schizophrenia is therefore a problem for further empirical research. As a starting point, however, we may take the *Diagnostic and Statistical Manual of Mental Disorders* (DSM III) published by the American Psychiatric Association (1986).

DSM-III diagnostic criteria for schizophrenic disorder

A At least one of the following during a phase of the illness:
1 bizarre delusions (content is patently absurd and has *no* possible basis in fact), such as delusions of being controlled, thought broadcasting, thought insertion, or thought withdrawal
2 somatic, grandiose, religious, nihilistic, or other delusions without persecutory or jealous content
3 delusions with persecutory or jealous content, if accompanied by hallucinations of any type

4 auditory hallucinations in which either a voice keeps a running commentary on the individual's behaviour or thoughts, or two or more voices converse with each other
5 auditory hallucinations on several occasions with contents of more than one or two words, having no apparent relation to depression or elation
6 incoherence, marked loosening of associations, markedly illogical thinking, or marked poverty of content of speech if associated with at least one of the following:
   (a) blunted, flat, or inappropriate affect
   (b) delusions or hallucinations

B Deterioration from a previous level of functioning in such areas as work, social relations, and self-care.

C Duration: Continuous signs of the illness for at least six months at some time during the person's life, with some signs of the illness at present. The six-month period must include an active phase during which there were symptoms from A, with or without a prodromal or residual phase.

It will be noted that while the symptoms represent distinctively psychotic alterations in mental activity, they cover a range of phenomena. In addition, 'B' and 'C' represent historical data, and thereby exclude from the diagnosis those experiencing a brief psychotic episode, and hence represent a shift in the United States towards the narrower conception of schizophrenia preferred in Western Europe. There is, however, a clear restriction on the data domain considered relevant to a diagnosis, in that clearly established behavioural, psychological, and psychophysiological correlates of these symptoms are excluded.

The emphasis of the above scheme is clearly on what have come to be referred to as positive symptoms, delusions, hallucinations and thought disorder. In contrast are the negative symptoms, which refer to the absence of a behaviour that would ordinarily exist in a person who is functioning and coping well. They include such abnormalities as poverty of speech, social withdrawal and affective flattening. Rating scales have been developed to assess these reliably and these have been shown to have prognostic value (e.g. Andreasen 1982). However, it is unclear whether the distinction represents (a) two underlying disorders, (b) differing severity of the same disorder, (c) individual differences in reaction to the same disorder, (d) different stages of the same disorder (acute versus chronic), or a combination of (b), (c) and (d).

The variability of schizophrenic symptomatology has, from the time of identification of the syndrome, led to a search for one or more psychological abnormalities from which the symptoms of schizophrenia might be derived. That is the attempt to specify the fundamental disturbance(s) of schizophrenia. In Bleuler's (1911/1950) view the symptoms resulted from a disturbance of the associative processes. The latter are the connections between ideas which enable normals to organize and inter-relate many single thoughts and exclude irrelevant thoughts. As will be seen below, this has intriguing similarities to more recent formulations. Bleuler also made the important distinction between primary and secondary symptoms, the former being those resulting directly from the organic disease that he presumed to underlie schizophrenia. On the other hand, secondary symptoms reflect the normal psychic processes or attempts at adaptation to the primary disturbance. More recent investigations have also viewed aspects of schizophrenic symptomatology as resulting from the interaction of the cognitively impaired individual with his environment (e.g. Hemsley 1977).

A major question concerning the abnormalities characteristic of schizophrenia is the extent to which they are continuous with normality. This has two aspects. The first is whether, for a given individual, the changes in behaviour/experience are gradual or abrupt. Both patterns may be observed, and correspond approximately to what has been referred to as the process-reactive dimension, the assessment of which is concerned mainly with the level of pre-morbid adjustment. Although the term 'process' schizophrenia has been taken to imply a distinct disease process, this is not justified; nor is it always possible to identify precipitants for 'reactive' schizophrenia (see below).

A related question concerns the extent to which psychiatric abnormalities are continuous with normality. As Bishop (1977) points out, this question is ambiguous, and at least three disinct interpretations are possible. The first, and most direct, is the claim that schizophrenia is continuous with normality at the level of clinical behaviour. This view was advanced by Claridge (1972). However, in his more recent review (Claridge 1985), he appears to take a more cautious position, arguing that schizophrenia shows 'a genuine continuity of behaviour, blending into a spectrum of illness which may manifest itself in varying degrees of disorder; thus making it virtually impossible to delineate an all-or-none category — *except at the very extreme where some degree of discontinuity does become apparent*' (ibid., p. 105). This view has led to the development of scales for rating psychotic and psychotic-like experiences as continua (Chapman & Chapman 1980). The type of experience at the high end of each hypothesized continuum is a psychotic symptom, the other types of experience on each scale having a similar theme but being to varying degrees less deviant. It appears likely that certain behaviours and experiences typical of schizophrenia are indeed continuous with normality, but it remains possible that certain experiences indicate a change to a qualitatively distinct state. If the latter is the case, then a new class of psychological models of schizophrenia may be necessary. In particular, it may be of interest to attempt to apply Catastrophe Theory to these phenomena. This is a mathematical method suitable for the description of situations where gradual changes on certain dimensions may produce discontinuous effects. Its potential application to psychology has been considered by Isnard & Zeeman (1976).

A weaker claim of continuity between schizophrenia and normality refers to continuity in indices of psychosis which are correlated with but not identical to clinical symptoms. This claim is of particular interest if one sees the index as reflecting a primary psychological disturbance from which the symptoms are derived.

The third and least controversial version of the continuity claim is that there exists a continuum of predisposition to schizophrenic symptoms. This brings us to a brief consideration of aetiological models of the disturbance. Most would now accept a vulnerability–stressor model of schizophrenia (e.g. Zubin & Spring 1977), vulnerability resulting both from genetic factors and acquired propensities. Thus certain characteristics of individuals may serve as vulnerability factors, environmental stressors precipitating psychotic episodes. It is further suggested that this vulnerability varies from one affected person to another so that for some only severe stress will suffice to produce schizophrenic symptoms, while in others minor stresses will do so. Maher (1983) points out that 'extreme vulnerability will mean that a constant and continuing schizophrenic syndrome is likely to arise early in life as minor stresses tend inevitably to be of frequent and repeated occurrence' (ibid., p. 13). Potential vulnerability factors considered by psychologists include information-processing deficits, anomalies of autonomic reactivity, and social competence and coping limitations. These will be discussed on p. 121. Stressors may take the form of discrete life events, but equally important is the need to consider the prevailing social environmental stress. There is thus increasing interest in the specification of the characteristics of environments tending to increase the likelihood of relapse. Despite this general agreement on a vulnerability–stressor model, the psychological processes which mediate the emergence of schizophrenic symptoms are far from clear.

METHODOLOGICAL PROBLEMS

There are numerous methodological problems associated with psychological research into schizophrenia. Among the most prominent are:

1 The selection of schizophrenic subjects. Until recently many studies have employed hospital case note diagnoses of unknown reliability to identify their samples. The introduction of more specific diagnostic criteria and the use of structured interviews have eased this problem, but they are still not employed routinely in psychological research.

2. The effects of anti-psychotic medication. The experimental study of schizophrenia has been greatly complicated by the widespread use of anti-psychotic drugs. Although their effects are generally in the direction of normalization of psychological functions, this cannot be assumed.

3. Control groups. Many investigators have employed normal subjects as controls. However, a psychiatric control group is also obviously necessary if the findings are to be seen as relating specifically to schizophrenia. An abnormality common to two psychiatric groups may be of interest.

However, if it is to be argued that certain forms of psychological dysfunction may be causally related to schizophrenic symptomatology the need for a psychiatric control group is apparent.

4. The stage of the disorder. Psychological research frequently omits a discussion of the clinical state of the patient at the time of assessment. As Cromwell (1984) points out, 'the premorbid ("high risk"), prodromal, acute and chronic phases of the disorder reveal themselves in different ways' (ibid., p. 16). To this one might add the stage of partial recovery, which for practical reasons is often that at which measures are taken. One cannot assume similar psychological correlates of these various stages.

In addition to the above, there are specific methodological problems associated with research into certain aspects of schizophrenic functioning. These will be considered in the relevant sections of this chapter.

PERCEPTUAL/COGNITIVE ABNORMALITIES

A disturbance of cognition has long been viewed as one of the most distinguishing features of schizophrenia. Thus on attention Kraepelin (1919) wrote: 'It is quite common for them to lose both inclination and ability on their own initiative to keep their attention fixed for any length of time . . . there is occasionally noticed a kind of irresistible attraction of the attention to casual external impressions.' (ibid., pp. 6 7). He also observed 'the patients lose in a most striking way the faculty of logical ordering of their trains of thought' (ibid., p. 19). More generally he noted: 'Mental efficiency is always diminished to a considerable extent' (ibid., p. 23). Such clinical observations are a necessary beginning to the understanding of schizophrenics' cognitive impairment.

Also influential have been reports by the patients themselves. McGhie & Chapman (1961) carried out an extended interview study of newly admitted schizophrenics, concentrating on changes in the patients' experiences, and presenting the findings in the form of selected quotations. Typical were the following: 'My thoughts get all jumbled up. I start thinking or talking about something but I never get there'; 'Things are coming in too fast. I lose my grip of it and get lost. I am attending to everything at once and as a result I do not attend to anything.' McGhie & Chapman argued that such reports indicated that the primary disorder in schizophrenia is a decrease in the selective and inhibitory functions of attention. They went on to suggest that many other cognitive, perceptual, affective and behavioural abnormalities could be seen as resulting from this primary attentional deficit.

The most ambitious aim of psychological research in this area is the attempt to specify a single cognitive dysfunction, or pattern of dysfunction, from which the various abnormalities resulting in a diagnosis of schizophrenia might be derived. There has been a considerable research effort directed at demonstrating psychological deficits specific to schizophrenia.

The results of such research are, however, often theoretically elaborated in two ways. As Oltmanns & Neale (1978) write: 'First, the single empirical measure which has been assessed is assumed to index a more general construct. Second, it is then postulated that the construct which is implicated in the deficit is causally related to schizophrenia and can account for a variety of schizophrenic behaviours. In other words it is held to be a primary symptom of schizophrenia' (ibid., p. 198).

The first stage of this elaboration is dependent on an agreed model of normal functioning, and the use of tasks which tap a particular function. Much of the early research on cognitive abnormalities either employed tasks, such as tests of 'overinclusion', unrelated to current models of normal cognition, or tasks which, although ostensibly tapping one aspect of cognition, were frequently open to alternative explanations. These issues are discussed more fully by Hemsley (1976).

More recently the information-processing approach has become dominant in research into adult cognitive processes and forms the basis for most current work on schizophrenics' cognitive abnormalities. The approach aims to 'make explicit the operations, stages, or processes that occur in the time between stimulation and the observed response' (Haber & Hershenson 1973, p. 158) and 'to describe the limits and characteristics of these processes' (Underwood 1978, p. 2). A feature of such models is the more specific relationship between observed task performance and inferred function; it was therefore seen as ideally suited to the description of schizophrenics' disturbances of cognition. The approach is, however, not without its difficulties. Although current models of human cognition share many important features, it cannot be claimed that there is an agreed model. They are constantly changing, and there are frequently opposing models to explain the same phenomena. A further problem is that schizophrenics tend to perform poorly on most cognitive tasks. In order to clarify the nature of their impairment, we need to demonstrate a greater deficit on one task than another, i.e. a differential deficit. However, it has been argued by Chapman & Chapman (1973) that a differential deficit may result for purely psychometric reasons, namely the discriminating power of the tests employed. These in turn are dependent on their reliability and difficulty level, and they claim that unless tasks are matched on these variables, the attribution of a differential deficit to the diagnostic variable may not be justified. However, Strauss (1978) points out that the matching of tasks for discriminating power (within the normal population) 'may remove the variance that must be studied in order to make valid inferences about the nature of the psychological processes that are involved in task performance' (ibid., p. 318). He claims that it is preferable to employ an experimental approach to eliminate alternative hypotheses about the specific processes which could account for an observed deficit in schizophrenics.

This section will draw upon several models of information processing. It will emphasize the utility of the following distinctions in considering the nature of schizophrenics' abnormalities: 'stimulus set' (filtering) versus 'response set' (pigeon-holing) in selective attention (Broadbent 1971); automatic versus controlled processing (Schneider & Shiffrin 1977); data-driven versus conceptually driven processing (Norman & Bobrow 1976). Also influential has been Sternberg's (1975) development of the stage model of choice reaction time performance.

Selective attention

Broadbent's (1958) model was most influential in early studies of schizophrenics' cognitive disturbance. A hypothetical 'filter' mechanism was seen as screening irrelevant stimuli from a limited-capacity decision channel. It was viewed as acting in an all-or-none fashion on the basis of the physical attributes of stimuli. This raised two possibilities as to the nature of schizophrenics' impairment: first, that they possess a defective 'filter' mechanism (e.g. McGhie & Chapman 1961); second, that schizophrenics are slow in processing information. Developments of the latter have largely been based on Sternberg (1975) and will be considered in a subsequent section. Broadbent's later probabilistic model of the methods by which the systematic selection of information takes place (1971) views filtering as a process of attenuation, and also makes the important distinction between stimulus set (filtering) and response set (pigeon-holing). The latter mechanism acts as a bias towards certain categories of response at the expense of others by allocating larger or smaller numbers of 'states of evidence' to each category state. An example may make this clearer. Consider a subject who is required to shadow a lengthy series of numbers against a white noise background: 9, 4, 1, 7, etc. If then the sound 'ee' is presented this 'evidence' may be sufficient to produce the response '3'. The subject is biased towards perception of digits rather than letters. Thus when the actual stimulus is unexpected, normal biases may act to impair performance. The mechanism may be seen as a way of making use of the redundancy and patterning of sensory input to reduce information-processing demands. As Broadbent (1977) writes, 'this kind of attention selects some of the possible interpretations that a man may hold about the world, and eliminates others as candidates to use in the particular situation' (ibid., p. 10).

Much of the evidence concerning a defective filter mechanism results from studies employing dichotic listening tasks. Unfortunately, the findings are inconsistent. Schizophrenics have typically made more errors in verbal shadowing of the relevant message, usually errors of omission, than normal subjects. However, the findings are less clear-cut when psychiatric control groups are employed (e.g. Straube & Germer 1979, Pogue-Geile & Oltmanns 1980). In addition, many such studies have not demonstrated an increased intrusion of the words of the irrelevant message into schizophrenics' repetition of the shadowed message. More recently, however, Spring and her colleagues (e.g. Spring 1985) have demonstrated that schizophrenics are more likely than psychiatric controls to interject phonemes from distractor words into their shadowing responses. This would suggest a deficit in filtering, albeit at a more subtle level. There is, however, a possible alternative explanation. Recall that in Broadbent's (1971) model the message from the irrelevant channel is attenuated rather than completely excluded. It might therefore reach awareness if the threshold for response is low — one is likely to hear one's own name in a dichotic listening task even if it is presented to the unattended ear. In dichotic listening tasks, thresholds for response are in part raised or lowered according to the nature of the preceding shadowed material. Thus the pigeon-holing mechanism is operative, and intrusions could be explicable in terms of an impairment at this stage of processing. This is a clear illustration of the problems discussed above.

A somewhat different approach to the assessment of inefficiency in filtering was adopted by Hemsley & Zawada (1976). They presented subjects with a series of lists of six digits read in alternation by a man and a woman. Two different recall conditions were imposed. In the pre-instruction condition subjects were told which set of digits they were later to report, and were thus able to ignore the digits spoken by the other voice. In the post-instruction condition they were informed following the presentation of the list. Normal subjects show a clear superiority with pre-instruction. An impairment in filtering should thus be reflected in a reduction in the discrepancy in performance between the two conditions. Schizophrenics, depressives and normals, matched on general intelligence, were assessed. Both psychiatric groups failed to benefit from pre-instruction. The authors suggested that the filter deficit 'may not be specific to schizophrenia but may rather be related to a "severity of illness" dimension not important causally in many of the behavioural abnormalities seen in schizophrenia' (ibid., p. 460).

The second method of selectivity of information within Broadbent's (1971) model, pigeon-holing, relies heavily on semantic cues. The relationship between this and the aetiology of disordered speech is intuitively more appealing, and Schwartz (1982) has reviewed findings supporting this position. However, direct evidence relating to a possible disturbance in pigeon-holing is scarce. Hemsley & Richardson (1980) employed a task based on an experimental paradigm devised by Treisman (1964). This required subjects to shadow one of two simultaneously presented prose passages, these being presented binaurally, at the same volume in the same voice, and at the same rate. The passage to be shadowed (extracts from a novel) was presented briefly, then the second (technical extracts) was superimposed. There is no possibility of the filter operating to distinguish between the passages. Instead, successful performance of the task requires subjects to use contextual variables in determining selection of the appropriate response. It is thus dependent on the pigeon-holing mechanism whereby category-state thresholds may be altered according to the preceding context. Normals, depressives and schizophrenics were assessed. These groups did not differ on shadowing ability without distraction, or verbal IQ. The schizophrenics performed significantly worse than both other groups with the superimposed technical extracts, consistent with a defect in pigeon-holing. However, as Knight (1982) points out, the group differences may reflect a generalized rather than specific deficit since the tasks of shadowing with and without distraction were not matched on discriminating power. Furthermore, much of the evidence seen by Schwartz (1982) as indicating a disturbance in pigeon-holing was designed to test other hypotheses. The suggestion that schizophrenics fail to establish appropriate response biases, and hence do not make use of temporal and spatial redundancy to reduce information-processing demands, merits further research.

A related formulation has been put forward by Maher (1983). He argues that in investigating attentional processes in schizophrenia, one should emphasize the failure of attentional focusing to respond to stimulus redundancy, features being redundant to the extent that they correlate with other features. He goes on to relate this to schizophrenics' language disturbances. In a general sense, most models of normal functioning accept that perception is dependent on an interaction between the stimulus presented and stored memories of regularities in previous input which result in expectancies or response biases and serve to reduce information-processing demands. It is also apparent that at different times either the stimulus or the expectation may exert the greater influence on perception. Thus Norman & Bobrow (1976) make a distinction between 'data-driven' processing and 'conceptually driven' processing. If schizophrenics are indeed less able to make use of the redundancy and patterning of sensory input, it should be possible to construct tasks where schizophrenics would be predicted to perform better than normals owing to the latter forming inappropriate expectancies. However, it is unlikely to be a straightforward endeavour to demonstrate such an effect, since its magnitude must be great enough to counteract the generally lowered performance of schizophrenics, resulting from such factors as poor motivation. It is also therefore of some interest to consider situations in which schizophrenics' performance is equivalent to that of normals.

There are few examples of schizophrenics' superior performance. An early finding of this kind was reported by Polyakov (1969). He demonstrated that in both visual and auditory modalities an ambiguous signal is identified by normals according to the probabilistic constraints of context more so than by schizophrenics. For example, in the following sentence 'The photographer made a pretty . . .' normals most frequently identified the ambiguous (partially masked by noise) term as 'picture'. If this was in fact the stimulus presented, their performance was superior to schizophrenics. If, however, an unlikely stimulus was presented, schizophrenics were correct significantly more often than normals. This is presumably because they are relying to a greater extent on the stimulus qualities of the signal, rather than prior expectancies, and is consistent with a disturbance in pigeon-holing.

An important study by Schwartz Place & Gilmore (1980) may also be linked to the present formulation. Schizophrenics and normal subjects were required to report the number of lines presented in a visual display. In one of their experiments, the perceptual organization or regularity of the arrays was manipulated by varying the proximity and similarity of the line elements. As the organization of the arrays became more complex the performance of the controls deteriorated, but the schizophrenics were not affected by the organization variable. Indeed, the average performance of the schizophrenics was superior to that of the controls, and the authors argue that this is consistent with the former subjects' failure to organize the information presented. Hemsley (1986) has argued that it may also be viewed as a situation where normal subjects' attempts to detect and make use of the minimal regularities present in the most complex array interfere with the counting of the lines. In contrast, the schizophrenics make little use of any spatial regularities present, hence performing worse when these might aid counting, but better when no such regularities are present.

Finally, mention should be made of a recent study (Brennan & Hemsley 1984) which indicated superior performance by non-paranoid schizophrenics. This made use of the phenomenon of 'illusory correlation', the report by observers of a correlation between two events which in reality are not correlated. It is particularly likely to occur when the two events have a strong associative connection, and it may be viewed as a way in which prior expectations influence, and in this case mislead, subjects. It was therefore predicted that non-paranoid schizophrenics would produce weaker illusory correlations than normals, i.e. their reports would more closely correspond to reality. Magaro (1980) has argued that the nature of the cognitive abnormality shown by non-paranoids is quite distinct from that of the paranoid. The latter is seen as relying on a rigid conceptual guiding of information processing, hence Magaro would predict stronger illusory correlations in paranoid subjects. In terms of Norman & Bobrow's (1976) distinction the non-paranoid might be seen as characterized by 'data-driven' processing. Across the three tasks employed by Brennan & Hemsley (1984), the non-paranoids showed the weakest and the paranoids the strongest tendency to report illusory correlations. The normals were in an intermediate position; such a pattern of results is not easily interpretable in terms of either a generalized deficit or lowered motivation.

Automatic versus controlled processing

The study of cognitive abnormalities in schizophrenia has recently become influenced by the distinction between automatic and controlled processing

(Schneider & Shiffrin 1977). Their theory attempted to integrate work in the related areas of selective attention, visual search and short-term memory search. Automatic processes are seen as involving the activation of a fixed sequence of mental operations in response to a particular input configuration. They involve direct access to long-term memory, require no processing capacity, and occur outside of conscious awareness. Extensive training results in the development of automatic processing, but once established it is relatively inflexible and difficult to suppress. In contrast, controlled processes are temporary sequences of mental operations under the control of the individual. They require attention, involve demands on limited processing capacity and are often serial in nature. Although relatively slow, and subject to interference by other simultaneous controlled processing, they can be flexibly adapted to task requirements.

Several authors have suggested that schizophrenics show a deficit in controlled processing but adequate or even superior automatic processing (e.g. Callaway & Naghdi 1982). It is clear that tasks with a high processing load are those on which schizophrenics' performance is likely to be most impaired, consistent with this view. However, Nuechterlein & Dawson (1984a) point out that the reduction in available processing capacity for task-relevant cognitive operations could result from several different factors:

> (1) the executive decision making or control function that allocates processing capacity is not responding appropriately to task demands despite a normal pool of processing capacity; (2) more processing capacity is devoted to task irrelevant external or internal stimuli; (3) conscious capacity demanding processing is required to complete cognitive operations that are usually completed automatically in parallel processing; (4) the total pool of processing capacity is smaller (ibid., p. 193).

The first of these would represent a strategic problem. The third possibility is of particular interest, since there is increased emphasis on the need to establish links between disturbances of cognition and schizophrenic symptoms. As Venables (1984) points out, a failure of automatic processing would result in activity proceeding at the level of consciously controlled sequential processing. Recall the study by McGhie & Chapman (1961) of patients' reports of their experiences. One said 'I have to do everything step-by-step, nothing is automatic now. Everything has to be considered' (ibid., p. 105). A disturbance of automatic processing would be consistent with those studies demonstrating greater decrements in schizophrenics' performance when processing load is increased, since automatic processes serve to expand capacity by reducing the load on controlled processes. Related to this proposal is Frith's (1979) suggestion that 'the basic cognitive defect associated with schizophrenia is an awareness of automatic processes which are normally carried out below the level of consciousness' (ibid., p. 233). This model will be considered in greater detail on p. 115.

Slowness of information processing

The generalized slowness of schizophrenics over a wide range of tasks is well established. It has been argued that studies of choice reaction time (CRT) may permit the precise specification of the stages of information processing that are impaired in schizophrenia. Within Broadbent's (1958) model, the concept of a limited-capacity decision channel was influenced by findings of a linear relationship between reaction time and the logarithm of the number of equiprobable stimulus alternatives. The slope of this function was seen as an inverse measure of the capacity of the decision channel. Such models have required considerable modification and Sanders (1980) has argued that six serial stages of information processing are necessary to account for the findings on CRT. His model represents a development of Sternberg's (1975) additive factor method for the isolation of processing stages. These approaches have an obvious appeal for experimental psychopathologists but this class of models is not without its critics. For example Rabbitt (1979) points out that it is often unjustified to assume linear, serial and independent processing stages.

Slowness of information processing at a particular stage is inferred from an increased slope of the function relating reaction time to variations in the level of a factor seen as influencing the demands on that stage. Many studies have employed CRT tasks in which stimulus and response uncertainty are manipulated. In reviewing these, Hemsley (1976b) argued that although at first sight the findings were inconsistent, they could be understood if account were taken of the stimulus–response compatibility of the task. S–R compatibility represents the degree of obviousness or naturalness of the response. The effect of prolonged practice on a given task is similar to that of high compatibility, the response selection stage being bypassed in favour of a direct S–R link. The degree of schizophrenic deficit on such tasks appears to increase mainly as a function of increasing response uncertainty, but this is apparent only on tasks of low S–R compatibility. This would be consistent with a disturbance at the level of response selection.

Sternberg's paradigm has also been applied to the study of schizophrenia. This requires subjects to memorize a short list of digits and then to respond 'Yes' or No' as to whether a test digit was a member of the memorized set. Checkosky (in Sternberg 1975) assessed chronic schizophrenics, acute schizophrenics and alcoholic controls; he varied stimulus intactness (implicating the encoding stage), memory set size (implicating the serial comparison stage) and presence vs. absence of the stimulus (implicating the decision stage). Although there were group differences in the intercepts of the functions relating reaction time to processing load, there were no differences in slope. This was seen as indicating no impairment at these stages of processing. More recently Russell et al (1980) employed a hybrid visual and memory search task requiring subjects to search displays of up to 15 letters for a target, which in different conditions was drawn from a memorized set of one, three or six letters. Although response times and intercepts of the schizophrenics exceeded those of the controls, no differences were found in rates of increase in response time as a function of the number of memorized or displayed items. This demonstrates the adequacy of the assessed processes, and Knight (1984) has argued that, in view of schizophrenics' generally poorer performance, this is a particularly valuable research strategy (ibid., p. 127). Russell et al (1980) suggest that the schizophrenics' generally slower performance on their task may be attributable to processes involved in response selection and production, consistent with Hemsley's (1976b) review of the effects of response uncertainty.

Impairment in 'perceptual organization'

The suggestion that schizophrenics show problems in perceptual organization derives from studies of early visual information processing. In particular the span of apprehension technique, which requires subjects to indicate which of two targets is present in a tachistoscopically flashed stimulus array, has demonstrated schizophrenics' greater decrement than normal controls as the number of irrelevant elements in the array increased (e.g. Neale 1971). Others have investigated the adequacy of schizophrenics' 'iconic memory' by means of the backward masking paradigm in which at various durations after the offset of a target stimulus, a masking stimulus is presented. Several such studies have found abnormalities in schizophrenics' iconic memory, most prominent being those of Saccuzzo and his colleagues (e.g. Saccuzzo & Braff 1981).

These findings have, however, proved difficult to interpret, and as Knight (1984) points out, they could result either from a deficient iconic storage, or inefficiency in the transfer of information from its spatial array on the icon to later verbal encoding. Knight (1984) argues that it is necessary to consider more recent work on normals' early visual information processing, which indicates two separate early memory stages. The first, susceptible to pattern masking, has a median duration of 100 ms or less; the second (STVM) can only be affected by a cognitive mask, i.e. one requiring the processing of new information. Knight goes on to suggest 'two possible explanations that could account for the backward masking deficit — either poor prognosis schizophrenics process the information in the pattern mask as meaningful (or at least they are not as efficient as normals at quickly determining the lack of meaning and terminating further processing) or they have an unstable STVM that is more easily disrupted than that of normals' (ibid., p. 105). He then draws upon the findings of Schwartz Place and Gilmore (1980), discussed above, to conclude that the most likely explanation is that schizophrenics show a deficiency in perceptual organization, resulting in a slowness in differentiating meaningless and meaningful information. Knight proposes that their perceptual organization deficit will be most apparent when the stimuli are less familiar, when the number of units to be processed is large, when limited time is available to process a unit, or when rapid organization is necessary. In attempting to link his formulation to other cognitive models Knight suggests that this deficit would constitute 'some deficiency in perceptual schema formation, in automaticity, or in the wholistic stage of processing' (ibid., p. 120). In view of Knight's emphasis on schizophrenics' problems in differentiating meaningful and meaningless information, it is worth recalling Garner's (1962) definition of both structure and meaning. The former was viewed as 'the amount of correlation between events' (ibid., p. 143) and meaning as 'the amount of structure which exists, and is perceived in a system of variables' (ibid., p. 145). The perceptual organization deficits might therefore be linked with the previous suggestion that schizophrenics fail to make use of the structure and patterning of sensory input to reduce processing demands. It would also be consistent with Cutting's (1985) concluding remarks, following his review of studies of schizophrenics' visual perception, that they 'concentrate on details at the expense of theme' (ibid., p. 300).

It is clear that in considering schizophrenics' disturbances of perception and cognition a number of theoretical models have been drawn upon. These often differ radically in their assumptions concerning the nature of normal information processing. It is therefore hazardous to attempt to interpret studies within a different framework from those in which they were designed. Nevertheless, this final section does indicate the possibility of a convergence of views as to the nature of schizophrenics' impairment. It is now necessary to consider ways in which these might relate to schizophrenic symptoms.

MODELS OF SCHIZOPHRENIA BASED ON PERCEPTUAL/COGNITIVE ABNORMALITIES

Spohn (1984) writes 'I consider it of some importance that information processing deficits such as Knight's "perceptual organization deficit" be shown to be related to more complex forms of psychopathology in schizophrenia, as a means for validating the deficit and demonstrating that it is not trivial' (ibid., p. 347). He goes on to recommend that relations between deficits and symptoms be predicted and tested. This is an important issue. Although the possible link between an information-processing disturbance and disordered thinking is easily understood, this is not the case for other important schizophrenic phenomena, such as hallucinatory experiences and delusional beliefs. Psychological approaches to these abnormalities will be considered in the following sections. First, however, we will consider examples of more general attempts to link a range of schizophrenic symptoms to a more basic abnormality of information processing.

Two areas of theorizing and related experimentation may be distinguished. The first approach seeks to account for the principal positive symptoms of schizophrenia, in terms of the cognitive impairment (e.g. Frith 1979). The second argues that certain aspects of schizophrenics' functioning may represent attempts to reduce the behavioural disorganization resulting from the cognitive disturbance (e.g. Hemsley 1977).

Frith's (1979) model relies heavily on the distinction between preconscious and conscious processing of information. He suggests that thought disorder, hallucinations and delusions may be seen as the result of a defect in the mechanism that controls and limits the contents of consciousness. Auditory hallucinations are thus viewed as an awareness of preconscious incorrect interpretations of auditory stimuli, and are therefore expected to increase in likelihood in conditions of ambiguous sensory input. Following earlier authors, Frith considers delusions as attempts to explain and understand the misperceptions resulting from the basic impairment. Unlike previous formulations his model can account for the occurrence of delusions in the absence of hallucinations. Percepts may achieve conscious awareness as a result of a disturbed process, but give rise to the correct interpretation of an event. The abnormality lies in the fact that normally such an aspect of the situation would not reach awareness, and its registration leads to a search for the reasons for its occurrence. Frith also notes that only certain people may be capable of constructing the complex belief system necessary to explain all the irrelevant percepts of which they become aware, and suggests that this may relate to such factors as premorbid intelligence. Hemsley (1977) also points out that it may be influenced by the severity of the cognitive abnormalities, it being possible to maintain a stable delusional system in the face of limited intrusions of percepts into awareness, but beyond a certain level they may be replaced by the more transient belief system characteristic of the non-paranoid schizophrenic. Finally, Frith suggests that thought disorder could result from a failure to inhibit awareness of alternative and irrelevant meanings and implications of words.

A similar view to that of Frith is presented by Maher (1983), who suggests that the pathology of schizophrenia 'involves an inability to exclude from intrusion into consciousness material from either external stimulation or internally stored associations, that would normally be excluded on the basis of its irrelevance to the task situation in which the patient is performing' (ibid., p. 35). He applies this model particularly to the abnormalities of schizophrenic speech. Intrusions into awareness are seen as attributable to a failure to make use of the redundancies of sensory input to permit the optimum deployment of attention. This is similar to Hemsley's (1982) suggestion that schizophrenics fail to make use of the structure and patterning of sensory input to reduce processing demands.

Hemsley (1977) argued that the pattern of cognitive deficits shown by schizophrenics might usefully be seen as resulting in a state of 'information overload' and that the strategies of processing employed by normal subjects in situations of experimenter-induced overload could be relevant to an understanding of schizophrenic behaviour. In particular, it was suggested that certain of the negative symptoms of schizophrenia, such as poverty of speech, social withdrawal and retardation might, for certain individuals, represent adaptive strategies, learnt over time, to minimize the effects of the cognitive impairment. Factors which might be expected to determine preferred strategies, and hence the form of behavioural abnormality, would include severity of impairment, personality factors independent of the psychosis, and environmental influences. It is possible that the most acceptable methods of adaptation within some institutions involve withdrawal and lowered responsiveness.

PSYCHOLOGICAL APPROACHES TO HALLUCINATIONS AND DELUSIONS

Hallucinations

Slade (1976) put forward a model of schizophrenic hallucinations which indicated three major areas of potential psychological research. Firstly, the investigation of factors within the individual predisposing to the development of hallucinations; secondly, the role of arousal in triggering the hallucinatory phenomena; thirdly, the influence of varying sensory input on the likelihood of hallucinatory experience. Relevant to these issues is the extensive research on sensory and/or perceptual deprivation in normal subjects. It appears to be the lack of structured input which is of importance in producing the abnormal perceptual experiences which Leff (1968) suggests 'overlap considerably with those of mentally ill patients' (ibid., p. 1507). Recently Jakes & Hemsley (1986) have examined individual differences in reaction to brief exposure to unpatterned visual stimulation. Significant relationships have been demonstrated between both a questionnaire measure purporting to assess hallucinatory predisposition and the Psychoticism (P) scale of the Eysenck Personality Questionnaire (Eysenck & Eysenck 1975), and reports of complex visual sensations such as meaningful objects or integrated scenes.

It has also proved possible to demonstrate the short-term manipulation of auditory hallucinations, in a group of schizophrenic patients, by means of variations in auditory input (Margo et al 1981). The greatest reduction in hallucinatory experiences occurred when a response was required of the subject; for the passive conditions, the experiences were inversely related to the structure and attention-commanding properties of the input. This is consistent with Frith's (1979) suggestion that hallucinations are dependent on the meaningfulness of sensory input. Such findings offer no direct explanation of the occurrence of schizophrenic hallucinations, only of the extent to which they may vary under short-term manipulations of sensory input. However, it is tempting to speculate, following Hartmann (1975, p. 73) that 'possibly something in the realm of ability to pattern sensory input or interact with it may be involved in the inhibitory factor' (for hallucinatory experience). On p. 114 it was suggested that schizophrenics may be less able to make use of the structure in presented material — one might therefore argue that hallucinations are related to a cognitive impairment which, even under normal conditions of sensory input, results in ambiguous messages reaching awareness.

Bentall & Slade (1985) have recently proposed that hallucinations result from a deficit in the metacognitive skill of reality testing. In two experiments, employing the methodology of signal detection theory, they have demonstrated that subjects either experiencing hallucinations, or highly disposed towards hallucination, show an increased willingness to believe that a stimulus is present, given a poor signal-to-noise ratio, and a reasonable expectation that a stimulus might be presented. They propose that this deficit relates to hallucinators' proneness to mistake internal events for external stimuli.

Perhaps the most ambitious attempt to explain hallucinatory phenomena has been put forward by Hoffman (1986). He presents a convincing case for considering the intendedness of imagery production as an important factor influencing the experience of hallucinations. It is of interest to recall James' (1890) distinction between the transitive and substantive aspects of conscious experience, the former linking the substantive parts together and giving consciousness its distinctive 'stream-like' attributes. A quality of the transitive parts of consciousness emphasized by James is that they are intentional or goal-directed, and he argues that personal identity is given to thought by (i) fundamental resemblance between phenomena forming part of the stream, and (ii) long-term continuity before the mind. Where the stream of consciousness is disrupted, psychopathology results. Collicutt & Hemsley (1985) suggested that unexpected internally generated experiences may be attributed to external events, and hence correspond to hallucinations. They went on to argue that the occurrence of such experiences might be related to an abnormality in Broadbent's (1971) pigeon-holing mechanism, such that the thresholds for inappropriate intrusions into awareness are not raised by the immediately preceding contents of consciousness. The use of the term 'inappropriate' of course raises the question 'inappropriate to what', and Hoffman's model provides the answer 'inappropriate to the intended imagery production'. In his article, Hoffman refers to 'expectations' being violated and hence the verbal imagery being experienced as alien. Pigeon-holing is viewed as a mechanism whereby expectancies influence perception, and a defect in this 'could result in highly improbable categorizations on the basis of minimal evidence' (Collicutt & Hemsley 1981, p. 204).

Delusions

Although in a general sense delusions may be viewed as abnormal beliefs, the definition of a delusion continues to present problems. Increasingly it is recognized that they may best be conceptualized as more or less extreme points along certain belief dimensions, such as conviction, preoccupation, fixity, bizarreness, etc. (Garety 1985). It appears necessary to distinguish between the establishment and maintenance of abnormal belief systems. The former may result from abnormal perceptual experiences, such as previously ignored and/or preconscious information becoming salient (cf. Frith 1979). Maher & Ross (1984) argue that the process whereby delusions are formed is the same as that used by normals to explain their experiences. This is seen as a five-stage process, beginning with the observation of something unusual, followed by a feeling of puzzlement. This may lead to a search for further information, and at some point subsequently there follows an explanatory insight where all becomes clear. Once this exploration has emerged, any further exploration is of a confirmatory nature, rather than a search for defects in the explanation in an impartial way.

Cameron (1951) has suggested that the processes in the maintenance of delusions are abnormal in that deluded individuals disregard information incongruent with the delusional system. However, it is clear that similar processes are operative in the maintenance of normal strongly held beliefs. It is apparent that a normative theory of how people should evaluate evidence relevant to their beliefs can provide a conceptual framework for a consideration of how they do in fact evaluate them. Fischoff & Beyth-Marom (1983) argue that Bayesian inference provides a general framework for evaluating hypotheses (beliefs) and that it may be used to describe a person's consistency with, or departures from, the model. They indicate a number of stages at which biases may occur in assessing evidence relevant to a hypothesis (belief). Hemsley & Garety (1986) have suggested that this approach may usefully be applied to the cognitive distortions shown by patients regarded as deluded. For a given belief, deluded subjects may demonstrate deviations from Bayesian inference at one or more of these stages. It is also necessary to explore the extent to which the distorted processing in the deluded individual is specific to material relevant to the belief, or represents a more generalized style of processing information.

PSYCHOPHYSIOLOGICAL ABNORMALITIES: 'AROUSAL' MODELS

Attempts to formulate models of schizophrenia based on disturbances of arousal mechanisms have been influenced both by the extremes of behavioural responsiveness which may be manifest during the disorder, and also by the effectiveness of the major tranquillizers in reducing many of the symptoms. However, a number of very different meanings have been attached to the term 'arousal'. It appears necessary either to abandon the use of the term or to replace it by a number of more specific concepts. Although there has been extensive research on psychophysiological abnormalities in schizophrenia, the findings are complex. In part this is attributable to the various measures employed; however, it is clear that the simple suggestions that schizophrenia represents either a state of heightened or reduced arousal are untenable. As Claridge (1972, p. 8) points out, 'they do not even get beyond the first stage of explaining why it is that neurotics also in varying states of arousal are not psychotic'. His own more elaborate formulation will be discussed later in this section.

Perhaps the most extensively investigated set of measures involves the assessment of electrodermal activity, particularly in response to mild innocuous stimuli. Variables of interest include tonic skin conductance level (SCL), non-specific skin conductance responses and the rate of habituation of the skin conductance response to a novel stimulus. The initial response to such a stimulus, part of the orienting response, is seen as related to a subject's attention to, and cognitive processing of, that stimulus. Findings on schizophrenics' electrodermal activity have been confusing and contradictory. Gruzelier & Venables (1975) argued that this was attributable to there being two distinct patterns of response to auditory stimuli that might be shown by schizophrenic subjects. One group, termed responders, exhibited high skin conductance levels, a high incidence of spontaneous fluctuations, high response amplitudes and slow habituation. The non-responder group demonstrated an absence of orienting responses, low skin conductance levels, and a low incidence of spontaneous fluctuations. Responders tended to display the more positive symptoms of schizophrenia, non-responders negative symptoms. The two groups do not appear to represent distinct disorders but rather two possible manifestations of a similar disturbance, since certain schizophrenics have been shown to alternate between these psychophysiological response patterns (Rubens & Lapidus 1978). These authors conclude that 'Overresponders react to the normal range of environmental stimuli . . . as though they were all potential danger signals . . . Underresponders on the other hand are in an unusually low state of baseline arousal. They have reduced their contact with the stimulus laden world and have ceased to exhibit the type of responsivity that is essential for adaptive functioning' (ibid., p. 209). The responders may be viewed as treating each stimulus as 'unexpected' and it is therefore tempting to link this with the failure to make use of the redundancy and patterning of sensory input to reduce processing demands, emphasized in the discussion of cognitive abnormalities. Of interest is a study by Straube (1979) which demonstrated, on a dichotic listening task, more errors of omission among non-responders.

Unfortunately, the situation is less straightforward than had initially appeared. Recent reviews (e.g. Ohman 1981) indicate that although there is a greatly increased incidence of non-responders among schizophrenics, there is less agreement about the course of habituation among those who respond to the initial stimulus. A further difficulty is that the patterns of skin conductance activity demonstrated are probably not specific to schizophrenia. For example, indices of autonomic activity have been widely employed in the investigation of depressive states. Byrne (1975) has shown that neurotic depressives exhibit higher skin conductance response amplitude to visual stimuli, and increased spontaneous fluctuations compared to control or psychotic depressive samples. The latter group were significantly lower than controls on both variables. Further, the neurotic sample showed significantly slower habituation rates than psychotic depressives. It is apparent that more elaborate models of arousal are required if they are to account for the differences between various forms of psychopathology. One such has been proposed by Claridge (1972), who argued that schizophrenics differ from others not in their absolute levels on given psychophysiological measures, but rather in the way in which different measures covary. In particular Claridge has been interested in the covariation of autonomic and perceptual functioning. The disequilibrium between these systems was seen as resulting in the maladaptive patterns of attention and perception observed in schizophrenia. While speculative, and in part relying on data from normal subjects following LSD administration, it provides an interesting explanation for the rapid onset of psychotic phenomena which may sometimes be observed. In normals, autonomic activity beyond a certain level is seen as reducing perceptual sensitivity. In contrast, for schizophrenics, beyond a certain level, increased autonomic activity is seen as increasing sensitivity, which in turn may feed back positively on the autonomic system; the system is thus an unstable one.

There has also been interest in the psychophysiological responses of schizophrenics to high and low Expressed Emotion (EE) relatives. Tarrier et al (1979) demonstrated that patients in remisson from low-EE homes showed physiological adaptation to an experimental situation in the presence of their key relative; those from high-EE homes did not. Skin conductance responses were also monitored in a study by Sturgeon et al (1984), who assessed acutely ill schizophrenic patients during a standardized interview, conducted with the patient's key relative present. Significant differences were demonstrated between patients whose relatives had high and low EE, the rate of skin conductance responses of the former being almost double that of the latter. It is of interest that MacCarthy et al (1986) have reported a relationship between critical comments, an important aspect of EE, and the unpredictability of the key relative's behaviour.

Mention should also be made of recent work attempting to identify cortical correlates of cognitive dysfunction in schizophrenia. This is based on the electrophysiological study of cortical activity, in particular event-related brain potentials. The most consistent finding among schizophrenics appears to be a reduction in the P300 component, a positive wave with a peak latency of about 300 ms following a stimulus. Hink et al (1978) have suggested, on the basis of work with normal subjects, that P300 is related to response set and this led Venables (1984) to speculate that the reduced P300 shown by schizophrenics is related to an inefficiency in pigeon-holing of the kind discussed on p. 107. A related point is made by Magaro (1984), who argues that the P300 effect 'supports the hypothesis that schizophrenia is a matter of not maintaining a strong conceptual organization or serial processing strategy . . . Schizophrenics can selectively attend to relevant stimuli (filter) [but not] organize stimuli extensively relative to others' (ibid., p. 202). It is clear that research of this kind may make it possible to link abnormalities of perception and cognition to disturbances at the level of neurophysiology.

ABNORMALITIES IN THE RELATIVES OF SCHIZOPHRENICS

Two related research strategies may be distinguished. The first attempts to identify variables or events early in the life span which are valid predictors of later onset of schizophrenia. Most commonly this involves a comparison of offspring with one schizophrenic parent and those with normal parents. These are frequently referred to as 'high-risk' studies in that the likelihood of occurrence of schizophrenia in the former group is 12–15%. The second approach involves the study of the healthy relatives of schizophrenics. As Cromwell (1984, p. 28) writes: 'When deviant factors are identified uniquely in this group, they serve as candidate hypotheses for either environmental or genetic vulnerability to schizophrenia.

The initial phase of a high-risk study aims to demonstrate group differences in the variables of interest, these usually being chosen because of their demonstrated abnormality in symptomatic patients. Subsequently one is interested in predicting which subjects within the high-risk group become schizophrenic. Measures employed include performance on a range of perceptual/cognitive tasks (e.g. Cornblatt & Erlenmeyer-Kimling 1985), psychophysiological indices (e.g. Mednick et al 1978) and behavioural assessments, such as ratings by peers and teachers of early school and social behaviour. The current status of these research programmes has been reviewed in a recent volume (Watt et al 1984), and there is space to consider only one or two examples of findings. Several investigators have demonstrated that children at risk for schizophrenia perform more poorly than do normal children on a variety of attentional measures. In a recent report (Cornblatt & Erlenmeyer-Kimling 1985) a subgroup of the high-risk children displayed extreme global deviance across attentional measures. Of particular interest was their finding that such deficits were related to subsequent behavioural disturbance in young adulthood. It remains to be seen whether such attentional disturbances are predictive of schizophrenia, since the subjects in the high-risk sample have yet to pass through the age of greatest risk for the disorder.

The first large-scale high-risk study was concerned primarily with psychophysiological predictors of breakdown (Mednick et al 1978). Their initial findings indicated larger skin conductance response, with shorter latencies and shorter recovery times in the high-risk group. This is similar to the pattern reported for 'responder' schizophrenics. Within the high-risk group, an index derived from the electrodermal measures was found to be predictive of future schizophrenia in males but not females. Subsequent studies, reviewed by Dawson & Nuechterlein (1984), have produced less consistent findings, and the authors suggest that rather than merely comparing group means, a more appropriate strategy may be 'to test for the existence of a disproportionately large extreme scoring subset of high risk subjects' (ibid., p. 217).

An example of a study illustrating interesting differences between the healthy relatives of schizophrenics and normal controls has recently been reported by Spring (1985). Using a dichotic listening task, subjects were required to shadow a message presented to one ear, ignoring distractions. By detailed analysis of the shadowing responses she was able to demonstrate that both schizophrenics and their relatives more frequently interjected phonemes from distractor words into their performance. Spring (1986) argues that a strategy for demonstrating a trait as a marker of vulnerability to schizophrenia should bring together three kinds of evidence: abnormalities found among first-degree biological relatives of schizophrenics; abnormalities demonstrated among schizophrenic individuals who are no longer highly psychotic; abnormalities present among individuals considered to be at risk for schizophrenia because of schizotypal personality features or biological characteristics associated with schizophrenia.

POSSIBLE LINKS WITH BIOLOGICAL MODELS OF SCHIZOPHRENIA

This section will attempt to indicate the way in which links might be forged between biological and psychological models of schizophrenia. To do so it will focus on one biochemical theory: that which emphasizes a disturbance in the dopamine system. This is not to imply acceptance of the theory, which is not without its critics. Rather, it will serve as an illustration of how different levels of explanation for schizophrenic phenomena might be related. The dopamine hypothesis suggests either that the neurotransmitter dopamine is produced in too great a quantity, or that its brain receptors are too sensitive to normal amounts. Two kinds of evidence have been put forward in support of this theory. First, the effective anti-psychotic drugs have in common the ability to block dopamine receptors in the brain. Second, amphetamine, which stimulates dopamine release in the brain can, in chronic abusers, induces symptoms similar to those encountered in schizophrenia (e.g. Angrist et al 1974). Several authors have attempted to relate this model to research on schizophrenics' cognitive impairment. For example, Joseph et al (1979) present a model which links abnormalities in the control of attention to dysfunctions in brain amine systems. More recently there has been a growth of interest in the effects of amphetamine on attention, and their possible implications for models of schizophrenia. Lubow et al (1982) have argued that the latent inhibition (LI) paradigm is an effective way of manipulating attention in animals and that this may provide a link with the attentional disturbance prominent in schizophrenia. In the first stage of the LI paradigm a stimulus is repeatedly presented to the organism. In the second stage, the pre-exposed stimulus is paired with reinforcement in any of the standard learning procedures, classical or instrumental. When the amount of learning is measured, relative to a group that did not receive the first stage of stimulus pre-exposure, it is found that the stimulus-pre-exposed group learn the new association much more slowly. This is interpreted as indicating a reduction in the deployment of attention to a predictable redundant stimulus. Lubow al et (1982) have shown in animals that LI is disrupted if amphetamine is administered in both the pre-exposure and test phase. They write: 'output is controlled, not like in the intact animal, by the integration of previous stored inputs and the prevailing situational conditions, but only by the latter' (ibid., p. 103). Recall the discussion on p. 109 of the distinction between 'data-driven' and 'conceptually driven' processing, optimal performance being dependent on an interaction between the stimulus presented and stored memories of regularities in previous inputs which result in expectancies or response biases. Lubow et al (1982) suggest that animals under the influence of amphetamine may be viewed as unable to utilize acquired knowledge in a newly encountered situation. They write: 'Not having the capacity to "use" old stimuli, all stimuli are novel. Therefore such an organism will find itself endlessly bombarded with novel stimulation, resulting perhaps in the perceptual inundation phenomena described in schizophrenia' (ibid., p. 104). There are intriguing similarities to the suggestion that schizophrenics fail to make use of the redundancy and patterning of sensory input to reduce information processing demands.

CONCLUSIONS

It is clear that there is no agreed psychological model for the abnormalities of behaviour and experience resulting in a diagnosis of schizophrenia. There is, however, some convergence of views as to the form of perceptual/cognitive abnormality characterizing the disorder. Clearly there are dysfunctions at a number of levels — social, cognitive, psychophysiological and biochemical — and a major task is to demonstrate how these are inter-related. A tentative model linking several of the topics discussed in this chapter has been put forward by Nuechterlein & Dawson (1984b). They argue that enduring vulnerability characteristics of individuals predisposed to schizophrenia include attentional disturbances, autonomic arousal anomalies and social competence deficits. These interact with stressful environmental stimuli to produce information overload, autonomic hyperarousal, and impaired processing of social stimuli. These in turn are viewed as resulting in disruptions in the individual's social and family network, and hence still further processing capacity overload and hyperarousal. The vicious cycle is seen as continuing until 'the individual's threshold point for the development of schizophrenic reality distorting psychotic symptoms' (ibid., p. 305) is reached. It is a highly plausible account of the relationship between social, cognitive and psychophysiological abnormalities. However, it is apparent from the preceding quotation that there remains much to be learnt concerning the way in which these are related to psychotic symptoms.

REFERENCES

American Psychiatric Association 1986 Diagnostic and Statistical Manual of Mental Disorders. Washington, DC
Andreasen N C 1982 Negative v. positive schizophrenia: definition and validation. Archives of General Psychiatry 39: 789–794
Angrist B M, Sathananthan G, Wilk S, Gershon S 1974 Amphetamine psychosis: behavioural and biochemical aspects. Journal of Psychiatric Research 11: 13–23
Bentall R P, Slade P D 1985 Reality testing and auditory hallucinations: a signal detection analysis. British Journal of Clinical Psychology 24: 159–169
Bishop D V M 1977 The P scale and psychosis. Journal of Abnormal Psychology 86: 127–134
Bleuler E 1950 Dementia praecox or the group of schizophrenias. International Universities Press, New York (originally published 1911)
Brennan H J, Hemsley D R 1984 Illusory correlations in paranoid and non paranoid schizophrenia. British Journal of Clinical Psychology 23: 225–226
Broadbent D E 1958 Perception and communication. Pergamon, London
Broadbent D E 1971 Decision and stress. Academic Press, London
Broadbent D E 1977 The hidden preattentive processes. American Psychologist 32: 109–118
Byrne D G 1975 A psychophysiological distinction between types of depressive states. Australian and New Zealand Journal of Psychiatry 9: 181–185
Callaway E, Naghdi S 1982 An information processing model for schizophrenia. Archives of General Psychiatry 39: 339–347
Cameron N 1951 Perceptual organization and behaviour pathology. In: Blake R R, Ramsey G V (eds) Perception: an approach to personality. Ronald, New York
Chapman L J, Chapman J P 1973 Disordered thought in schizophrenia. Appleton-Century-Crofts, New York
Chapman L J, Chapman J P 1980 Scales for rating psychotic and psychotic-like experiences as continua. Schizophrenia Bulletin 6: 476–489
Claridge G S 1972 The schizophrenias as nervous types. British Journal of Psychiatry 121: 1–17
Claridge G S 1985 Origins of mental illness. Blackwell, Oxford
Collicutt J R, Hemsley D R 1981 A psychophysical investigation of auditory functioning in schizophrenics. British Journal of Clinical Psychology 120: 199–204
Collicutt J R, Hemsley D R 1985 Schizophrenia: a disruption of the stream of thought. Unpublished manuscript.
Cornblatt B A, Erlenmeyer-Kimling L 1985 Global attentional deviance as a marker of risk for schizophrenia: specificity and predictive validity. Journal of Abnormal Psychology 94: 470–486
Cromwell R L 1984 Preemptive thinking and schizophrenia research. In: Spaulding W D, Cole J K (eds) Theories of schizophrenia and psychosis. University of Nebraska Press, London
Cutting J 1985 The psychology of schizophrenia. Churchill Livingstone, London
Dawson M E, Nuechterlein K H 1984 Psychophysiological dysfunctions in the development course of the schizophrenic disorders. Schizophrenia Bulletin 10: 204–232
Eysenck H J, Eysenck S B G 1975 Manual of the Eysenck personality questionnaire. Hodder & Stoughton, London
Fischoff B, Beyth-Marom R 1983 Hypothesis evaluation from a Bayesian perspective. Psychological Review 90: 239–260

Frith C D 1979 Consciousness, information processing and schizophrenia. British Journal of Psychiatry 134: 225–235
Garety P A 1985 Delusions: problems in definition and measurement. British Journal of Medical Psychology 58: 25–34
Garner W R 1962 Uncertainly and structure as psychological concepts. Wiley, New York
Gruzelier J H, Venables P H 1975 Evidence of high and low arousal in schizophrenics. Psychophysiology 12: 66–73
Haber R N, Hershenson M 1973 The psychology of visual perception. Holt, Rinehart & Winston, New York
Hartmann E 1975 Dreams and other hallucinations: an approach to the underlying mechanisms. In: Siegel R K, West L J (eds) Hallucinations: behavior, experience and theory. Wiley, New York
Hemsley D R 1976a Problems in the interpretation of cognitive abnormalities in schizophrenia. British Journal of Psychiatry 129: 332–335
Hemsley D R 1976b Stimulus uncertainly, response uncertainty and stimulus–response compatibility as determinants of schizophrenic reaction time performance. Bulletin of the Psychonomic Society 8: 425–427
Hemsley D R 1977 What have cognitive deficits to do with schizophrenic symptoms? British Journal of Psychiatry 130: 167–173
Hemsley D R 1982 Cognitive impairment in schizophrenia. In: Burton A (ed) The pathology and psychology of cognition. Methuen, London
Hemsley D R 1987 Schizophrenia: concepts, vulnerability and intervention. In: Straube E, Hahlweg K (eds) Schizophrenia: models and intervention. Springer Verlag, Heidelberg
Hemsley D R, Garety P A 1986 The formation and maintenance of delusions: a Bayesian analysis. British Journal of Psychiatry 149: 51
Hemsley D R, Richardson P H 1980 Shadowing by context in schizophrenia. Journal of Nervous and Mental Disease 168: 141–145
Hemsley D R, Zawada S L 1976 'Filtering' and the cognitive deficit in schizophrenia. British Journal of Psychiatry 128: 456–461
Hink R F, Hillyard S A, Benson P J 1978 Event related brain potentials and selective attention to acoustic and phonetic cues. Biological Psychology 6: 1–16
Hoffman R E 1986 Verbal hallucinations and language production processes in schizophrenia. Behavioural and Brain Sciences 9: 503–548
Isnard C A, Zeeman E C 1976 Some models from catastrophe theory in the social sciences. In: Collins L (ed) Use of models in the social sciences. Tavistock, London
Jakes S, Hemsley D R 1986 Individual differences in reaction to brief exposure to unpatterned visual stimulation. Personality and Individual Differences 7: 121–123
James W 1890 The principles of psychology. Macmillan, London
Joseph M H, Frith C D, Waddington J L 1979 Dopaminergic mechanisms and cognitive deficit in schizophrenia: a neurological model. Psychopharmacology 63: 273–280
Knight R A 1984 Converging models of cognitive deficit in schizophrenia. In: Spaulding W D, Cole J K (eds) Theories of schizophrenia and psychosis. University of Nebraska Press, London
Knight R G 1982 Language disorder and hemispheric asymmetries in schizophrenia. Behavioural and Brain Sciences 5: 603–604
Kraepelin E 1919 Dementia praecox and paraphrenia. Livingstone, Edinburgh (translated by Barclay R M)
Leff J P 1968 Perceptual phenomena and personality in sensory deprivation. British Journal of Psychiatry 114: 1499–1508
Lubow R E, Weiner J, Feldan J 1982 An animal model of attention. In: Spiegelstein M Y, Levy A (eds) Behavioural models and the analysis of drug action. Elsevier, Amsterdam
MacCarthy B, Hemsley D R, Schrank-Fernandez G, Kuipers E, Katz R 1986 Unpredictability as a correlate of expressed emotion in the relatives of schizophrenics. British Journal of Psychiatry 148: 727
McGhie A, Chapman J 1961 Disorders of attention and perception in early schizophrenia. British Journal of Medical Psychology 34: 103–116
Magaro P A 1980 Cognition in schizophrenia and paranoia. Lawrence Erlbaum, Hillside, NJ
Magaro P A 1984 Psychosis and schizophrenia. In: Spaulding N D, Cole J K (eds) Theories of schizophrenia and psychosis. University of Nebraska Press, London

Maher B A 1983 A tentative theory of schizophrenic utterance. In: Maher B A, Maher W B (eds) Progress in experimental personality research. Vol 12 Psychopathology. Academic Press, New York

Maher B, Ross J S 1984 Delusions. In: Adams H E, Sutker P (eds) Comprehensive handbook of psychopathology. Plenum, New York

Margo A, Hemsley D R, Slade P D 1981 The effects of varying auditory input on schizophrenic hallucinations. British Journal of Psychiatry 139: 122–127

Mednick S A, Schulsinger F, Teasdale T W, Schulsinger H, Venables P H, Rock D R 1978 Schizophrenia in high risk children: sex differences in predisposing factors. In: Serban G (ed) Cognitive defects in the development of mental illness. Brunner/Mazel, New York

Neale J M 1971 Perceptual span in schizophrenia. Journal of Abnormal Psychology 77: 196–204

Neale J M, Oltmanns T F 1980 Schizophrenia. Wiley, New York

Norman D A, Bobrow D G 1976 On the role of active memory processes in perception and cognition. In: Cofer C N (ed) The structure of human memory. Freeman, San Francisco

Nuechterlein K H, Dawson M E 1984a Information processing and attentional functioning in the development course of the schizophrenic disorders. Schizophrenia Bulletin 10: 160–203

Nuechterlein K H, Dawson M E 1984b A heuristic vulnerability/stress model of schizophrenic episodes. Schizophrenia Bulletin 10: 300–312

Ohman A 1981 Electrodermal activity and vulnerability to schizophrenia: a review. Biological Psychology 12: 87–145

Oltmanns T F, Neale J M 1978 Abstraction and schizophrenia: problems in psychological deficit research. In: Maher B A (ed) Progress in experimental personality research, Vol 8. Academic Press, New York

Pogue-Geile M F, Oltmanns T F 1980 Sentence perception and distractibility in schizophrenic, manic, and depressed patients. Journal of Abnormal Psychology 89: 115–124

Polyakov V F 1969 The experimental investigation of cognitive functioning in schizophrenia. In: Cole M, Maltzman J (eds) Handbook of contemporary social psychology. Basic Books, New York

Rabbitt C P 1979 Current paradigms and models in human information processing. In: Hamilton V, Warburton D M (eds) Human stress and cognition: an information processing approach. Wiley, New York

Rubens R L, Lapidus L B 1978 Schizophrenic patterns of arousal and stimulus barrier functioning. Journal of Abnormal Psychology 87: 199–211

Russell P N, Consedine C E, Knight R G 1980 Visual and memory search by process schizophrenics. Journal of Abnormal Psychology 89: 109–114

Saccuzzo D P, Braff D L 1981 Early visual information processing deficit in schizophrenia: new findings using schizophrenic subgroups and manic control subjects. Archives of General Psychiatry 38: 175–179

Sanders A F 1980 Stage analyses of reaction processes. In: Stelmach E, Requin J (eds) Tutorials in Motor behaviour. North Holland, Amsterdam

Schneider W, Shiffrin R M 1977 Controlled and automatic human information processing: I. Detection, search, and attention. Psychological Review 84: 1–66

Schwartz S 1982 Is there a schizophrenic language? Behavioural and Brain Sciences 5: 579–626

Schwartz Place E J, Gilmore G C 1980 Perceptual organization in schizophrenia. Journal of Abnormal Psychology 89: 409–418

Slade P D 1976 Towards a theory of auditory hallucinations: outline of a hypothetical 4-factor model. British Journal of Social and Clinical Psychology 15: 415–423

Spohn H E 1984 Discussion. In: Spaulding N D, Cole J K (eds) Theories of schizophrenia and psychosis. University of Nebraska Press, London

Spring B 1985 Distractibility as a marker of vulnerability to schizophrenia. Psychopharmacology Bulletin 21: 509–512

Spring B 1986 Cognitive alterations as markers of vulnerability to schizophrenia. In: Perez V, Chiodo J (eds) Biological and psychological correlates of psychopathology. Texas Technical University Press, Lubbock

Sternberg S 1975 Memory scanning: new findings and current controversies. Quarterly Journal of Experimental Psychology 27: 1–32

Straube E R 1979 On the meaning of electrodermal non responding in schizophrenia. Journal of Nervous and Mental Disease 167: 601

Straube E R, Germer C K 1979 Dichotic shadowing and defective attention to word meaning in schizophrenia. Journal of Abnormal Psychology 88: 346–353

Strauss M E 1978 The differential and experimental paradigms in the study of cognition in schizophrenia. Journal of Psychiatric Research 14: 316–326

Sturgeon D, Turpin G, Kuipers L, Berkowitz R, Leff J 1984 Psychophysiological responses of schizophrenic patients to high and low expressed emotion relatives: a follow-up study. British Journal of Psychiatry 145: 62–69

Tarrier N, Vaughn C E, Lader M H, Leff J P 1979 Bodily reactions to people and events in schizophrenics. Archives of General Psychiatry 36: 311–315

Treisman A M 1964 Verbal cues, language, and meaning in selective attention. American Journal of Psychology 77: 206–219

Underwood G 1978 Attentional selectivity and behavioural control. In: Underwood G (ed) Strategies of information processing. Academic Press, London

Venables P H 1984 Cerebral mechanisms, autonomic responsiveness and attention in schizophrenia. In: Spaulding W D, Cole J K (eds) Theories of schizophrenia and psychosis. University of Nebraska Press, Nebraska

Watt N F, Anthony E J, Wynne L C, Rolf J E (eds) 1984 Children at risk for schizophrenia: a longitudinal perspective. Cambridge University Press, New York

Zubin J, Spring B 1977 Vulnerability — a new view of schizophrenia. Journal of Abnormal Psychology 86: 103–126

7   Ivy M. Blackburn

Psychological processes in depression

INTRODUCTION

Depression is probably the most intensively researched topic in psychiatry, if not in clinical psychology. This is rightly so, as depression is the commonest of psychological disorders, affecting both children and adults. It has sometimes been called the 'common cold of mental illness' (Miller & Seligman 1973) and 'the bread and butter' of the general psychiatrist. It affects, in its various forms, about 4% of males and twice as many females at any one time in the general population (Boyd & Weissman 1982) and makes up about 14% of hospital admissions (Scottish Home & Health Department 1978 admission figures).

This chapter will forcibly exclude more than it includes. Depression research has been conducted from sociological, biological and psychological points of view and the plan here is to review selectively research pertaining only to psychological factors of depression. In the first section, depression will be described and defined, giving a short summary of classificatory systems, without going into the vast literature in the controversies relating to this area (Kendell 1976, Eysenck 1970). In the second section, studies of the psychological phenomena of depression will be reviewed — these will include intellectual function, psychomotor speed, learning and memory, motivation, personality, different aspects of thinking style and psychophysiology. In the last section, psychological theories which attempt to account for these phenomena will be discussed. These will be restricted to behavioural and cognitive theories and to attempts at psychobiological integration. There have been other approaches to the understanding of depression which will not be reviewed here as they relate less directly to the psychological processes which are dealt with in this chapter, for example psychodynamic theories (Freud 1917, Abraham 1911) and psychosocial theories (Bandura 1977, Brown & Harris 1978).

DEFINITION OF DEPRESSION

The general term depression is a confusing one as it encompasses a whole variety of conditions, which can vary from a simple transient mood change with no other accompanying symptoms to different types of depressive illnesses with different degrees of severity. Although it is outside the scope of this chapter to review the controversies which still surround the classification of depressive illness, it will be necessary to define the subcategories used in the research literature as these terms will recur later.

The seeds of the modern debate about the boundaries between depressive illness and normality and depressive illness and other psychiatric disorders were sewn by Kraepelin (1921), who grouped all depressive syndromes together under the single heading of *manic-depressive psychosis*, to be distinguished from *dementia praecox* or schizophrenia on the basis of course of the illness, age, type of onset, presumed heredity and clinical symptoms. Since then, controversies have centred around the issue of how many different types of depression there are, whether they form a continuum from normality or whether they are disease entities. These issues continue to generate an abundance of research using multivariate statistical analyses of symptoms and rating scales, response to different treatments, biological variables and psychological variables in support of one or other school of thought. Since no clear system of classification based on aetiological principles has emerged so far, for research purposes, diagnosis is made by checking recognized diagnostic criteria met by the symptoms elicited from standard interviews. These criteria, mostly evolved in the USA, circumvent controversies by making no causal assumptions, but ensure that research findings are more easily interpretable and reproducible because the type of patients studied are so clearly specified. Table 7.1 describes the main distinctions made by the Research Diagnostic Criteria (RDC) of Spitzer et al (1978), one of the most widely used classificatory systems.

The 'major depression' category includes the main symptoms which make up the depressive syndrome as compared to a 'minor depression' category which might include none of the symptoms in group B, and show no more than two symptoms, such as tearfulness, pessimistic attidues, being broody, preoccupation with feelings of inadequacy, irritability, demandingness or clinging dependency, self-pity and excessive somatic complaints. The subgroups of major depression listed in Table 7.1 (endogenous, psychotic, unipolar and bipolar) have shown major differences in research findings, particularly in biological and personality research and in treatment response, so that it would now be considered inadequate to group together all depressive syndromes as Kraepelin once did.

Table 7.1 also indicates that the symptoms of depression affect a whole gamut of functions, both biological and psychological. It would be useful to look at a functional analysis of depression, regardless of diagnostic subcategories, before reviewing the studies which have looked at the psychological processes underlying the functional deficits. Table 7.2 presents such an analysis.

The change in *mood* or affect has traditionally been considered the central feature of depressive illness, hence the term affective illness is used as the

Table 7.1 Main diagnostic distinctions in depression according to the Research Diagnostic Criteria (Spitzer et al 1978)

Categories	Symptoms
1. Major Depressive Disorder (A + 5 symptoms from B)	A (1) Dysphoric mood or pervasive loss of interest (duration at least 2 weeks)
	B (1a) Poor appetite or weight loss (1b) or increased appetite or weight gain (2) Sleep difficulty or sleeping too much (3) Loss of energy, fatiguability (4) Psychomotor agitation or retardation (5) Loss of interest or pleasure in usual activities (6) Feelings of self-reproach or excessive guilt (7) Diminished ability to concentrate (8) Suicidal thoughts or behaviour
2. Endogenous Major Depressive Disorder (6 symptoms from C + D, with at least one from C)	C (1) Distinct quality of depressed mood (2) Lack of reactivity to environmental change (3) Mood is regularly worse in the morning (4) Pervasive loss of interest or pleasure
3. Psychotic Major Depressive Disorder (with delusions and/or hallucinations)	
4. Bipolar depression (with a history of mania or hypomania)	D (1) Feelings of self-reproach or excessive guilt (2) Early morning or middle insomnia (3) Psychomotor retardation or agitation (4) Poor appetite (5) Severe weight loss (6) Loss of interest or pleasure or decreased sexual drive
5. Recurrent unipolar major depression (never met criteria for a manic disorder)	

Table 7.2 Functional analysis of depression

Psychological Symptoms	
Mood	Sadness, anxiety, irritability
Thinking	Loss of concentration, slow and muddled thinking, pessimistic outlook, self-blame, indecisiveness, low self-esteem
Motivation	Lack of interest in work and hobbies, avoidance of social or work activities, wish to escape, increased dependency
Behaviour	Inactivity, pacing, crying, complaining
Biological Symptoms	Loss of appetite/increased appetite Loss of libido Disturbed sleep Retardation/agitation

generic term to describe the different subtypes. Although sadness and a gloomy feeling are often reported, anxiety and increased irritability are also often present. Patients do not always describe their mood as depressed. They may use metaphors as 'it's like a black cloud' or 'it's like having cotton wool in my head'. This is often an attempt by the sufferer to describe 'the special quality' of the depressed mood mentioned in Table 7.1. Some authors have described the change in *thinking* style as the most striking feature in depressed patients (for example, Beck 1967, 1976). There is a subjective feeling of slow and inefficient thinking, of poor concentration, of poor memory and of inability to make decisions. The observer is struck by the negative tone of the content of thought relating to the self, the environment and the future. Beck has described this as the negative cognitive triad. *Motivational* changes also predominate, expressed as loss of interest in work and leisure activities, avoidance behaviour which often leads to a wish to die, suicidal ideas and suicidal behaviour. The risk of suicide in depression is at least 100 times the general population risk. Loss of self-confidence and feelings of inadequacy lead to an increased dependency on others. *Behavioural* changes are also notable; the depressed person can become very inactive, sitting for hours on end, or he may fidget and pace about, unable to fix his attention on any one task. On the other hand, some passive behaviours, such as crying and complaining, are increased.

All the symptoms and signs described so far are psychological in nature, while some other symptoms have traditionally been considered biological or 'vital' (Van Praag et al 1965) or endogenous (see Table 7.1), implying physical underlying mechanisms. These biological symptoms are changes in appetite (loss or increase), in weight (loss or increase), and in sleep (again, loss or increase) and loss of sexual interest. These symptoms lead to the hypothesis of a reversible abnormality in the hypothalamic–pituitary–adrenal axis, and a wealth of studies have been conducted to clarify the nature, extent and specificity of neurotransmitter and neuroendocrine changes in this system (Post & Ballenger 1984). This promising and important aspect of depression will not be reviewed here, but where possible some link will be made between biological and psychological aspects of depression.

Thus, although there is complete consensus about the presence of psychological deficits in depression, there has not been a corresponding agreement about the role of these deficits, their importance, their mode of interaction or the primacy of one class of variables over another.

PSYCHOLOGICAL PROCESSES

Intellectual level

Most reported studies have found no differences in intellectual performance between depressed patients and normal controls. Grannick (1963) compared 50 psychotically depressed patients and 50 normal controls, matched for age, sex, race, education and religion on the Wechsler Adult Intelligence Scale (WAIS) subtests of Information and Similarities and on the Thorndike–Gallup Vocabulary Test. He failed to find any significant difference in performance between the two groups. Friedman (1964) compared 55 depressed patients and 65 normal controls, matched for age, sex, education, vocabulary score and race, on a battery of 33 cognitive, perceptual and psychomotor tests. The patients obtained lower scores on only 4% of the 82 test scores derived, a finding which could be due to chance. Friedman concluded that actual ability and performance during severe depression is not consistent with the depressed patient's unrealistically low image of himself.

On the other hand, Payne (1968) in a review of several studies concluded that affectively ill patients may show more deterioration than schizophrenics who do not differ in IQ when ill, whereas the affective patients have a higher pre-morbid IQ. Such a conclusion is unwarranted as many of the studies reviewed used timed tests, which put depressed patients at a disadvantage, and in addition, the groups studied were often not properly defined, different groups of patients, such as unipolars, bipolars, psychotics and non-psychotics being included under the general term of 'affectively ill' or 'manic-depression'. Miller (1975), in his review article, concluded that deterioration in manic-depression and endogenous depression (again, undefined) is reversible with improvement in clinical state.

Intellectual and psychomotor speed

Slowness and retardation are well-recognized clinical signs of depression, when subjectively or objectively rated, yet experimental demonstration of this phenomenon has not always been consistent. As early as 1945, Rapaport reported a significant lowering of digit-symbol scores in a depressed group as compared with a schizophrenic group. He concluded that performance on this test was sensitive to retardation, as seen clinically in depression. However, Jastak (1949) re-analysed Rapaport's data and noted that the schizophrenic group had a mean age of 31 years and the depressed group a mean age of 49 years. When age was held constant, the depressed patients failed to show the consistently lower test score. Fisher (1949) reported that depressed patients who were rated as improved following electroconvulsive therapy (ECT) obtained significantly higher mean digit-symbol scores than a group of unimproved patients. Payne & Hewlett (1960) compared groups of normals, dysthymic neurotics, hysterics, endogenous depressed patients and schizophrenics, matched for age, education and pre-morbid intelligence. They found that the depressed patients were consistently slower both on intellectual speed tests (as tested by the Nufferno Speed Tests, Furneaux 1956) and on motor-speed tests (as tested by the Babcock-Levy 1940 test). Foulds (1952) found that on a maze-drawing task, the introduction of a distraction (repeating numbers) temporarily obscured the pattern of disturbance in depressed patients and resulted in an increased speed, whereas no such effect was obtained in non-depressed patients. The same effect was obtained after ECT. Foulds concluded that distraction may achieve the effect of speeding up performance 'by drawing the attention away from the affective disturbance, whilst

ECT in some way reduces the intensity of the unpleasant affect and thus enables the activity with which it is competing to dominate consciousness more frequently than had been possible'.

Two inconsistent findings were obtained in a follow-up study by Shapiro et al (1958), who found that depressed patients, after recovery, did not show any improvement in their performance on a battery of psychomotor tests when compared with a control group, and by Beck et al (1962), who controlled for age and intelligence in a group of 78 psychiatric patients and found no relationship between digit-symbol scores and depression.

Thus, early studies of retardation in depression have produced equivocal results, again probably because of the heterogeneous nature of the groups studied and possibly because of the disparate nature of the studies.

Recent studies more carefully specify patient groups and, because of the advent of new instrumentation, they have been able to provide more detailed measures of different aspects of retardation. As Greden & Carroll (1981) note: 'Psychomotor functions are multifaceted, complex and difficult to isolate into measurable segments'. Blackburn (1975) compared unipolar and bipolar depressed patients, ill and recovered, in a cross-sectional design, on intellectual speed (Nufferno Speed Tests) and motor speed (Gibson's spiral maze 1965). Very different results were obtained for the two types of depression. Intellectual speed tests, given in stressed and unstressed conditions, did not differentiate the two ill groups. Intellectual speed, under unstressed but not stressed conditions, differentiated ill and recovered bipolar patients, but did not differentiate between ill and recovered unipolar patients. Motor speed differentiated the two depressed groups and only the bipolars gained speed when a distraction stimulus (listening to a tape-recorded story) was present. Motor speed also differentiated between ill and recovered bipolar patients, but not between ill and recovered unipolar patients. She concluded that retardation could only be demonstrated in bipolar patients and that external distraction and stress to work quicker interfered in some way with the process or mechanism causing retardation and thus resulted in temporary increase in speed. Kupfer and his associates (Kupfer et al 1972, 1974) largely supported this conclusion by recording activity patterns in unipolar and bipolar depressed patients with specially designed motor-activated electronic equipment and by monitoring body activity around the clock. They found that unipolar depressed patients exhibited significantly more motor activity before treatment than bipolar patients. These differences disappeared when both groups improved, and activity levels measured in this way were very useful in monitoring the course of bipolar illness; they tended to increase with mania and decrease with depression.

Speech rate measurement, using a polygraph, has also provided a reliable and sensitive measure of retardation. Szabadi et al (1976) measured phonation time and pause time in the automatic speech (counting one to ten) of healthy controls and depressed patients (apparently unipolar). The oscilloscope tracings showed that phonation and pause times were constant in normal controls over a period of two months. In depressed subjects, the pause times were significantly elongated compared with controls and reverted to normal after recovery following treatment with antidepressant medication.

The conclusion from these studies is that clinically observed retardation can be measured experimentally and that reliable evidence of retardation can be obtained, even when not observable clinically (Greden & Carroll 1981). Some diagnostic subgroups of depressed subjects do not show retardation, and different profiles of retardation may be present in different individuals, for example, motor, mental, speech and bodily functions can be selectively affected.

Learning and memory

A number of early studies have found memory deficits in depressed patients compared to controls on word-learning tasks (for example, Walton et al 1959, Kendrick et al 1965, Post 1966). More recently, the actual nature of the deficit has been studied more closely, taking into consideration type of patients, effects of medication, the memory task and different components of learning and memory, i.e. attention, encoding, retrieval, short- and long-term memory processes.

Weingartner and his colleagues at the National Institute of Mental Health have produced an important series of papers on some aspects of memory deficits in depression. Henry et al (1973) found that a group of unipolar and bipolar patients showed no impairment in short-term memory, i.e. on the first trial of an eight-word learning task. However, they showed an impairment on later trials, thus indicating an inability to shift information from short- to long-term storage. Similar deficits were shown on a free-recall task. Greater deficit was associated with higher depression scores, confirming other findings (Miller 1975, Murphy et al 1973). They interpreted the results as indicating a deficit in the ability to organize stimuli by association, which could be due to a lack of motivation or to a disturbance in catecholamines (neurotransmitters implicated in biological studies of depression) in the brain with consequent changes in brain state activation and arousal (Weingartner et al 1976).

In a later study, Weingartner et al (1977) found in repeated testing of bipolar patients fluctuating in mood between mania, normal mood and depression that episodic events generated from semantic memory can be recalled more completely in a similar mood state than in a different mood state. They concluded that a simple relation between disturbance in mood and deficits in learning could not adequately account for the results, because the associations produced while a patient was manic or depressed were more effectively reproduced during a period of congruent mood than during a period of disparate mood. They found the paradigm of state-dependent learning more plausible in explaining their results. This effect has been shown in studies of drug effects on a variety of learning–memory procedures. Learning that has occurred in one drug state is retrieved better when the subject is similarly drugged than when the subject is in an undrugged (or different) drug state. Mood states, in the same way as drugs, determine not only how events are encoded (state-dependent learning), but also how memory is searched (state-dependent retrieval). Parallel findings have been observed in depressed patients and normal volunteers subjected to alteration in mood through sleep deprivation (Weingartner & Murphy 1977, Macht et al 1977). The same group (Reus et al 1979) listed ways in which the effects of state-dependent learning and state-dependent retrieval can be prevented. Dissociative phenomena are not seen when subjects are given retrieval strategies as in cued recall; 'overlearning' of items at the time of storage also prevents the phenomenon, and information which is highly encodable is less likely to be lost than subtle, less saliently encoded information.

These findings have implications for the psychotherapeutic treatment of depressed patients, who generally show difficulty in remembering past pleasant events or envisioning future mood improvement. Weingartner et al (1981) investigated further the structure of the strategies used by depressed patients to process information. All subjects satisfied RDC for major depression, unipolar subtype. In three experiments, subjects were asked first to attend and respond to either the meaning or the sounds of words that were to be recalled either freely or in the presence of cues; secondly, to recall words which had first been grouped or sorted into categories; thirdly, to process sets of words which varied according to how much organization they contained. Thus, in each experiment, a different approach was used to control how encoding strategies might later influence the recall of information. Relative to normal controls, depressed patients were not able to take advantage of the more elaborate strategy using semantic processing to enhance recall; they showed a deficit in the recall of random words which needed more elaborate processing, but not in the recall of highly structured information which required less elaborate processing; and they showed a relative inability to impose structure on lists of words when the form of presentation required an active restructuring. Unlike Willner (1984), who interpreted this body of data as indicating an inability to sustain effort and concentration, Weingartner et al evoked a psychobiological mechanism relating to brain state arousal and activation under cholinergic and/or noradrenergic control.

A different set of studies have looked at the accessibility of different types of memories in different mood states in patient populations or normal controls in whom contrasting mood states have been induced. Lishman (1972) found that depressed in-patients relative to non-depressed patients showed less of the established bias in recall of pleasant over unpleasant material. Lloyd & Lishman (1975) tested 38 in-patients for time taken to retrieve pleasant and unpleasant experiences in response to a series of standard stimulus words. They found that the ratio of time taken to recall pleasant memories to time taken to recall unpleasant memories increased with increased depression. This did not seem related to the previous experience of more unpleasant life events, or to the recent occurrence of more unpleasant events. The authors interpreted the results as being due to the greater intensity of hedonic tone attached to unpleasant experiences, to the mental set of depressed patients which would direct the recall process towards unpleasant experiences and perhaps to more mental rehearsal of the memories.

Teasdale and his colleagues have conducted a number of experiments to elucidate this process further. Teasdale & Fogarty (1979) used the mood manipulation technique developed by Velten (1968) to induce elated and depressed mood in depressed volunteers. The technique involves the reading of mood-relevant self-statements. In each mood state, neutral cue words were presented and subjects were asked to retrieve memories of real-life experiences, specified as pleasant or unpleasant, associated with the cue word. They found that time to retrieve pleasant experiences was significantly longer in depressed than in elated mood, suggesting that their accessibility was reduced. By contrast, time taken to retrieve unpleasant memories was very similar in the two mood states. In a second study (Teasdale et al 1980), a similar experimental procedure was used, but it was not specified whether the memory retrieved should be pleasant or unpleasant. At the end of the experiment, subjects categorized their memories as pleasant or unpleasant, to ensure that the memories retrieved in the two induced moods could be confidently interpreted in terms of differences in accessibility rather than in terms of the effects of mood on rating. The results indicated this time that depressed mood not only decreased the accessibility of pleasant memories but also increased the accessibility of unpleasant memories. Teasdale & Taylor (1981) showed the same effect when using a different mood-inducing procedure from the previous experiments, by removing all references to the subjects' life in the self-statements. Teasdale & Russell (1983) conducted a more conventional learning experiment by presenting a list of positive, negative and neutral personality trait words in a neutral mood state to student volunteers. Depressed and elated mood were then induced, and in a within-subject design the results again indicated that positive trait words were recalled more in elated mood than in depressed mood, and the converse was true for negative trait words. Neutral personality words were not recalled differentially in the two mood states. Clark & Teasdale (1982) were able to reproduce the same results of differential accessibility of pleasant and unpleasant memories elicited by neutral cue words in a group of depressed in-patients showing the endogenous symptom of diurnal variation.

The effect of mood on the retrieval of differently toned material has also been shown by Bower (1981) in a series of experiments, using hypnotic suggestions to induce mood. Subjects learned two lists of words — one while happy, the other while sad — and were then tested for recall of a given list while in the same or the opposite mood. Retention was assessed as the percentage of items learned in the first list that were recalled on a later test in a congruent or disparate mood. A mood-state-dependent effect was clearly obtained in free recall, with no main effect of the type of emotion on learning. The same effect was obtained for real-life incidents experienced in the previous week when subjects were in an induced mood state, as well as for remote childhood incidents and for the interpretation of ambiguous figures.

To sum up, early studies of learning and memory processes in depression showed a deficit which was interpreted mostly as a deficit in sustaining motivation to perform well, rather than a deficit in information processing (Miller 1975). Later studies have tended to refute this in more detailed investigations which have shown that the deficit is in the transfer of material to long-term memory and that short-term memory is not affected. These studies have also demonstrated state-dependent learning and retrieval and the differential accessibility of material whose hedonic tone is congruent with or disparate from the prevailing mood. While biogenic amines in brain activation have been implicated in one model, other workers have elaborated psychological theories, which will be described later in this chapter.

Motivation

A deficit in motivation or drive in depression is posited from clinical observations as described in the first section. Avoidance behaviour, inactivity, increased dependency and unwillingness to initiate behaviour contribute to the general picture of a motivational change. Motivational change has also been assumed to underlie lower performance on intellectual tests (Friedman 1964, Miller 1975) and memory deficits (Willner 1984). However, direct tests of motivational deficits have not been prominent in the literature.

Cohen et al (1982) reported an experiment particularly designed to allow for direct comparison between motor effort and cognitive performance. In a group of drug-free depressed patients meeting RDC for major affective disorder and a group of normal volunteers, subjects were required to squeeze a dynamometer with the right and left hand alternately, first to reach a peak and then to maintain half their individual pressure for as long as possible. They were also given a memory task involving the learning of trigrams (nonsense syllables of three different consonants) at different rates of presentation, and mood was measured on various rating scales. The results indicated that all behavioural ratings were negatively related to motor performance and to memory performance, indicating that the more depressed performed worst on all tasks. Motor and memory performance were positively correlated. When subjects were divided according to severity of depression and compared with normals, there was only a trend towards a difference in peak motor performance, but the difference in sustained effort was highly significant. Despite the reduction in peak, the depressed subjects could not hold at half-maximum as long as normal subjects. There was a significant time effect on the memory tests, i.e. performance decreased with time between presentation and recall. This effect was more pronounced in the more severely depressed patients. Thus, the impairment on both motor and cognitive tasks appeared to be most noticeable on tasks that required more sustained effort. Cognitive performance in general requires little motor activation or effort and simple motor tasks require little in the way of cognitive process. Cohen et al (1982) thus concluded that, if there is a close relationship between the deficits in both these functions, the most parsimonious explanation would be one based on a single deficit in the area of the central motivational state. The results of memory experiments which show more deficit when more effortful encoding strategies are required, therefore, support the hypothesis of a central deficit in motivation. In summary, memory studies may, in Cohen's view, help to demonstrate the specific sites for the physiological and neurochemical substrata which influence the interaction of the central motivational state with the specific processes that are part of memory. Motivational deficits have also been shown by studies indicating that depressed individuals engage in fewer activities than controls, find less activities as potentially pleasant and give lower enjoyability ratings to potentially pleasant events (Lewinsohn et al 1979).

Personality

Although aspects of personality of depressed patients have been mentioned from the early descriptive and classificatory studies, there have been very few systematic studies in this area. Kraepelin (1921) devoted a special chapter of his textbook on manic-depressive disorders to what he called 'fundamental' states. He described these as relatively enduring characteristics of the manic-depressive temperament that are evident even when the patient is well. He differentiated between the 'depressive temperament', the 'manic temperament', the 'irritable temperament' and the 'cyclothymic temperament'. He stated that the cyclothymic temperament was without doubt the most frequent and several clinical investigators have since supported this opinion (Kretschmer 1936, Henderson & Gillespie 1956, Astrup et al 1959). Winokur et al (1969) found that 80% of their bipolar patients had a cyclothymic or hypochondriacal pre-morbid personality, whereas only 29% of unipolar patients were considered cyclothymic or hypomanic. The psychoanalysts (Freud 1908, Abraham 1954) have emphasized the 'anal' (obsessional) features of depressed patients, i.e. the rigid, dependent, obsessional traits.

Systematic studies, using validated scales or standard interviews, have tended to support the early impressionistic reports. Unfortunately, many studies have not differentiated between subgroups of patients or they have assessed patients when ill, when self-report of long-standing traits is likely to be biased by current state (Perris 1966, Metcalfe 1968). Becker (1960) compared 24 recovered bipolar patients with matched controls on scales derived from McClelland's work on achievement motivation (McClelland et al 1953) to measure two types of achievement orientation. 'Need achievement' is said to characterize people whose concern is to live up to an internalized standard of achievement, whereas 'value achievement' characterizes people who value achievement for achievement's sake as a response to excessive parental stress on achievement. Cohen et al (1954), working within the psychoanalytic concept, had identified the latter type as typical of their bipolar patients. Becker (1960) was able to support this observation, which had been made during psychotherapy. He found that the scores of the bipolar patients on the value achievement scale were significantly higher than those of controls and that they also scored higher on a scale measuring rigidly conventional authoritarian attitudes, conformity, intolerance of ambiguity and social imperceptiveness. Their scores did not differ from the controls on need achievement measures.

Perris (1966) compared two well-defined groups of recovered unipolar and bipolar patients on a multi-dimensional scale derived from the work of the Swedish psychiatrist Sjobring, discussed in English by Coppen (1966). He found that the bipolars scored significantly higher on the dimension of 'sub-stability', i.e. as cycloid or cyclothymic, while the unipolars scored significantly higher on the dimension of 'sub-validity' i.e. as insecure, obsessional and sensitive. Murray & Blackburn (1974), using the sixteen personality factor (16PF) (Cattell & Eber 1957), compared recovered unipolars and bipolars and anxious patients. When ill, all the groups deviated from normal on several primary factors and on the two second-order factors, indicating high anxiety (similar to the neuroticism factor of the MPI, Eysenck 1959) and high introversion, but did not differ from each other, except that the ill bipolars were less tense than the other groups. When recovered, the unipolars were more anxious (second-order factor of neuroticism) and more introverted (second-order factor) than the bipolars and were more similar to the chronically anxious patients. These findings substantially support Perris's findings, although different scales were used in the two studies.

Several studies have used Eysenck's dimensional concepts of neuroticism and extroversion/introversion. Coppen & Metcalfe (1965) tested 39 severely depressed patients on the MPI just after admission to hospital and again after recovery. They found a significant drop in neuroticism (N) and significant increase in extroversion (E) and that recovered patients obtained scores within normal limits. Perris (1971), using the same measure, found that recovered bipolars had higher E and lower N scores than unipolars (as Murray & Blackburn 1974 later found using the 16PF) and that E scores increased and N scores decreased as both groups recovered.

However, Metcalfe (1968) reported that even though the neuroticism score of recovered depressed patients did not differ from normal, when the individual items are examined differences are obtained on eight items, indicating 'a tense, worrying attitude to life' and 'a denial of fantasy and imagination and a rigid, limited, habit-bound personality'. Kendell & DiScipio (1970) also found the same characteristics by showing similarities between the personality structure of unipolar depressed patients and obsessive-compulsive neurotics. This description closely resembles some psychoanalytic observations and Perris's account of the 'sub-valid' personality in recovered unipolar depressed patients.

Clinical descriptions have often been supported by psychometric findings from different scales. However, there is little evidence at the moment for a depression-prone personality type. More studies, in particular prospective studies, are needed to establish the validity of the concept of a vulnerable personality to depression.

Cognitive style

With the upsurge of interest in the role of thought patterns in depression and the development of cognitive therapies for the emotional disorders (Beck 1967, 1976, Ellis 1962), a number of studies have investigated the content and, to a lesser extent, the form and process of thought in depression. Most of these studies have investigated the role of negatively toned cognitions in the maintenance of depression, although some have investigated the role of these cognitions in the onset of depression. There have been several reviews of these studies (Blaney 1977, Hollon & Beck 1979, Rush & Beck 1978, Blackburn 1984) and only examples of the different types of studies will be given here.

Content of thought and attitudes

There is evidence that depressive states correlate with negative cognitions. For example, Weintraub et al (1974) demonstrated that negative perception of self, the world and the future are intercorrelated and covary over time with self-rated depression. Minkoff et al (1973) reported a high positive relationship between depression and hopelessness and an even higher relationship between hopelessness and intent to commit suicide, although this relationship also held in a schizophrenic group. Nekanda-Trepka et al (1983), using the Hopelessness Scale (Beck et al 1974), found high levels of hopelessness in a large depressed group compared to normative data (Greene 1981) and that greater hopelessness was associated with an increase in suicidal wishes and with more negative expectations about real-life problems. Using self-esteem ratings to assess the self-evaluative aspect of depressive cognitions, Hammen & Krantz (1976) found that depressed women were significantly more self-critical than non-depressed women. Several studies have shown that depressed and non-depressed populations differ on measures of dream content, with depressed subjects reporting more themes of personal loss and failure (Beck & Ward 1961, Hauri 1976).

Several questionnaires have now been developed to measure negative thought content and negative attitudes in depressed patients as compared to controls. Nelson (1977) reported highly significant correlations between the Beck Depression Inventory (BDI) (Beck et al 1961), a widely used self-report measure of severity of depression, and the Irrational Belief Test (IBT) (Jones 1968), an inventory designed to assess belief in the types of irrational attitudes considered by Ellis (1962) to cause emotional distress. Krantz & Hammen (1979) developed a Cognitive Bias Questionnaire (CBQ) designed to assess the biased manner of evaluating situations that emphasize negative, self-critical or pessimistic interpretations that are not warranted by the events themselves. They found a consistent positive relationship between the BDI and negative cognitive bias across samples of college students, depressed out-patients and non-depressed psychiatric patients. Another questionnaire of negative content of thought was developed by Hollon & Kendall (1980) to measure the frequency of automatic negative thought, the Automatic Thoughts Questionnaire (ATQ). This measure has been widely used in several recent studies. Hollon & Kendall (1980) reported high correlations between the ATQ and the BDI, but also with a measure of trait anxiety. The ATQ differentiated significantly between depressed and non-depressed college students. Eaves & Rush (1984) found that endogenous and non-endogenous unipolar depressed patients did not differ on the ATQ, but scored significantly higher than non-depressed subjects. The scores of the depressed patients reverted to normal levels on remission. Simons et al (1984), in a treatment trial of major depression, found elevated ATQ scores in patients entering treatment, which decreased to normal levels after treatment. Blackburn et al (1986) found significantly higher ATQ scores in a group of depressed patients compared to normal controls and recovered depressed patients; there were no significant differences between normal controls and recovered depressed patients.

A different type of scale, the Dysfunctional Attitude Scale (DAS), was developed by Weissman & Beck (1978) to measure the basic attitudes and beliefs which are assumed to be relevant to depression. Again, significant differences have been found between depressed and recovered depressed populations (Hamilton & Abramson 1983, Eaves & Rush 1984, Simons et al 1984, Silverman et al 1984, Blackburn et al 1986). Hamilton & Abramson (1983) compared a group of unipolar major depressed patients at admission to hospital and at discharge with normal controls and a non-depressed psychiatric group. They found a large decrease in score on remission in the depressed group, while the recovered depressed group did not differ from controls. The depressed patients scored significantly higher than the psychiatric controls, but not all depressed patients scored highly. Blackburn et al (1986) also found a degree of specificity in that the depressed subjects scored significantly higher than a group of anxious patients. Simons et al (1986) found that a low DAS score in combination with a low BDI score at the end of treatment was predictive of non-recurrence of illness in a one-year post-treatment follow-up. Reda (1984) reported that although the total score of recovered depressed patients on the DAS reverted to normal, scores on some individual items did not change with recovery, and differentiated recovered depressed patients from normal controls. This persistent depressogenic cognitive style indicated a pessimistic view towards reality, the need for complete control over situations and feelings, excessive attention towards other people's judgement, and the idea that need for effort relating to problems indicates some sort of inferiority.

Wilkinson & Blackburn (1981) and Blackburn et al (1986) have developed a scale, the Cognitive Style Test (CST), to measure negative thinking relating to the self, the world and the future, the three elements labelled by Beck (1976) as the negative cognitive triad, in relation to negative and positive events. Wilkinson & Blackburn (1981) found significant differences between depressed and recovered depressed patients, but the latter did not differ from patients recovered from other psychiatric disorders. In the more recent study, Blackburn et al (1986), using an updated version of the CST, replicated these findings in part, in that all the different components of CST differentiated depressed and normal controls and depressed and recovered depressed patients, except for some indication that negative thinking relating to the self might be more stable when age was covaried. Depressed and anxious patients were differentiated on total score and on negative thinking relating to the world, again only when age was covaried.

Negative content of thought and maladaptive attitudes have been well demonstrated in depressed subjects but not in recovered depressed patients. The specificity of these deficits to depression is not well established and there is only tentative indication from Reda's and Blackburn's work described above that more detailed item analysis of the scales in use may indicate an aspect of depressive thinking which is not state-bound and may reflect a depressogenic style of thinking.

Thought process

Depressed patients differ from non-depressed controls not only in *what* they think, but also in *how* they think. The findings on selective memory in depression, reviewed above, are relevant to the process of thought because they demonstrate the bias in information processing.

Depressed subjects underestimate their performance on a laboratory task compared to non-depressed controls. For example, De Monbreun & Craighead (1977), Wener & Rehm (1975) and Nelson & Craighead (1977) have found that depressed subjects underestimate the amount of reinforcement received when different rates of positive and negative feedback are given. These differences are seen at later recall rather than immediately and may arise because non-depressed subjects underestimate the amount of punishment received at a high rate of negative feedback, a phenomenon sometimes called the 'self-serving bias'. They may also be due to the depressed subjects underestimating the amount of positive feedback at a high rate of positive reinforcement. Alloy & Abramson (1979) and Abramson et al (1981) also observed that in laboratory contingency tasks where depressed and non-depressed subjects have to estimate the degree of control that they exert on outcome, depressed subjects underestimate their personal control on outcomes. The difference between groups is due to depressed subjects being relatively accurate, whereas non-depressed subjects overestimate their degree of control.

Seligman and colleagues (Klein & Seligman 1976, Miller & Seligman 1973, 1975) have found differences between depressed and non-depressed subjects in change in expectations following outcomes on chance and skill tasks. Depressed subjects did not change their expectations on the basis of feedback on previous trials for skilled tasks. Abramson et al (1978) found the same insensitivity to outcome in a group of unipolar depressed in-patients, but not in schizophrenic patients.

Questionnaire methods have also been used to investigate the attributional styles of depressed patients and of controls. Most studies have used one of several versions of the Attributional Style Questionnaire (ASQ), recently validated by Peterson et al (1982), to provide subjects with a list of hypothetical events with good and bad outcomes. Seligman et al (1979) reported that depressed students made more internal, stable and global attributions for bad outcomes than non-depressed students. For good outcomes, the only difference was that the non-depressed made more stable attributions. Similar findings were reported by Raps et al (1982), Blaney et al (1980) and Golin et al (1981). Metalsky et al (1982) found a significant correlation between low mood and internal and global attributions for negative events. Several studies have, however, failed to replicate these results in patient populations (e.g. Manly et al 1982, Miller et al 1982).

Other questionnaire studies have investigated the type of logical errors made by depressed patients. Lefebvre (1981) developed the Cognitive Error Questionnaire to measure four types of cognitive errors: catastrophizing (maximizing the negative aspects of events and minimizing the positive aspects), overgeneralization (generalizing from one negative incident), personalization (relating negative events to oneself) and selective abstraction (interpreting situations on the basis of one selective negative aspect). Four groups of subjects were compared: depressed in-patients, depressed and non-depressed low back pain patients, and normal controls. Depressed subjects obtained higher Cognitive Error scores than did non-depressed subjects, but a relatively low, although significant, correlation ($r = 0.39$) was obtained with the BDI.

Watkins & Rush (1983) developed the Cognitive Response Test (CRT) to measure rational and irrational responses to open-ended vignettes. They reported that depressed out-patients, as compared with normal controls, non-depressed psychiatric out-patients and non-depressed medical controls, reported more irrational-depressed responses (such responses contain a negative statement not justified by the stem) and fewer rational responses. Interestingly, a deficit in logical reasoning was also found by Silberman et al (1983) in a discrimination laboratory task testing for logic and strategy in abstract reasoning (Levene 1966). Thirteen in-patients meeting criteria for major depression and 11 normal controls took part in the study. The results indicated that two types of errors — inability to narrow down the set of possible solutions (poor 'focusing') and perseveration on disconfirmed hypotheses — were related to the poorer performance of the depressed patients. While logic, memory and attention were intact at an elementary level, an inability to co-ordinate these functions in more complex tasks appeared to be an important feature of the depressive impairment.

Fennell & Campbell (1984) developed the Cognitions Questionnaire (CQ) to identify specific formal errors in thinking in response to negative, positive and neutral events. The scale measures emotional impact, attribution of causality, generalization across time and across situations and perceived uncontrollability. They found a strong positive association between degree of depression and overall level of cognitive distortion; negative events discriminated more sensitively between different levels of depression than positive or neutral events, there were significant differences between currently depressed and never-depressed individuals on all response dimensions, except for emotional impact, and generalization was not consistently sensitive to differences in depression level. The authors identified two possible markers of vulnerability to depression in recovered depressed patients: generalization from negative events and responses to the question describing the expression of depression itself.

A different approach to the analysis of the organization of thoughts in depression has been the use of the repertory grid technique (Fransella & Bannister 1977) derived from personal construct theory (Kelly 1955). Central to Kelly's personal construct theory account of depression are the related processes of *construction* and *pre-emption*. The former occurs when a person minimizes apparent contradictions among his cognitive subsystems by reducing aspects of the environment to which he attends. Constriction is often accompanied by pre-emptive thinking, in which the person limits the number of constructs which he applies to each aspect of the environment ('elements' in Kelly's terms), thus dealing with events in an unvarying, stereotyped way. For example, he may decide to 'concentrate exclusively on his job' (constriction) and think of it 'only as a means of proving his personal worth' (pre-emptive). Ashworth et al (1982) tested 20 depressed in-patients (major depression), 10 manic, 10 schizophrenic, 10 alcoholic, 10 physically ill non-depressed patients, and 10 recovered depressed patients who were administered repertory grids where 10 elements were role titles; for example, self, father, mother, friend. Principal component analysis of each grid indicated that depressed patients were characterized by grids showing relative 'cognitive simplicity' and 'monolithic' but 'inarticulated' structure, a large perceived distance between self and others and low self-esteem. The authors argued that these repertory grid measures reflected constriction and pre-emptive thinking because they portray an undifferentiated structure characterized by few components and a single large cluster. Ashworth et al (1986) retested 16 of the depressed patients on recovery and found that, for the most part, the cognitive abnormalities and features identified during illness disappeared after recovery.

In conclusion, depressed individuals show different types of processing errors in their thinking. The specificity of these errors to depression is only partly established, and there is only tentative evidence in the work of Fennell & Campbell that some types of processing errors persist in recovered patients, as in the case of thought content and basic attitudes.

Psychophysiology

Psychophysiological studies of depression have investigated both peripheral and central indices of arousal. Among the 'traditional' *peripheral measures*, electrodermal activity (EDA) has been the most studied. Christie et al (1980) reviewed various studies and pointed out that early studies unfortunately made no distinction between subtypes of depressive illness. Some studies introduced unclear diagnostic terms, often used differently. Martin (1963) subdivided depressed patients using a retarded/agitated classification and found no difference in EDA between each subgroup and normal controls and no difference in sedation threshold (the time taken to induce sleep after intravenous administration of sodium amytal). A group of agitated depressed patients were reported by Lader & Wing (1969) not to show any habituation of the skin conductance response (SCR), while retarded depressed patients showed so little reactivity that habituation could not be measured. Low skin conductance level (SCL) has been associated with severity of depression and, in particular, with an endogenous pattern of symptoms (Noble & Lader 1971, 1972), while high SCL has been associated with neurotic depression (Byrne 1975).

Cardiac activity has been little studied in depression. Lader & Wing (1969) and Kelly & Walter (1969) showed higher pulse rates in agitated than non-agitated depressed patients, but Martin (1963) and Byrne (1975) did not show any difference in heart rate between psychotic and neurotic depressed patients and normal controls. Dawson et al (1977) looked at psychophysiological variables in depressed patients before and after ECT. The main findings were that, before treatment, patients had a higher heart rate and lower SCL. Patients who made a good recovery after ECT were, before treatment, more like normals than those patients who did not respond to ECT. Blackburn & Bonham (1980) also found a relationship between depressed mood and heart rate in single-case experiments where patients were asked to use different cognitive coping strategies.

The most consistent finding using electromyographic measures (EMG) has been the increase in the corrugator supercilii muscle activity with depression or after thinking unhappy thoughts (Schwartz 1975, Teasdale & Bancroft 1977, Blackburn & Bonham 1980, Teasdale & Rezin 1978a). This muscle has sometimes been described as the grief muscle.

Recent hypotheses about brain lateralization in psychiatric illness have proposed that schizophrenia is associated with dysfunction of the dominant cerebral hemisphere, and depression is related to dysfunction of the non-dominant hemisphere (Flor-Henry 1969, 1984). Support for these hypotheses has been provided by Gruzelier & Venables (1974), who found that SCR was lower in amplitude on the right side for depressed patients and higher on the right side for schizophrenic patients. Tucker et al (1981) observed that college students who reported greater depression also reported less vivid imagery (indicating a dysfunction of right hemisphere) and, after induced depressed mood in the laboratory, students showed an auditory attentional bias (by discriminating sounds in the right ear as louder in a dichotic listening task) and impaired imagery during the depression condition, while their arithmetic performance (a left hemisphere function) was unchanged. In a second experiment, depressed mood was associated with asymmetrical electroencephalogram (EEG) activation over the frontal lobes with relatively greater activity in the right frontal region. The authors suggested that anterior regions of the brain modulate the differential effects of emotional arousal on information processing. Schwartz et al (1975) have emphasized the emotional capacities of the right hemisphere and the non-emotional characteristics of the left hemisphere; however, in persons with high anxiety trait, the left hemisphere appears particularly activated (Tucker 1981).

Using *central measures* of arousal, D'Elia & Perris (1973) showed that the mean integrated amplitude of the EEG was lower on the dominant than on the non-dominant side in a group of 18 depressed patients and that, on recovery, no differences between the two sides were apparent. Several studies using EEG measures have shown faster cortical activity in depressed patients relative to controls (Kiloh & Osselton 1964, Shagass & Schwartz 1962, Whybrow & Mendels 1969). Studies of the alpha-blocking response (ABR) or 'arousal response' to photic stimulation have also been consistent in showing a longer ABR in depressed patients as compared to controls, a reduction in ABR after treatment, and a positive correlation with retardation scores (Paulson & Gotlieb 1961, Wilson & Wilson 1961, Perris 1980). Sleep studies have also consistently shown shortened REM (rapid eye movement) latency in depressed patients, associated with a deficiency in stage 4 sleep (Kupfer 1976, Hartmann 1980). More recently, investigators have used the average evoked response (AER) to different modalities of stimulation (visual, auditory or somatosensory) as measures of cortical activity. While the EEG reflects spontaneous brain electrical activity, the AER represents the response of the central nervous system to specific extrinsic stimuli in the first few hundred milliseconds post-stimulation. The responses are measured in terms of latency and amplitude of the averaged evoked wave components or peaks. A number of studies have reported asymmetry in amplitude of certain evoked potential components, with lower voltage on the left. This asymmetry decreases after successful treatment (Flor-Henry 1984). Perris (1974) found a greater amplitude of visual AER from the right hemisphere and Roemer et al (1978) confirmed this finding, while also finding unusually low variability of AER in the right hemisphere. Buchsbaum et al (1981a) examined the effects of sleep deprivation on mood in depressed patients and normal controls. Previous work had shown that sleep deprivation can produce improvement in depressed patients. With visual evoked potentials, they found that the positive peak at 100 ms (P100) changed in different directions: a decrease in amplitude for normal controls, but an increase in amplitude in depressed patients, which paralleled an improvement in mood and other symptoms of depression. Shagass et al (1980) investigated somatosensory, visual and auditory evoked potentials in psychotic depressed, neurotic depressed and schizophrenic patients as compared to normal controls. They found little difference between the two depressed groups but a number of topographic differences between depressed and schizophrenic subjects and between depressed and control subjects, which they interpreted as of possible diagnostic value.

Psychophysiological research, in particular new methods of investigating central nervous system reactivity, is promising, although still patchy and largely inconclusive. Such research has considerable potential for studies of possible links between mood, cognitive and behavioural changes on the one hand, and biochemical changes and abnormalities in physiological mechanisms and neuronal pathways on the other.

PSYCHOLOGICAL THEORIES

Several psychological theories of depression have sought to account, within a general framework, for the many phenomena described above. While behavioural theories have stressed motivational factors, cognitive theories have emphasized cognitive factors in the causation and maintenance of symptoms.

Behavioural theories

Since Skinner (1953) described depression as a weakening of behaviour and loneliness due to the interruptions of established sequences of behaviour which have been positively reinforced in the past, the conceptualization of depression as an *extinction phenomenon* has been central to all behavioural positions. Ferster (1973, 1974, 1981) outlined the applicability of an operant model of conditioning to depression in detailed functional analyses in terms of antecedents and consequences and the function of behaviours. Depression is defined as (1) retardation of psychomotor and thought processes and (2) reduction or absence of previously reinforced behaviours. The essential observable characteristic of a depressed person is a reduced frequency of emission of positively reinforced behaviour, which can be due to several environmental contingencies: sudden environmental changes; punishment and aversive control; shifts in reinforcement contingencies; restricted source of reinforcement because of a restriction in the range of persons with whom an individual interacts.

The functional analyses also stressed the marked passivity of the depressed person. This passivity leads to the depressed person reacting to external sources, i.e. to prompts and commands from others, rather than initiating behaviour, so that reinforcers in social interactions are more likely to be appropriate to others than to the depressed person. Passivity also leads to inadequate behaviour relative to aversive situations and, therefore, to more negative experience. Finally, passivity leads to many of the cognitive features stressed by the cognitive theorists: a *limited view of the world* because of restricted activity; a *'lousy' view of the world* because of the consequences of not avoiding aversive situations; an *unchanging view of the world* because diminished normal exploration of the environment and avoidance behaviour lead to lack of clarification and a restricted behavioural repertoire.

Lewinsohn and his colleagues (Lewinsohn 1974, Lewinsohn et al 1979, 1982) have developed this operational approach further and conducted numerous studies commented on above in the section on motivational deficits (see p. 138). His theoretical approach is summarized in Figure 7.1.

A low rate of positive reinforcement constitutes the eliciting stimulus (unconditioned stimulus) for depressive behaviours: low mood, inactivity, avoidance behaviour, negative thinking, fatigue and other physical symptoms. The depressive behaviours are positively reinforced by the environment which provides sympathy, concern and interest and are therefore increased. However, the depressive behaviours are aversive for most people, who will then withdraw from the depressed person, thus decreasing his rate of positive reinforcement further and accentuating the depression. The eliciting stimulus in depression, the total amount of positive reinforcement, is presumed to be a function of three variables: (1) the number and type of potentially reinforcing situations, this variable being influenced by biological (genetic factors and central brain mechanisms) and experiential (learned) factors; (2) the availability of potentially reinforcing events in the environment, this variable being influenced by life circumstances, for example, poverty, employment, marital status etc.; (3) the instrumental skill of the individual, i.e. the extent to which he possesses the skills which will provide reinforcement. In this context, social skill is considered to be of crucial importance.

Lewinsohn's operant model of depression

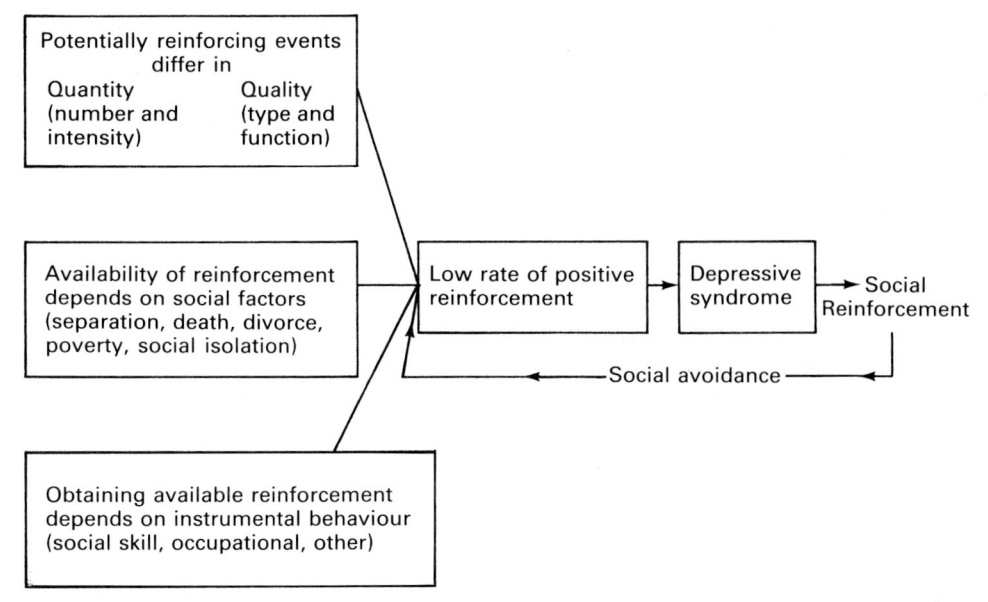

```
┌─────────────────────────────┐
│ Potentially reinforcing     │
│    events differ in         │
│ Quantity      Quality       │
│ (number and   (type and     │
│ intensity)    function)     │
└─────────────────────────────┘
                    ↓
┌─────────────────────────┐   ┌──────────────────┐   ┌────────────┐
│ Availability of         │   │ Low rate of      │   │ Depressive │ → Social
│ reinforcement depends   │ → │ positive         │ → │ syndrome   │   Reinforcement
│ on social factors       │   │ reinforcement    │   │            │
│ (separation, death,     │   └──────────────────┘   └────────────┘
│ divorce, poverty,       │        ↑
│ social isolation)       │        └──── Social avoidance ────┘
└─────────────────────────┘
                    ↑
┌─────────────────────────────────────┐
│ Obtaining available reinforcement   │
│ depends on instrumental behaviour   │
│ (social skill, occupational, other) │
└─────────────────────────────────────┘
```

Fig. 7.1 Lewinsohn's operant model of depression.

Empirical studies have shown a significant association between mood and the number and kind of pleasant activities in which an individual engages (Lewinsohn & Amenson 1978, Lewinsohn & Graf 1973, Lewinsohn & Libet 1972). Other studies have shown that depressed individuals, as compared to controls, engage in fewer activities, rate fewer activities as pleasant and give lower enjoyability ratings to activities which are rated as pleasant (Lewinsohn et al 1979, MacPhillamy & Lewinsohn 1973).

Social skill deficits have been demonstrated in group and family interactions where depressed individuals interact with an increasingly limited number of people, elicit fewer reactions from others, and give shorter messages which are often timed wrongly (Libet & Lewinsohn 1973). The emphasis put on the importance of social interactions in the development of depression derives support from sociological studies; for example, the vulnerability factors identified by Brown & Harris (1978) in depressed women all appear to indicate a depleted social network. These are: low intimacy or not having a valued confidant; not having a job outside the house; having three or more children at home under the age of 14 and having suffered the loss of mother before the age of 11. Lewinsohn et al (1984) have developed a systematic treatment approach derived from this theory but, in the author's opinion, this has not been adequately tested yet in clinical populations.

Lazarus (1968) described depression in the same operant terms as Ferster and Lewinsohn, i.e. as elicited by a loss of reinforcement. However, Costello (1972) maintained that it is not the loss of reinforcers but the loss of reinforcer effectiveness which is important in the precipitation of depression. Reinforcers may lose their effectiveness either because of endogenous biochemical and neurophysiological change or because of the disruption of a chain of behaviour, maybe through the loss of an important discriminative stimulus. This variation of the operant model has clinical appeal, as many depressed patients have no evidence of loss of reinforcers in that objectively nothing has changed in their life, and it also allows a link with potential biological factors, for example a change in neurotransmitter levels, particularly in the so-called reward system of the brain (Olds & Milner 1954, Routtenberg 1978). Klinger (1975, 1977) also saw depression as outcome mediated or due to operant factors, but the important motivational process for him is disengagement from incentives. The commitment to incentives or goals gives meaning to life and these are largely personally determined. When incentives become more difficult to obtain, or become unobtainable, there is an increase in behaviour, an invigoration, with an accompanying increase in anger and aggression. However, if invigorated behaviour fails to secure the incentive, there is a downswing into depression, which may be mild or prolonged and severe. Klinger also invokes possible cognitive and biological factors as mediators of the depressive syndrome. Unfortunately, his theory has attracted little empirical interest.

Other behavioural theories propose an affect-mediated (or classical) approach (Wolpe 1971, 1979) by focusing on the role of classically conditioned anxiety. Certain stimuli come to elicit conditioned anxiety and are, therefore, avoided; when those stimuli are also related to major sources of gratification, for example social events, members of the opposite sex or job interviews, the individual is effectively devoid of major sources of reinforcement and thus becomes depressed. Wolpe also suggests that prolonged anxiety can develop into depression. There has been little testing of this approach and the behavioural treatment techniques derived from it, for example desensitization, the elicitation of incompatible affect (like anger) and flooding, have not been satisfactorily tried in controlled studies. Rehm (1977) has put forward a different behavioural approach to the understanding of depression and depressive behaviour developed from self-control theory as described by Kanfer (1970). Self-control refers to those processes by which an individual alters the probability of a response in the relative absence of immediate external supports. Three processes are postulated in a feedback loop model: self-monitoring, self-evaluation and self-reinforcement. There may be defects in any one or all of these processes in depression.

1. Self-monitoring: depressed patients tend to attend selectively to immediate versus delayed outcomes of their behaviour.
2. Self-evaluation: (a) depressed patients fail to make accurate internal attributions of causality; (b) they set over-stringent criteria for self-

evaluation; (c) they perceive themselves as lacking in ability to obtain positive consequences.
3. Self-reinforcement: depressed patients have low rates of self-reward and high rates of self-punishment.

These concepts can be easily incorporated within Beck's cognitive theory, as described below, although they are couched in more behavioural, operational terms. This model obtains support from the studies derived from both Beck's and Seligman's models. Studies showing deficits in monitoring success and failure support the idea of defective monitoring; studies in attributional style support the notion of defective self-evaluation, while defective self-reinforcement is evident in the underestimation of performance and the measurement of automatic thoughts and negative thinking shown on various questionnaires. Fuchs & Rehm (1977) and Rehm et al (1979) have evaluated a treatment programme based on the self-control model, involving the use of both behavioural and cognitive techniques not unlike those described by Beck et al (1979). This approach was shown to be superior to waiting-list controls and non-specific treatment controls.

Cognitive theories

Unlike the behavioural theories described above, which emphasize change in motivation with their accompanying activity deficits, cognitive theories have stressed the changes in thinking as pivotal in the understanding of depressive phenomena.

Most studies summarized in the cognitive style section above have been inspired by the theoretical work of Beck (1967, 1976) and Seligman (1975, 1981).

Beck's theory

Beck proposed that depression is the result of a negative cognitive set, a negative view of the self, the world and the future (the negative cognitive triad), which is maintained by typical information-processing errors. The negative content of thought and processing errors are related to maladaptive basic attidues (or schemata) which are activated at the onset of a depressive illness by events, situations and perceptions which act as cues. Cognitive theory proposes that these negatively biased changes in patterns of thought logically lead to depressed mood and the behavioural deficits observed in depression.

The negative cognitive triad involves a low opinion of self, seeing oneself as inadequate and unworthy, and as not possessing the necessary qualities to obtain desired goals. The world and the environment are seen as unsympathetic, frustrating and as putting barriers in one's way. Difficulties are seen as likely to last for ever and, consequently, the future is hopeless. This negative cognitive set leads the depressed individual to show motivational symptoms such as loss of interest, increased dependency on others, wishes to avoid situations and suicidal behaviour, behavioural symptoms such as inactivity, retardation and agitation and vegetative symptoms such as loss of sleep, loss of appetite and loss of libido. Processing errors maintain the negative content of thought by emphasizing the negative aspect of situations or by distorting reality. These have been detailed as: *selective abstraction* (a stimulus set, defined above p. 143), *arbitrary inference* (a response set which leads to drawing a conclusion in the absence of evidence); *overgeneralization* (a response set, defined above); magnification and minimization (a response set defined above as catastrophizing); *all-or-none thinking* (a response set which leads to the tendency of thinking in absolute terms) and personalization (a stimulus set defined above). Deep cognitive structures or schemata allow for an integration of the thematic content of depressive cognitions and the particular transformations that stimuli are subjected to (Kovacs & Beck 1978). Schemata (Piaget 1950, Neisser 1967) are organized representations of earlier experience which both facilitate recall and systematically distort new constructions. Hollon & Kriss (1984) comment that schemata make information processing more economical and coherent as they lead to *heuristics* or short-cuts which reduce complex judgemental tasks to a set of simple operations. These schemata are typically rigid, undifferentiated and overinclusive in depression and, according to the theory, although they can be relatively dormant during periods of health, they become progressively more prepotent during illness and become applicable to a wider set of stimuli. Table 7.3 shows a schematic account of how a schema could become activated and how Beck's theory of a primary shift in cognition can account for many of the deficits described above: negatively biased selective recall, negative expectations of outcome, evidence of distorted thinking on cognitive questionnaires and differential attributions for success and failure and for outcome on skilled and chance tasks.

A different approach to the validation of the theory has been the use of cognitive induction procedures to induce mood states. Velten (1968) had subjects read self-referent depressing, elating or neutral statements and found that subjects reading negative statements reported an increase in depressed mood. Similar results were reported by Coleman (1975), Strickland et al (1975), Hale & Strickland (1976) and Natale (1977a,b). Teasdale & Bancroft (1977) reported similar mood changes after thinking unhappy thoughts and, in addition, found increased electromyographic activity (EMG) of the corrugator supercilii muscle. Blackburn & Bonham (1980) tested the immediate effect on mood and physiological variables in six depressed patients of two ways of dealing with a sad thought, involving oneself with it and examining the thought logically by using the technique of 'distancing' derived from cognitive therapy (Beck et al 1979). They found that 'distancing' had a significantly alleviating effect on mood and that heart

Table 7.3 An example of the cognitive development of depression

		Thinking error
Event ↓	Two friends do not attend your party because of unforeseen circumstances	
Perception	People ignored my invitation	Selective abstraction
Interpretation ↓	My friends don't like me any more Nobody likes me any more I am not worth knowing	Arbitrary inference Overgeneralisation Personalisation
Idiosyncratic schema ↓	If people do not like me, I am worthless	Undifferentiation globality, rigidity
Mood	Sadness	
Event ↓	Not greeted by colleague in the street	
Perception	He ignored me	
Interpretation ↓	It is true that nobody wants to know	Arbitrary inference Overgeneralisation
Mood ↓	Increasing depression	
Negative cognitive triad	I am not worth knowing	Negative view of self
	People are selfish and do not appreciate me	Negative view of the world
↓	I will never have friends	Negative view of the future
Full depressive syndrome		

rate, corrugator EMG and mood were all significantly correlated. Thus, manipulation of thought has been shown to have an effect on mood and physiology. Teasdale & Rezin (1978b) found that the presentation of external information at high rate (repeating letters of the alphabet presented randomly through earphones) reduced the frequency of negative thoughts in some patients, with a corresponding decrease in depressed mood. Teasdale & Fennell (1982) have also compared two techniques of dealing with depressive thoughts — exploring and modifying — in five depressed patients and found that modifying thoughts, again a technique derived from cognitive therapy, consistently produced more change in belief in the identified thoughts, accompanied by a greater reduction in depressed mood. Raps et al (1980) found that Velten's mood-elation procedure reduced depressed affect in a group of depressed patients, whereas the mood-neutral procedure produced no affective change. Blackburn et al (1979), using cross-lagged correlations, demonstrated that in a group of depressed inpatients treated by physical methods (antidepressant medication or ECT), changes in negative attitudes preceded changes in mood.

The cognitive theory of depression has also obtained support from the efficacy of treatment methods derived from the theory. Although treatment studies offer less direct evidence for a theory in that treatment packages like cognitive therapy (Beck et al 1979) include not only a variety of specific change methods but also general therapeutic factors which are common to all therapies, it stands to reason that an adequate theory of a disorder should generate effective therapeutic procedures. Several outcome studies compare the efficacy of cognitive therapy with antidepressant medication or other psychological treatments in the treatment of major depressives, unipolar and non-psychotic subtype. For exhaustive reviews, the interested reader should refer to Rush & Giles (1982) and Blackburn (1985). These studies have consistently shown cognitive therapy to be at least as effective as a standard antidepressant medication, and often superior. Similar findings have been obtained when cognitive therapy has been compared with behaviour therapy, although these studies are less methodologically adequate than the drug comparison studies, as the groups compared have been small and have tended to consist of depressed volunteers instead of clinic patients.

Weaknesses in the cognitive theory of depression have been pointed out lately (Coyne & Gotlib 1983) from two points of view.

Firstly, there has been little support for the concept of negative cognitions as vulnerability factors in depression. Some promising results were obtained by Golin et al (1981), Reda (1984), Fennell & Campbell (1984) and Blackburn et al (1986), but largely negative results have been found, as reported above (for example, Wilkinson & Blackburn 1981, Hamilton & Abramson 1983). Further, Lewinsohn et al (1981) and Peterson et al (1981) failed to predict subsequent depression from current cognition.

Secondly, the causal priority of cognition over affect has also been called into question. Zajonc (1980), in a provoking paper on the primacy of affect, argued that 'affective judgements may be fairly independent of and precede in time the sorts of perceptual and cognitive operations commonly assumed to be the basis of these affective judgements and that affect and cognition are under the control of separate and partially independent systems'. In this he follows Wundt (1907), who argued that objects need 'to be cognized very little — in fact, minimally' to arouse affect. Affective responses are said to be effortless, inescapable, irrevocable, holistic, instantaneous, dominant, primary and precognitive. By contrast, cognitions require substantial effort, are refutable, verbal, justifiable and take longer to form. In other words, they are 'cold' compared to the 'hot' affects. Rachman (1981), in a critical appraisal of Zajonc's paper, commented that he exaggerated the irrevocable quality of affective reactions in view of the successes of behavioural therapies and, in this author's opinion, in view of the successes of the cognitive therapies. He also exaggerates the independence of affect and cognition, in view of the successful manipulation of mood through cognition, as described earlier.

The approaches of Bower (1981) and Teasdale (1983) are much more satisfactory in their explanations of the processes discussed in the previous sections. Bower interpreted his data on state-dependent learning and retrieval (see p. 136) within an associative network theory of memory (cognition) and emotion. This is an elaboration of general semantic-network theory of long-term memory (Collins & Loftus 1975), whereby each distinct emotion, for example sadness, has a specific node or unit of memory which collects together many other aspects of the emotion that are connected to it by associative pointers. Each emotion unit is linked with propositions describing events from one's life during which that emotion was aroused. Activation of an emotion node spreads activation (as in an electrical network) throughout the memory structures to which it is connected, creating subthreshold excitation at those event nodes. A weak cue that partially describes an event, for example 'bus', may combine with activation from an emotion unit and raise the total activation of a relevant memory above the threshold of consciousness. Thus, a sad person, given the cue 'bus' will recall a sad event related to buses. This recall reactivates a sad memory and sends feedback excitation to the sadness node, which will maintain activation of that emotion and thus again influence later memories retrieved. Teasdale (1983) interpreted his data on induction of mood and memory in the same way, suggesting that there is good evidence that negative cognitions can produce and maintain the state of depression and also that depression increases the probability of just those cognitions which will cause further depression. He proposes, therefore, that there is a reciprocal relationship between depression and cognition which may form the basis of a vicious cycle which perpetrates and intensifies depression.

Learned helplessness

The learned helplessness theory of depression (Overmeir & Seligman 1967, Seligman & Maier 1967) was derived from animal experiments where dogs were exposed to unavoidable shock. Dogs were placed in a Pavlovian harness and mild electric shocks contingent on a conditioned stimulus (CS) were presented. When the dogs were subsequently released and allowed to learn an appropriate escape response, a large majority of the animals showed considerable difficulty in learning how to avoid the shock. Mowrer & Viek (1948) had also shown that rats pre-treated with inescapable shock demonstrated subsequent deficits in escape-avoidance learning. In addition, they showed passivity which was difficult to extinguish and appeared dejected. Seligman postulated that instead of not learning in the inescapable situation, these animals actually learned that their responses were ineffective. Thus, a cognitive factor, expectation that outcomes are uncontrollable, lead to motivational, cognitive and emotional deficits. This finding was found to be reproducible in a variety of species (Seligman 1974, 1975) and was subsequently offered as an explanatory model of depression which would account for the deficit in performance of humans exposed to experiment-induced failure (see p. 142).

This approach has generated much research which showed generalization of effect of learned helplessness to other behaviours (for example, problem solving after experience of unsolvable problems), the similarities between experimentally induced learning deficits and deficits seen in clinical depression and the effect of uncontrollable situations on mood (Miller & Seligman 1973, 1975, Hiroto & Seligman 1975, Klein et al 1976). These studies have been well reviewed by Blaney (1977) and Costello (1978), who pointed out the shortcomings of the theory to account for human depression. Alternative explanations, for example loss of self-esteem, are possible as many of the experimental manipulations also involve manipulations of self-esteem. Also, people who become depressed have often not experienced uncontrollable trauma and the theory would lead to the predictions of blame directed outwards at uncontrollable outcomes (external attribution), whereas clinically, the observation is that depressed patients blame themselves (internal attribution).

Seligman and his colleagues (Abramson et al 1978) have since proposed a *reformulated learned helplessness theory* based on attribution theory. Attribution theory was developed by social psychologists (Heider 1958, Rotter 1966) to explain causal perceptions, especially for success and failure in achievement-related tasks. Seligman (1981) summarizes the reformulated learned helplessness theory in four premises:

Premise 1 (expected aversiveness). The individual expects that highly aversive outcomes are probable or that highly desired outcomes are improbable.

Premise 2 (expected uncontrollability). The individual expects that no response in his or her repertoire will change the likelihood of these events.

Premise 3 (attributional style). The individual possesses an insidious attributional style that governs the duration and breadth of the deficits related to depression and whether self-esteem is lowered. The depressive attributional style consists of a tendency to make internal attribution for failure, but external attributions for success; stable attributions for failure, but unstable attributions for success; and global attributions for failure, but specific attributions for success. Internal attributions for failure (and external ones for success) produce long-lasting depressive deficits, and global attributions for failure (and specific ones for success) produce depressive deficits over a variety of situations.

Premise 4 (severity). The strength of the motivational and cognitive deficits of depression depends jointly on the strength (that is, the certainty) of the expectation of the aversive outcome (premise 1) and the strength of the uncontrollability expectancy (premise 2). The severity of the affective and self-esteem deficits is governed by the importance of the uncontrollable outcome.

According to Seligman (1981), these few premises and their co-occurrence are deemed sufficient but not necessary to account for the four sets of deficits seen in depression; that is, motivational, cognitive, affective-somatic and self-esteem. Abramson et al (1980) stressed that it is the *expectation* of helplessness which is critical in depression. Although the formation of attributions is the most potent way of bringing this expectation about, other sources of information, such as verbal persuasion, modelling and physiological changes, may also affect expectations.

The research literature in attributions (see p. 143) has not always supported the hypothesis derived from the theory and no systematic treatment strategies have been derived from it. The theory does not account for attitudes (schemata) found in depressed patients and could perhaps be seen as one aspect of a more comprehensive theory, perhaps like Beck's model. In this regard, since it stresses the primacy of cognitive factors, the reservations regarding Beck's model, as described above, also apply to the learned helplessness model.

Synthesis

The preceding short review of psychological theories of depression suggests that many of the processes which are affected in depressive illness can be understood from diametrically opposed approaches. Cognitive theories account more easily for cognitive changes while behavioural theories account more easily for motivational changes, although both approaches can accommodate other phenomena. What is needed now are broader-based models which can take into account neurochemical and neurophysiological changes as well as psychological changes. Unfortunately, it has proved difficult to build such conceptual bridges, most researchers feeling more comfortable within the mind–body dichotomy. Several stimulating attempts at synthesis have, however, been made (Akiskal & McKinney 1973, 1975, Gilbert 1984, Siever & Davis 1985). Akiskal & McKinney view depressive illness as a psychobiological final common pathway which is the culmination of processes converging in those areas of the diencephalon which modulate arousal, mood, motivation and psychomotor function. The specific form in which the depressive syndrome will express itself will depend on the interaction of several factors. These include *genetic vulnerability*, which has been convincingly demonstrated in both bipolar and unipolar illness (Perris 1966, Winokur et al 1969, Gershon et al 1971, Baker et al 1972); *developmental events*, for example loss of a parent in childhood, which appear to have a sensitizing effect to later losses (Brown & Harris 1978, Bowlby 1980, Granville-Grossman 1968); *psychosocial events*, which have been described as severe or threatening (Brown & Harris 1978) or exit events (Paykel 1978); *physiological stressors*, such as the drug reserpine, childbirth and hypothyroidism, which have been shown to affect diencephalic function, as evidenced by the symptoms shown; and *personality traits*, which may determine or modify the reactivity of the individual to stress (see pp 138–140 for a review of personality studies). One might add to this list, provided by

Akiskal & McKinney (1975), other factors as described in the above sections, for example: basic attitudes (Beck 1976), which would also have been learned from early childhood, or attributional style (Abramson et al 1978), which might be conditioned by developmental history; an impoverished reinforcement situation (Lewinsohn et al 1979) or a history of uncontrollable adverse situations leading to learned helplessness (Seligman 1975).

The interaction of all these diverse factors would be expected to result in a variety of biochemical alterations in the central nervous system. Catecholamines (Schildkraut 1965), indoleamines (Coppen 1967), false neurotransmitters (Murphy 1972), sodium metabolism (Whybrow & Mendels 1969) and neuroendocrine disturbance (Carroll et al 1978) have all been incriminated in the biochemical aetiology of depressive illness. Akiskal & McKinney (1975) propose that a diencephalic final common pathway may provide a neurophysiological system where different biochemical events converge, thus accounting for the common features (Table 7.2) shared by the various forms of depressive disorders.

Evidence for a diencephalic involvement comes from animal experiments, which suggest that lesions that interfere with the anatomical or chemical integrity of the reinforcement system in the diencephalon impair the ability of the organism to respond to environmental reinforcers (Olds & Milner 1954). Pharmacological experiments in animals have shown that both the catecholamines and the indoleamines play a significant role in modulating the function of the medial forebrain bundle (MFB) and the periventricular system (PVS), the neuroanatomical substrates of 'reward' and 'punishment' (Wise et al 1973). It is, therefore, presumed that psychological events and processes which precipitate and maintain depression would act on the MFB and the PVS which establish feedback connections with other systems in the brain. Functional impairment in one system would, then, result in functional shifts in one or more systems.

Gilbert (1984) offers a psycho-evolutionary perspective which links cognitive-behavioural and biological data. Starting from the basis of the probable innate predisposition to depression, he concludes, after reviewing data from various fields, that it is not only genetic variations which may facilitate brain-behaviour response patterns, but also psychological processes which are concerned with structuring reality, interpreting external and internal stimuli meaningfully and planning actions. He suggests that negatively biased cognitive distortions do not cause depression, but evoke brain-behaviour patterns of responding which have an innate basis. Thus, like Akiskal & McKinney (1975), he proposes a view of depression as the activation of multiple response systems.

Siever & Davis (1985) proposed a dysregulation hypothesis of depression which suggests that it is not simply increases and decreases in neurotransmitters which are associated with depression, but a dysregulation caused by the failure in one or more neurotransmitter homeostatic regulatory mechanisms which confers a trait vulnerability. Such a dysregulated neurotransmitter system would lead to less selectivity in the organism's responsiveness to environmental stimuli. Various studies have shown that depressed patients, relative to normal controls, show a more variable response to stressors, as reflected by noradrenergic output and cortisol secretion. For example, 3-methoxy-4-hydroxyphenylethylene glycol (MHPG, the major metabolite of noradrenaline in human brain) excretion following a series of mild shocks, has been reported to be significantly less in control subjects than in controls (Buchsbaum et al 1981b), and similarly lower and more variable responses in plasma noradrenaline were observed after a cold pressor test (immersing the hand in cold water) or a cognitive stressor (mental arithmetic) (Le Blanc et al 1979). On the other hand, physical exercise, which produces minimal changes in urinary MHPG excretion in normal subjects, leads to increases in MHPG excretion in depressed patients (Ebert et al 1972). Frankenhaeuser & Patkai (1965) also reported a low adrenaline secretion in depressed subjects relative to controls during stressful tests, while cortisol production is highly increased in experimentally induced depressed state through learned helplessness or uncontrollable situations (Weiss 1972).

Depressive illness, in its many forms, is a complex phenomenon. Its frequency of occurrence in the population indicates the likelihood of divergent causes leading to a common functional deficit of varying severity, probably via a final common pathway. It seems, therefore, that more satisfactory theories of depression will be reached when multi-factorial approaches are developed which take into consideration neurochemical, neurophysiological and psychological processes and clarify their relative role and mode of interaction in different subtypes of the illness.

ACKNOWLEDGEMENTS

I am very grateful to Dr L. J. Whalley for his careful reading of the first draft of this chapter and to Norma Brearly for her patience in typing the manuscript.

REFERENCES

Abraham K 1911 Notes on the psychoanalytic investigation and treatment of manic-depressive insanity and allied conditions. In: Abraham K (ed) Selected papers on psychoanalysis. Hogarth Press, London (1927)

Abraham K 1954 A short study of the development of the libido, viewed in the light of mental disorders. In: Selected papers of Karl Abraham, 5th edn, pp 418–502. Hogarth Press, London

Abramson L Y, Seligman M E P, Teasdale J D 1978 Learned helplessness in humans: critique and reformulation. Journal of Abnormal Psychology 87: 49–74

Abramson L Y, Garber J, Seligman M E P 1980 Learned helplessness: An attributional analysis. In: Garber J, Seligman M E P (eds) Human helplessness: Theory and Applications. Academic Press, New York

Abramson L Y, Alloy L B, Rosoff R 1981 Depression and the generation of complex hypotheses in the judgement of contingency. Behaviour Research and Therapy 19: 75–86

Akiskal H S, McKinney W T 1973 Depressive disorders: towards a unified hypothesis. Science 182: 20–29

Akiskal H S, McKinney W T 1975 Overview of recent research in depression: integration of ten conceptual models into a comprehensive clinical frame. Archives of General Psychiatry 32: 285–305

Alloy L B, Abramson L Y 1979 Judgement of contingency in depressed and non-depressed students: sadder but wiser? Journal of Expermental Psychology: General 108: 441–485

Ashworth C M, Blackburn I M, McPherson F M 1982 The performance of depressed and manic patients on some repertory grid measures: A cross-sectional study. British Journal of Medical Psychology 55: 247–255

Ashworth C M, Blackburn I M, McPherson F M 1986 The performance of depressed and manic patients on some repertory grid measures: A longitudinal study. British Journal of Medical Psychology 58: 337–342

Astrup C, Fossum A, Holmboe R A 1959 Follow-up study of 270 patients with acute affective psychoses. Acta Psychiatrica et Neurologica Scandinavica 34: Suppl 135

Babcock H, Levy L 1940 The measurement of efficiency of mental functioning. Stoelting, Chicago

Baker M, Dorzab J, Winokur G et al 1972 Depressive disease: Evidence favouring polygenic inheritance based on an analysis of ancestral cases. Archives of General Psychiatry 27: 320–327

Bandura A 1977 Social learning theory. Prentice-Hall, Englewood Cliffs, NJ

Beck A T 1967 Depression: clinical experimental and theoretical aspects. Harper & Row, New York

Beck A T 1976 Cognitive therapy and the emotional disorders. International Universities Press, New York

Beck A T, Ward C H 1961 Dreams of depressed patients: characteristic themes in manifest content. Archives of General Psychiatry 5: 462–467

Beck A T, Ward C H, Mendelson M, Mock J E, Erbaugh J K 1961 An inventory for measuring depression. Archives of General Psychiatry 4: 561–571

Beck A T, Feshback S, Legg D 1962 The clinical utility of the digit-symbol test. Journal of Consulting Psychology 26: 263–268

Beck A T, Weissman A, Lester D, Trexler L 1974 The measurement of pessimism: The Hopelessness Scale. Journal of Consulting and Clinical Psychology 42: 861

Beck A T, Rush A J, Shaw B F, Emery G 1979 Cognitive therapy of depression. Wiley, New York

Becker J 1960 Achievement related characteristics of manic-depressives. Journal of Abnormal and Social Psychology 60: 334–339

Blackburn I M 1975 Mental and psychomotor speed in depression and mania. British Journal of Psychiatry 126: 329–335

Blackburn I M 1984 Cognitive approaches to clinical psychology. In: Nicholson J, Beloff H (eds) Psychology survey, Vol 5, pp 290–319. British Psychological Society

Blackburn I M 1985 Depression. In: Bradley B P, Thompson C (eds) Psychological applications in psychiatry, pp 61–93 Wiley, Chichester

Blackburn I M, Bonham K G 1980 Experimental effects of a cognitive therapy technique in depressed patients. British Journal of Social and Clinical Psychology 19: 353–363

Blackburn I M, Lyketsos G, Tsiantis J 1979 The temporal relationship between hostility and depressed mood. British Journal of Social and Clinical Psychology 18:227–235

Blackburn I M, Jones S, Lewin R J P 1986 Cognitive style in depression. British Journal of Clinical Psychology 25: 241–251

Blaney P H 1977 Contemporary theories of depression: critique and comparison. Journal of Abnormal Psychology 86: 203–223

Blaney P H, Behar V, Head R 1980 Two measures of depressive cognitions: their association with depression and with each other. Journal of Abnormal Psychology 89: 678–682

Bower G H 1981 Mood and memory. American Psychologist 36: 129–148

Bowlby J 1980 Loss: sadness and depression. Attachment and loss, Vol 3. Hogarth Press, London

Boyd J H, Weissman M M 1982 Epidemiology. In: Paykel E S (ed) Handbook of affective disorders, pp 109–125. Guilford Press, New York

Brown G W, Harris T 1978 Social origins of depression. Tavistock, London

Buchsbaum M S, Gerner R, Post R M 1981a The effects of sleep deprivation on average evoked responses in depressed patients and in normals. Biological Psychiatry 16: 351–363

Buchsbaum M S, Muscettola G, Goodwin F K 1981b Urinary MHPG, stress response, personality factors and somatosensory evoked potentials in normal subjects and patients with major affective disorders. Neuropsychobiology 7: 212–224

Byrne D G 1975 A psychophysiological distinction between types of depressive states. Australian and New Zealand Journal of Psychiatry 9: 181–185

Carroll B J, Greden J F, Rubin R T, Haskett R, Feinberg M, Schteingart D 1978 Neurotransmitter mechanism of neuroendocrine disturbance in depression. Acta Endocrinologica Supplement, Part 220, 14

Cattell R B, Eber H W 1957 Handbook for the sixteen personality factor questionnaire. Institute for Personality and Ability Testing, Champaign, Ill

Christie M J, Little B C, Gordon A M 1980 Peripheral indices of depressive states. In: Von Praag H M (ed) Handbook of biological psychiatry Part II, pp 145–182. Dekker, New York

Clark D M, Teasdale J D 1982 Diurnal variation in clinical depression and accessibility of positive and negative experiences. Journal of Abnormal Psychology 91: 87–95

Cohen M B, Baker G, Cohen R A, Fromm-Reichmann F, Weigert E 1954 An intensive study of 12 cases of manic depressive psychosis. Psychiatry 17: 103–137

Cohen R M, Weingartner H, Smallberg S A, Pickar D, Murphy D L 1982 Effort and cognition in depression. Archives of General Psychiatry 39: 593–597

Coleman R E 1975 Manipulation of self-esteem as a determinant of mood of elated and depressed women. Journal of Abnormal Psychology 84: 693–700

Collins A M, Loftus E F 1975 A spreading-activation theory of semantic processing. Psychological Review 82: 407–428

Coppen A 1966 The Marke–Nyman temperament scale. An English translation. British Journal of Medical Psychology 39: 55–59

Coppen A 1967 The biochemistry of affective disorders. British Journal of Psychiatry 113: 1237–1264

Coppen A, Metcalfe M 1965 Effect of a depressive illness on MPI scores. British Journal of Psychiatry 111: 236–239

Costello C G 1972 Depression: loss of reinforcers or loss of reinforcer effectiveness? Behaviour Therapy 3: 240–247

Costello C G 1978 A critical review of Seligman's laboratory experiments on learned helplessness and depression in humans. Journal of Abnormal Psychology 87: 21–31

Coyne J C, Gotlib I H 1983 The role of cognition in depression: a critical appraisal. Psychological Bulletin 94: 472–505

Dawson M E, Schell A M, Catania J F 1977 Autonomic correlates of depression and clinical improvement following electroconvulsive shock therapy. Psychophysiology 14: 569–578

D'Elia G, Perris C 1973 Cerebral functional dominance and depression. An analysis of EEG amplitude in depressed patients. Acta Psychiatrica Scandinavica 49: 191–197

De Monbreun B G, Craighead W E 1977 Distortion of perception and recall of positive and neutral feedback in depression. Cognitive Therapy and Research 1: 311–330

Eaves G, Rush A J 1984 Cognitive patterns in symptomatic and remitted major depression. Journal of Abnormal Psychology 93: 31–40

Ebert M H, Post R M, Goodwin F K 1972 Effect of physical activity on urinary MHPG excretion in depressed patients. Lancet 2: 766

Ellis A 1962 Reason and emotion in psychotherapy. Lyle Stuart, New York

Eysenck H J 1959 The manual of the Maudsley Personality Inventory. London University Press, London

Eysenck H J 1970 The classification of depressive illness. British Journal of Psychiatry 117: 241–250

Fennell M J V, Campbell E A 1984 The cognitions questionnaire: specific thinking errors in depression. British Journal of Clinical Psychology 23: 81–92

Ferster C B 1973 A functional analysis of depression. American Psychologist 28: 857–870

Ferster C B 1974 Behavioural approaches to depression. In: Friedman R J, Katz M M (eds) The psychology of depression: contemporary theory and research, pp 29–45. Winston/Wiley, New York

Ferster C B 1981 A functional analysis of behaviour therapy. In: Rehm L P (ed) Behavior therapy of depression, pp 181–196. Academic Press, New York

Fisher K A 1949 Changes in test performance of ambulatory depressed patients undergoing electric shock therapy. Journal of General Psychology 41: 195–232

Flor-Henry P 1969 Psychosis and temporal lobe epilepsy. A controlled investigation. Epilepsia 10: 363–395

Flor-Henry P 1984 Hemisphere laterality and disorders of affect. In: Post R M, Ballenger J C (eds) Neurobiology of mood disorders, pp 467–480. Williams & Wilkins, Baltimore

Foulds G A 1952 Temperamental differences in maze performance part 2. The effect of distraction and electroconvulsive therapy on psychomotor retardation. British Journal of Psychology 43: 33–41

Frankenhaeuser M, Patkai P 1965 Interindividual differences in catecholamine excretion during stress. Scandinavian Journal of Psychology 6: 117–123

Fransella F, Bannister D 1977 A manual repertory grid technique. Academic Press, London

Freud S 1908 Character and eroticism. In: Strachey J (ed) The standard edition, pp 167–175. Hogarth Press, London, 1957

Freud S 1917 Mourning and melancholia. In: Collected papers, vol 4. Hogarth Press, London

Friedman A S 1964 Minimal effects of severe depression on cognitive functioning. Journal of Abnormal and Social Psychology 69: 237–243

Fuchs C Z, Rehm L P 1977 A self-control behaviour therapy programme for depression. Journal of Consulting and Clinical Psychology 45: 206–215

Furneaux W D 1956 Manual of Nufferno speed tests. National Foundation for Education Research

Gershon E, Dunner D, Goodwin F K 1971 Toward a biology of affective disorders: genetic contributions. Archives of General Psychiatry 25: 1–15

Gibson H B 1965 Manual of the Gibson spiral maze. University of London Press, London

Gilbert P 1984 Depression: from psychology to brain state. Lawrence Erlbaum Associates, London

Golin S, Sweeney P D, Schaeffer D E 1981 The causality of causal attributions in depression. A cross-lagged panel correlational analysis. Journal of Abnormal Psychology 90: 14–22

Grannick S 1963 Comparative analysis of psychotic depressives with matched normals on some untimed verbal intelligence tests. Journal of Consulting Psychology 27: 439–443

Granville-Grossman K L 1968 The early environment in affective disorder. In: Coppen A, Walk A (eds): Recent developments in affective disorders, pp 65–79. Royal Medical Psychiatric Association, Ashford, Kent

Greden J F, Carroll J B 1981 Psychomotor function in affective disorders: an overview of new monitoring techniques. American Journal of Psychiatry 138: 1441–1448

Greene S M 1981 Levels of measured hopelessness in the general population. British Journal of Clinical Psychology 20: 11–14

Gruzelier J, Venables P H 1974 Bimodality and lateral asymmetry of skin conductance orienting activity in schizophrenics. Replication and evidence of lateral asymmetry in patients with depression and disorders of personality. Biological Psychiatry 8: 55–73

Hale W D, Strickland B R 1976 Induction of mood states and their effect on cognitive and social behaviors. Journal of Consulting and Clinical Psychology 44: 55

Hamilton E W, Abramson L Y 1983 Cognitive patterns and major depressive disorder: a longitudinal study in a hospital setting. Journal of Abnormal Psychology 92: 173–184

Hammen C L, Krantz S 1976 Effect of success and failure on depressive cognitions. Journal of Abnormal Psychology 85: 577–586

Hartmann E L 1980 Sleep and sleep disorders. In: Van Praag H M (ed) Handbook of biological psychiatry, Part II, pp 331–358. Dekker, New York

Hauri P 1976 Dreams in patients remitted from reactive depression. Journal of Abnormal Psychology 85: 1–10

Heider F 1958 The psychology of interpersonal relations. Wiley, New York

Henderson D, Gillespie R D 1956 A textbook of psychiatry for students and practitioners, 8th edn. Oxford University Press, London

Henry G M, Weingartner H, Murphy D L 1973 Influence of affective states and psychoactive drugs on verbal learning and memory. American Journal of Psychiatry 130: 966–971

Hiroto D S, Seligman M E P 1975 Generality of learned helplessness in man. Journal of Personality and Social Psychology 31: 311–327

Hollon S D, Beck A T 1979 Cognitive therapy of depression. In: Kendall P C Hollon S D (eds) Cognitive behavioural interventions. Theory, research and procedures, pp 153–203. Academic Press, New York

Hollon S D, Kendall P C 1980 Cognitive self-statements in depression: development of an automatic thoughts questionnaire. Cognitive Therapy and Research 4: 383–395

Hollon S D, Kriss M R 1984 Cognitive factors in clinical research and practice. Clinical Psychology Review 4: 35–76

Jastak J 1949 Problems of psychometric scatter analysis. Psychological Bulletin 46: 177–197

Jones R G 1968 A factored measure of Ellis' irrational belief system. Test Systems, Wichita, Kan

Kanfer F H 1970 Self-regulation. Research issues and speculations. In: Neuringer C, Michael J L (eds) Behaviour modification in clinical psychology, pp 178–220. Appleton-Century-Croft, New York

Kelly D H W, Walter C J S 1969 A clinical and physiological relationship between anxiety and depression. British Journal of Psychiatry 115: 401–406

Kelly G A 1955 The psychology of personal constructs. Norton, New York

Kendell R E 1976 The classifications of depressions: a review of contemporary confusion. British Journal of Psychiatry 129: 15–28

Kendell R E, DiScipio W J 1970 Obsessional symptoms and obsessional personality traits in patients with depressive illness. Psychological Medicine 1: 65–72

Kendrick D C, Parboosingh R, Post F 1965 A synonym learning test for use with elderly psychiatric subjects: a validation study. British Journal of Social and Clinical Psychology 4: 63–71

Kiloh L G, Osselton J W 1964 Clinical Electroencephalography. Butterworth, London

Klein D C, Seligman M E P 1976 Reversal of performance deficits and perceptual deficits in learned helplessness and depression. Journal of Abnormal Psychology 85: 11–26

Klein D C, Fencil-Morse E, Seligman M E P 1976 Learned helplessness, depression and the attribution of failure. Journal of Personality and Social Psychology 33: 508–516

Klinger E 1975 Consequences and commitment to aid disengagement from incentives. Psychological Review 82: 1–24

Klinger E 1977 Meaning and void. University of Minnesota Press, Minneapolis

Kovacs M, Beck A T 1978 Maladaptive cognitive structures in depression. American Journal of Psychiatry 135: 525–535

Kraepelin E 1921 Manic-depressive insanity and paranoia, 8th edn. Churchill Livingstone, Edinburgh

Krantz S, Hammen C L 1979 Assessment of cognitive bias in depression. Journal of Abnormal Psychology 88: 611–619

Kretschmer E 1936 Physique and character. Harcourt, New York

Kupfer D J 1976 REM latency: a psychobiologic marker for primary depressive disease. Biological Psychiatry 11: 159–174

Kupfer D J, Detre T P, Foster F G, Tucker G J, Delgado J 1972 The application of Delgado's telemetric mobility recorder for human studies. Behavioural Biology 7: 585–590

Kupfer D J, Weiss B L, Foster F G, Detre T P, Delgado J, McPartland R 1974 Psychomotor activity in affective states. Archives of General Psychiatry 30: 765–768

Lader M H, Wing L 1969 Physiological measures in agitated and retarded depressed patients. Journal of Psychiatric Research 7: 89–100

Lazarus A A 1968 Learning theory and the treatment of depression. Behaviour Research and Therapy 6: 83–89

Le Blanc J, Cote J, Jobin M, La Brie A S 1979 Plasma catecholamines and cardiovascular responses to cold and mental activity. Journal of Applied Physiology 47: 1207–1211

Lefebvre M F 1981 Cognitive distortion and cognitive errors in depressed psychiatric and low back pain patients. Journal of Consulting and Clinical Psychology 49: 517–525

Levene M 1966 Hypothesis behavior by humans during discrimination learning. Journal of Experimental Psychology 71: 331–338

Lewinsohn P M 1974 Clinical and theoretical aspects of depression. In: Calhoun K S, Adams H E, Mitchell K M (eds) Innovative treatment methods in psychopathology, pp 63–120. Wiley, Chichester

Lewinsohn P M, Amenson C 1978 Some relations between pleasant and unpleasant mood-related activities and depression. Journal of Abnormal Psychology 87: 644–654
Lewinsohn P M, Graf M 1973 Pleasant activities and depression. Journal of Consulting and Clinical Psychology 41: 261–268
Lewinsohn P M, Libet J 1972 Pleasant events, activity schedules and depression. Journal of Abnormal Psychology 79: 291–295
Lewinsohn P M, Youngren M A, Grosscup S J 1979 Reinforcement and depression. In: Depue R A (ed) The psychobiology of the depressive disorders: implications for the effect of stress, pp 291–316. Academic Press, New York
Lewinsohn P M, Steinmetz J L, Larsen D W, Franklin J 1981 Depression, elated cognitions: antecedent or consequence? Journal of Abnormal Psychology 90: 212–219
Lewinsohn P M, Sullivan J M, Grosscup S J 1982 Behavioural therapy: clinical implications. In: Rush A J (ed) Short-term psychotherapies for depression, pp 50–87. Wiley, Chichester
Lewinsohn P M, Antonuccio D O, Steinmetz J L, Teri L 1984 The coping with depression course. Castalia, Eugene, Ore
Libet J, Lewinsohn P M 1973 The concept of social skill with special references to the behaviour of depressed persons. Journal of Consulting and Clinical Psychology 40: 304–312
Lishman W A 1972 Selective factors in memory. Psychological Medicine 2: 248–253
Lloyd G G, Lishman W A 1975 Effect of depression on the speed of recall of pleasant and unpleasant experiences. Psychological Medicine 5: 173–180
McClelland D C, Atkinson J W, Clark R A, Lowell E L 1953 The achievement motive. Appleton-Century-Croft, New York
Macht M L, Spear N E, Lewis D 1977 State dependent retention in humans induced by alterations in affective state. Bulletin of the Psychonomic Society 10: 415–418
MacPhillamy D J, Lewinsohn P M 1973 A scale for the measurement of positive reinforcement. Unpublished mimeograph, University of Oregon
Manly P C, McMahon R J, Bradley C F, Davidson P O 1982 Depressive attributional style and depression following childbirth. Journal of Abnormal Psychology 91: 245–254
Martin I 1963 The measurement of autonomic activity in depressive patients during sodium amytal sedation. In: Votava K (ed) Psychopharmacological methods, pp 321–325. Pergamon, Oxford
Metalsky G I, Abramson L Y, Seligman M E P, Semmel A, Peterson C 1982 Attributional styles and life events in the classroom: vulnerability and invulnerability to depressive mood reactions. Journal of Personality and Social Psychology 43: 612–617
Metcalfe M 1968 The personality of depressive patients. In: Coppen A, Walk A (eds) Recent developments in affective disorders, pp 97–104. Royal Medical Psychiatric Association, Ashford, Kent
Miller I W, Klee S H, Norman W H 1982 Depressed and nondepressed inpatients' cognitions of hypothetical events, experimental tasks and stressful life events. Journal of Abnormal Psychology 91: 78–81
Miller W R 1975 Psychological deficit in depression. Psychological Bulletin 82: 238–260
Miller W R, Seligman M E P 1973 Depression and the perception of reinforcement. Journal of Abnormal Psychology 82: 62–73
Miller W R, Seligman M E P 1975 Learned helplessness, depression and the perception of reinforcement. Behaviour, Research and Therapy 14: 7–17
Minkoff K, Bergman E, Beck A T, Beck R 1973 Hopelessness, depression and attempted suicide. American Journal of Psychiatry 130: 455–459
Mowrer O H, Viek P 1948 An experimental analogue of fear from a sense of helplessness. Journal of Abnormal Psychology 43: 193–200
Murphy D L 1972 Amine precursors, amines and false neurotransmitters in depressed patients. American Journal of Psychiatry 129: 41–48
Murphy D L, Henry G M, Weingartner H 1973 Catecholamines and memory: Enhanced verbal learning during L-dopa administration. Psychopharmacologia 27: 319–326
Murray L G, Blackburn I M 1974 Personality differences in patients with depressive illness and anxiety neurosis. Acta Psychiatrica Scandinavica 50: 183–191
Natale M 1977a Effects of induced elation-depression on speech in the initial interview. Journal of Consulting and Clinical Psychology 45: 45–52

Natale M 1977b Induction of mood states and their effect on gaze behavior. Journal of Consulting and Clinical Psychology 45: 717–723
Neisser U 1967 Cognitive psychology. Appleton-Century-Croft, New York
Nekanda-Trepka C J S, Bishop S, Blackburn I M 1983 Hopelessness and depression. British Journal of Clinical Psychology 22: 49–60
Nelson R E 1977 Irrational beliefs in depression. Journal of Consulting and Clinical Psychology 45: 1190–1191
Nelson R E, Craighead W E 1977 Selective recall of positive and negative feed-back, self-control behaviors and depression. Journal of Abnormal Psychology 86: 379–388
Noble P, Lader M H 1971 The symptomatic correlates of the skin conductance changes in depression. Journal of Psychiatric Research 9: 61–69
Noble P, Lader M H 1972 A physiological comparison of endogenous and reactive depression. British Journal of Psychiatry 120: 541–542
Olds J, Milner P 1954 Positive reinforcement produced by electrical stimulation of septal area and other regions of rat brain. Journal of Comparative Physiology and Psychology 47: 419–427
Overmeir J B, Seligman M E P 1967 Effects of inescapable shock upon subsequent escape and avoidance learning. Journal of Comparative and Physiological Psychology 63: 28–33
Paulson G W, Gottlieb G 1961 A longitudinal study of the electroencephalographic arousal response in depressed patients. Journal of Nervous and Mental Diseases 133: 524–528
Paykel E S 1978 Contribution of life events to causation of psychiatric illness. Psychological Medicine 8: 245–253
Payne R W 1968 Cognitive abnormalities. In: Eysenck H J (ed) Handbook of Abnormal Psychology: 193–261. Pitman, London
Payne R W, Hewlett J H G 1960 Thought disorder in psychotic patients. In: Eysenck H J (ed) Experiments in personality, Vol 2, pp 3–104. Routledge & Kegan Paul, London
Perris C 1966 A study of bipolar (manic depressive) and unipolar (recurrent depressive) psychoses. Acta Psychiatrica Scandinavica 42 Suppl 194: 7–189
Perris C 1971 Personality patterns in patients with affective disorders. Acta Psychiatrica Scandinavica, Suppl 221: 43–51
Perris C 1974 Averaged evoked responses (AER) in patients with affective disorders. A pilot study of possible hemispheric differences in depressed patients. Acta Psychiatrica Scandinavica, Suppl 255: 89–98
Perris C 1980 Central measures of depression. In: Von Praag H M (ed) Handbook of biological psychiatry, Part II, pp 183–223. Dekker, New York
Peterson C, Schwartz S M, Seligman M E P 1981 Self-blame and depressive symptoms. Journal of Personality and Social Psychology 41: 253–259
Peterson C, Semmel A, Von Baeyer C, Abramson L Y, Metalsky G, Seligman M E P 1982 The attributional style questionnaire. Cognitive Therapy and Research 6: 287–299
Piaget J 1950 The psychology of intelligence. Harcourt Brace, New York
Post F 1966 Somatic and psychic factors in the treatment of elderly psychiatric patients. Journal of Psychosomatic Research 10: 13–19
Post R M, Ballenger J C (eds) 1984 Neurobiology of mood disorders. Williams & Wilkins, Baltimore
Rachman S 1981 The primacy of affect: some theoretical implications. Behaviour Research and Theory 19: 279–290
Rapaport D 1945 Diagnostic psychological testing: the theory, statistical evaluation and diagnostic application of a battery of tests, Vol 1. Chicago Yearbook
Raps C S, Reinhard K E, Seligman M E P 1980 Reversal of cognitive and affective deficits associated with depression and learned helplessness by mood elevation in patients. Journal of Abnormal Psychology 89: 342–349
Raps C S, Peterson C, Reinhard K E, Abramson L Y, Seligman M E P 1982 Attributional style among depressed patients. Journal of Abnormal Psychology 91: 102–108
Reda M A 1984 Cognitive organisation and antidepressants: attitude modification during amitriptyline treatment in severely depressed individuals. In: Reda M A, Mahoney M J (eds) Cognitive psychotherapies. Recent developments in theory, research and practice, pp 119–140. Ballinger, Cambridge, Mass
Rehm L P 1977 A self-control model of depression. Behaviour Therapy 8: 787–804
Rehm L P, Fuchs C Z, Roth D M, Kornblitz S J, Romano J M 1979 A comparison of self-control and assertion skills treatments of depression. Behaviour Therapy 10: 429–442

Reus V I, Weingartner H, Post R M 1979 Clinical implications of state dependent learning. American Journal of Psychiatry 136: 927–931

Roemer R A, Shagass C, Straumanis J J, Amadeo M 1978 Pattern evoked potential measurements suggesting lateralized hemispheric dysfunction in chronic schizophrenics. Biological Psychiatry 13: 185–202

Rotter J B 1966 Generalized expectancies for internal versus external control of reinforcement. Psychological Monographs 80: No 609

Routtenberg 1978 The reward system of the brain. Scientific American, November: 122–132

Rush A J, Beck A T 1978 Cognitive approaches to depression and suicide. In: Serban G (ed) Cognitive defects in the development of mental illness, pp 201–219. Brunner-Mazel, New York

Rush A J, Giles D E 1982 Cognitive therapy, theory and research. In: Rush A J (ed) Short-term psychotherapies for depression, pp 143–181. Wiley, Chichester

Schildkraut J 1965 Catecholamine hypothesis of affective disorders. American Journal of Psychiatry 122: 509–522

Schwartz G E 1975 Biofeedback, self-regulation, and the patterning of physiological processes. American Scientist 63: 314–324

Schwartz G E, Davidson R F, Maer F 1975 Right hemisphere lateralization for emotion in the human brain. Interaction with cognitions. Science 190: 286–288

Seligman M E P 1974 Depression and learned helplessness. In: Friedman R J, Katz M M (eds) The psychology of depression: contemporary theory and research, pp 83–113. Winston/Wiley, New York

Seligman M E P 1975 Helplessness: on depression, development and death. Freeman, San Francisco

Seligman M E P 1981 A learned helplessness point of view. In: Rehm L P (ed) Behavior therapy of depression, pp 123–141. Academic Press, New York

Seligman M E P, Maier S F 1967 Failure to escape traumatic shock. Journal of Experimental Psychology 74: 1–9

Seligman M E P, Abramson L Y, Semmel A, Von Baeyer C 1979 Depressive attributional style. Journal of Abnormal Psychology 88: 242–247

Shagass C, Schwartz G E 1962 Cerebral cortical reactivity in psychotic depressions. Archives of General Psychiatry 6: 235–242

Shagass C, Roemer R A, Straumanis J J, Amadeo M 1980 Topography of sensory evoked potentials in depressive disorders. Biological Psychiatry 15: 183–207

Shapiro M B, Campbell D, Harris A, Dewsbury J P 1958 Effects of ECT upon psychomotor speed and the distraction effect in depressed psychiatric patients. Journal of Mental Science 104: 681–695

Siever L J, Davis K L 1985 Overview: toward a dysregulation hypothesis of depression. American Journal of Psychiatry 142: 1017–1031

Silberman E K, Weingartner H, Post R M 1983 Thinking disorder in depression. Logic and strategy in an abstract reasoning task. Archives of General Psychiatry 40: 775–780

Silverman J S, Silverman J A, Eardley D A 1984 Do maladaptive attitudes cause depression? Archives of General Psychiatry 41: 28–30

Simons A D, Garfield S L, Murphy G E 1984 The process of change in cognitive therapy and pharmacotherapy for depression. Changes in mood and cognition. Archives of General Psychiatry 41: 45–51

Simons A D, Murphy G E, Levine J L, Wetzel R D 1986 Cognitive therapy and pharmacotherapy for depression. Sustained improvement over one year. Archives of General Psychiatry 43: 43–48

Skinner B F 1953 Science and human behaviour. Macmillan, New York

Spitzer R L, Endicott J, Robins E 1978 Research diagnostic criteria for a selected group of functional disorder, 3rd edn. Biometrics Research, New York State Psychiatric Institute, New York

Strickland B R, Hale W D, Anderson L K 1975 Effect of induced mood states on activity and self-reported affect. Journal of Consulting and Clinical Psychology 43: 587

Szabadi E, Bradshaw C M, Besson J A O 1976 Elongation of pause-time in speech: a simple objective measure of motor retardation in depression. British Journal of Psychiatry 129: 592–597

Teasdale J D 1983 Negative thinking in depression: cause, effect, or reciprocal relationship? Advances in Behaviour Research and Therapy 5: 3–25

Teasdale J D, Bancroft J 1977 Manipulation of thought content as a determinant of mood and corrugator electromyographic activity in depressed patients. Journal of Abnormal Psychology 86: 235–241

Teasdale J D, Fennell M J V 1982 Immediate effects on depression of cognitive therapy intervention. Cognitive Therapy and Research 6: 343–351

Teasdale J D, Fogarty S J 1979 Differential effects of induced mood on retrieval of pleasant and unpleasant events from episodic memory. Journal of Abnormal Psychology 88: 248–257

Teasdale J D, Rezin V 1978a Effect of thought-stopping on thoughts, mood and corrugator EMG in depressed patients. Behaviour Research and Therapy 16: 97–102

Teasdale J D, Rezin V 1978b The effects of reducing frequency of negative thoughts on the mood of depressed patients, tests of a cognitive model of depression. British Journal of Social and Clinical Psychology 17: 65–74

Teasdale J D, Russell M L 1983 Differential effects of induced mood on the recall of positive, negative and neutral words. British Journal of Clinical Psychology 22: 163

Teasdale J D, Taylor R 1981 Induced mood and accessibility of memories: An effect of mood state or of mood induction procedure? British Journal of Social and Clinical Psychology 20: 39–48

Teasdale J D, Taylor R, Fogarty S J 1980 Effects of induced elation-depression on the accessibility of memories of happy and unhappy experiences. Behaviour Research and Therapy 18: 339–346

Tucker D M 1981 Lateral brain function, emotion, and conceptualization. Psychological Bulletin 89: 19–46

Tucker D M, Stenslie C E, Roth R S, Shearer S L 1981 Right frontal lobe activation and right hemisphere performance. Decrement during a depressed mood. Archives of General Psychiatry 38: 169–174

Van Praag H M, Uleman A M, Spitz J C 1965 The vital syndrome interview. Psychiatrica Neurologica et Neurochirurgica 68: 329–346

Velten E 1968 A laboratory task for induction of mood states. Behaviour Research and Therapy 6: 473–482

Walton D, White J G, Black D, Young A J 1959 The modified word-learning test: a cross-validation study. British Journal of Medical Psychology 32: 213–220

Watkins J T, Rush A J 1983 Cognitive response test. Cognitive Therapy and Research 7: 425–435

Weingartner H, Murphy D L 1977 Brain states and memory. Psychopharmacological Bulletin 13: 66–67

Weingartner H, Hall B, Murphy D L, Weinstein W 1976 Imagery, affective arousal and memory consolidation. Nature 263: 311–312

Weingartner H, Miller H, Murphy D L 1977 Mood-state-dependent retrieval of verbal associations. Journal of Abnormal Psychology 86: 276–284

Weingartner H, Cohen R, Murphy D L, Martello J, Gerdt C 1981 Cognitive processes in depression. Archives of General Psychiatry 38: 42–47

Weintraub M, Segal R M, Beck A T 1974 An investigation of cognition and affect in the depressive experiences of normal men. Journal of Consulting and Clinical Psychology 42: 911

Weiss J M 1972 Psychological factors in stress and disease. Scientific American 226: 104–113

Weissman A, Beck A T 1978 Development and validation of the Dysfunctional Attitude Scale. Paper presented at the Annual Meeting of the Association for Advancement of Behaviour Therapy

Wener A E, Rehm L P 1975 Depressive affect: a test of behavioural hypothesis. Journal of Abnormal Psychology 84: 221–227

Whybrow P C, Mendels J 1969 Towards a biology of depression. Some suggestions from neurophysiology. American Journal of Psychiatry 125: 1491–1500

Wilkinson I M, Blackburn I M 1981 Cognitive style in depressed and recovered patients. British Journal of Clinical Psychology 20: 283–292

Willner P 1984 Cognitive functioning in depression: a review of theory and research. Psychological Medicine 14: 807–823

Wilson W P, Wilson N J 1961 Observations on the duration of photically elicited arousal responses in depressive psychoses. Journal of Nervous and Mental Diseases 133: 438–440

Winokur G, Clayton P, Reich T 1969 Manic-depressive illness. Mosby, St Louis

Wise C, Berger B, Stein L 1973 Evidence of alpha-noradrenergic reward receptors and serotonergic punishment receptors in the rat brain. Biological Psychiatry 6: 3–21

Wolpe J 1971 Neurotic depression: experimental analogue, clinical syndromes and treatment. Journal of Psychotherapy 25: 362–368

Wolpe J 1979 The experimental model and treatment of neurotic depression. Behaviour Research and Therapy 17: 555–565

Wundt W 1907 Outlines of psychology. Englemann, Leipzig

Zajonc R B 1980 Feeling and thinking. Preferences need no inferences. American Psychologist 35: 151–175

Current perspectives on anxiety

THE NATURE OF ANXIETY

Anxiety is a complex emotional reaction which cannot accurately be characterized as a unitary phenomenon. Lang (1968) identifies three basic sources of data from which anxiety may be inferred: physiological, behavioural and verbal indices. There is good evidence that these indices do not necessarily correlate highly with one another except during episodes of intense fear (Hodgson & Rachman 1974, Rachman & Hodgson 1974). Indeed, Lehrer & Woolfolk (1982) have recently shown that they emerged as three orthogonal dimensions when a pool of anxiety-related symptoms were factor analysed. Failure to distinguish between these three aspects of anxiety has led to some confusion in the literature, with supposedly general models of anxiety being constructed on the basis of studying only some components of the anxiety response. In this chapter each of the major theoretical formulations will be discussed in turn, and it will be seen that each is primarily successful in accounting for a particular subsection of the empirical data. An attempt will be made to integrate these accounts to yield a more complete and, hopefully, more powerful model.

The somatic symptoms of anxiety reflect physiological arousal, associated largely with the consequences of increased adrenaline and noradrenaline secretion. This 'fight or flight' response (Cannon 1929) prepares the body for activity by increasing the rate and strength of the heart's contractions, redirecting blood flow from the skin and viscera to the muscles and brain, converting the liver's glycogen resources to sugar, and so on. The behavioural component of anxiety seems, at least partly, to be mediated by prior learning experiences. The most pervasive feature is a pattern of avoidance behaviour which may in the past have served to reduce anxiety, but which often generalizes far beyond any originally adaptive level. Cognitive aspects of anxiety include characteristic patterns of thinking. The most obvious such manifestation is termed worry, which may itself arise from more fundamental changes in the way information is processed.

Anxiety disorders

While a certain degree of anxiety is part of the normal coping process in everyday life (Lader & Marks 1971), when this is excessive or is experienced in inappropriate situations, it can handicap the everyday functioning of the individual, and constitute a clinical problem. Such clinical problems have a diverse range of manifestations depending, in part, upon the relative contribution made by each of the three major component sets of symptoms. Avoidance behaviour may or may not be present, and may be specific to certain stimuli, as in phobic states. Specific phobias can develop at any time of life, although they frequently begin in early childhood, and typically involve little or no anxiety outside of the phobic situation (Marks 1969). Less specific phobias, including agoraphobia and social phobia, tend to develop after puberty but before the age of 30 years and often form part of a more general anxiety problem.

At the extreme, however, anxiety can be so general that avoidance behaviour apparently plays little part in the disorder. Generalized, or free-floating, anxiety is one of the commonest neurotic disorders, affecting an estimated 3% of the general population (Marks & Lader 1973), and onset typically occurs around the mid-twenties. While avoidance behaviour is not obvious, the relative contribution of somatic and cognitive symptoms appears to vary with different individuals (e.g. Buss 1962, Barrett 1972, Schwartz et al 1978). Recent research suggests that the efficacy of particular treatment approaches is not equivalent for subgroups of generalized anxious disorders associated with predominantly somatic or predominantly cognitive symptoms (Schwartz et al 1978). Positive findings have been described recently for phobic disorders, with better results when symptoms are matched with treatment (Öst et al 1981), although some negative results have also been reported (Jerremalm et al 1986).

Before examining the various theoretical approaches to anxiety, we will briefly address another general issue that has led to disagreement about the nature of disorders. This is the question of whether anxiety disorders are qualitatively different from normal emotional states, or whether they differ only in a dimensional sense, such as in generality or severity. The former view would lead us to look for some discrete aetiological process, often conceptualized as a disease by psychiatric researchers. Psychologists, on the other hand, are more inclined to look on anxiety as dimensional in nature. Individuals are thought to vary from being emotionally stable at one extreme, to being highly unstable at the other, as assessed by measures such as neuroticism or trait anxiety. Given appropriate circumstances or life events (Finlay-Jones & Brown 1981) high trait anxiety individuals may become sufficiently disturbed to meet the diagnostic criteria for anxiety states. Presumably, the higher the pre-existing level of trait anxiety, the less the intensity of stressful life events required to produce clinical levels of mood disturbance. Although surprisingly sparse, some evidence is available to support this view. For example, McKeon et al (1984) found that obsessive-compulsive patients rated as having a highly anxious personality prior to the disorder, had experienced fewer life events than did those with lower previous trait anxiety. By implication, a relatively high number of life events were required to produce breakdown in those with low trait anxiety, while only a few were necessary in the case of highly anxious individuals.

The discontinuous view of anxiety disorders is sometimes maintained on the basis of the argument that clinical phenomena, such as apparently unprovoked panic attacks, never occur in the normal population. Whether unprovoked panic attacks actually occur in the non-clinical population is of course an empirical question, and one that has not been examined in any detail. Examination of other supposed pathological phenomena, such as intrusive obsessional thoughts, has found them to be surprisingly common in the normal population (Rachman & De Silva 1978). Even if it were possible to demonstrate the existence of phenomena in the clinical population that never occur among normals, this would not demonstrate that the same underlying processes are not distributed across both groups. To take a medical example, steadily increasing levels of blood pressure may eventually result in a catastrophic cerebral vascular accident, but clearly this does not indicate that the aetiology of strokes is unrelated to normal variations in blood pressure. Similarly, it is quite plausible that increasing levels of either physiological (e.g. autonomic arousal) or cognitive (selective attention to threat) components of anxiety may eventually culminate in an apparently discontinuous panic attack.

BIOLOGICAL BASIS OF ANXIETY

Theories of anxiety have tended to polarize into those that emphasize psychological concepts, and those that focus more on biological processes and structures. Abnormal anxiety states may be seen as the product of psychological processes such as maladaptive conditioning or irrational thinking on the one hand, or on the other, as the result of biological events such as neuroendocrine or neurotransmitter dysfunction. This dichotomy would appear both unnecessary and unhelpful, since it seems obvious that any given psychological event could also be redescribed in terms of its underlying biological basis; while equally any change in the central nervous system is also a psychological event. Although a dichotomy is thus inappropriate, the fact remains that the language and methods of biological research have been quite different from those associated with psychological inquiry.

Peripheral psychophysiological changes are particularly marked in anxiety states, with increases in heart rate, blood pressure, muscle blood flow, palmar sweating and and muscular tremor all being obvious features. These autonomic reactions may sometimes be simulated by physical pathology, as in cases of thyrotoxicosis. Such observations have tended to suggest to medical researchers that a single pathological lesion may underly states of generalized anxiety or panic disorder. As a result, there has been a search for biological markers: physiological or biochemical tests that will reliably distinguish anxious from non-anxious individuals. For example, Lader & Wing (1966) showed that in comparison with normal controls, anxious patients failed to show habituation of skin conductance responses to repeated neutral stimuli. As a result it was suggested that, whatever neural mechanism is normally responsible for dampening down reactions to unimportant or irrelevant stimuli, this mechanism must be defective in anxious patients. Pitts & McLure (1967) found that injections of calcium lactate tended to precipitate panic attacks in anxious patients, but did so rarely in normal individuals. More recently, Carr & Sheehan (1984) have suggested that lactate infusion, inhalation of carbon dioxide and acute hyperventilation all produce panic via a common mechanism involving alkalosis and its effects on neural regulatory processes. As a final example, Reiman et al (1984) report evidence of asymmetrical blood flow (greater on the right) in the parahippocampal gyrus of patients with a history of panic attacks. This allowed the authors to conclude that they have demonstrated a focal brain abnormality related to a specific anxiety disorder.

These examples show how medically oriented research continues to favour aetiological explanations of anxiety disorders based on simple biological pathology. As indicated earlier, in our view this approach is limited and misleading. First, it implies a dichotomy between anxiety-disordered individuals and the normal population, whereas in fact trait anxiety measures show a continuous normal distribution, and mild symptoms of anxiety are quite widespread even among non-clinical populations (cf. Taylor & Chave 1964). Secondly, aetiological factors include social and other environmental influences such as life events (Finlay-Jones & Brown 1981) which are ignored in purely biological accounts. Lastly, there seems no scope in simple biological theories for explaining individual differences in the type of situations that provoke anxiety. However, phobias can develop to many different stimuli, including those which can hardly be seen as being biologically significant (Rachman & Seligman 1976). Even so-called generalized forms of anxiety are not completely undifferentiated; both high-trait normals and anxious patients may vary in the extent to which they react to social versus physical types of threat (Mathews & MacLeod 1985).

Neuropsychology of the limbic brain

The data considered above argue for a neuropsychological rather than a pathophysiological theory of anxiety, and for one that is capable of addressing individual differences in trait anxiety, as well as differences in the types of situation capable of evoking fear. Two such theories will be considered here: those of Hans Eysenck (1967) and Jeffrey Gray (1982), both of which are concerned with the role of mid-brain structures in regulating anxiety.

Eysenck suggests that neuroticism, which is highly correlated with trait anxiety measures, depends on the function of the limbic system of the brain. High-neuroticism individuals are supposed to demonstrate greater reactivity in the limbic system, and thus greater emotionality. Anxiety responses to specific stimuli are the joint function of emotionality levels and personal conditioning history, with introverts being generally more conditionable than are extroverts. Evidence for Eysenck's position is largely limited to questionnaire measures of personality, rather than being based on direct assessment of limbic system function. Nonetheless, there is general agreement that the limbic system is involved in the expression of emotions, and perhaps also in their initiation. As indicated earlier, patients complaining of panic attacks can be distinguished from normal controls by asymmetrical blood flow to the hippocampal area of the brain. Other recent research has implicated a number of specific brain sites, either within the limbic system or having projections to that area, which produce behavioural signs of anxiety when electrically stimulated. Stimulation of the locus coeruleus in monkeys produces behavioural signs of fear and alarm (Redmond & Huang 1979), which can be reduced by tranquillizers or other drugs which block noradrenaline-mediated transmission from this site. Stimulation of the periaqueductal grey matter in the brain-stem can also produce fear-like behaviour, but this reaction is reduced by simultaneous stimulation of the nearby raphe nucleus (Kiser et al 1980). This latter area is predominantly innervated by serotonin-containing neurones, and like the locus coeruleus also projects onto the septo-hippocampal area. To make clear the significance of these observations we turn now to Gray's theory, which provides the most detailed and integrated account of such neuropsychological findings.

Gray and the behavioural inhibition system

In Gray's theoretical approach, it is assumed that a description of the brain areas and psychological processes that are affected by anti-anxiety drugs is essentially equivalent to a description of anxiety itself. This heuristic assumption can of course be questioned, since (by analogy) the action of aspirin may not tell us everything we need to know about the processes underlying headache. However, it may still provide a useful beginning, and in the case of anxiety leads to a remarkably simple formulation of the behavioural components of anxiety, and of the types of stimuli that elicit them. The effects of anxiolytic drugs are limited to selective blocking of three main classes of response: (a) inhibition of behaviour (e.g. passive avoidance); (b) increments of arousal; and (c) enhanced attention. The stimuli that are capable of eliciting these three classes of response are also highly specific: (a) signals of punishment; (b) signals of non-reward; and

(c) novel or unfamiliar stimuli. The hypothetical brain system that responds to such stimuli to produce anxiety is termed the behavioural inhibition system (BIS).

A number of considerations implicate the limbic brain and specifically the septo-hippocampal system (SHS) as being involved in the function of the BIS. As indicated earlier, sites such as the locus coeruleus or the raphe nucleus, which when stimulated can increase or decrease anxious behaviour, have important projections to the SHS. Lesions in the SHS have effects that are related although not identical to those of anxiolytic drugs. Electrical activity in the SHS (in particular the θ or 7.7 Hz rhythm) is blocked by tranquillizers, while electrical driving to enhance θ rhythm produces effects opposing those of anxiolytic drugs. In sum, this evidence is taken to suggest that the SHS, together with the noradrenergic and serotonergic inputs from other areas, provides at least part of the neural machinery of the BIS, and that the operation of the BIS constitutes anxiety itself.

Rather than dwell further on the postulated neural machinery, however, it may be helpful at this stage to consider in greater detail the psychological functions which the BIS is said to perform. In information-processing terms, the heart of the BIS is a comparator: a device for comparing one set of information with another and deciding whether the two sets are the same or different. A comparator is required by the BIS because the function of the system is to check whether the organism's environment is as expected and planned, or whether an unexpected (and potentially threatening) situation has developed. Information flow to the comparator thus comes from perceptual representations of the environment on the one hand, and from an internal prediction generator, which takes account of plans and expected regularities in the environment, on the other. The comparator's job is to search for a mismatch between expected and actual events, with special reference to any events that have important consequences, such as stimuli associated with punishment. On detection of a mismatch, the BIS takes control of behaviour, stops ongoing activity, increases arousal, and directs attention towards the unexpected event. Furthermore, the system is supposed to tag the behavioural activity that led up to this unexpected event as suspect, and to direct the organism towards alternatives in the future.

This theoretical model fits with evidence from other sources concerning hippocampal function, which indicates that the hippocampus selectively responds to important or previously reinforced stimuli, while habituating to irrelevant input. The theory thus accounts well enough for the organism's response to unfamiliar situations, while being less specific about how certain classes of events may come to elicit BIS activity in one individual but not in another. Gray simply suggests that the sensitivity of the BIS varies from individual to individual in such a way as to account for differences in trait anxiety. He also adds that certain innate fear stimuli may selectively activate the system, and thus account for phobic states.

While powerfully integrating a great deal of neurophysiological and neuropsychological data, the theory clearly remains incomplete at the psychological and particularly at the cognitive level. If differences in anxiety are determined only by differences in the sensitivity of the BIS, then it remains unclear why some individuals worry more about (say) social events and others more about physical dangers, even given the same objective environment. Indeed, it is not even clear whether the concepts of cognitive appraisal and worry fit into Gray's theory at all. Cognitive theorists assume that knowledge and experiences are represented and stored in long-term memory, and may be used in deciding whether or not ambiguous situations are interpreted as threatening. However, such high-level processes are barely referred to in Gray's theory, other than the suggestion that some verbally encoded information may be available to the SHS via forebrain structures.

While therefore incomplete, Gray's theory represents a significant advance towards an integrated theory of anxiety, and one that leads to important predictions concerning treatment. For example, within the theory, tranquillizing drugs are thought to reduce the noradrenergic and serotonergic signals reaching the SHS, with the consequence that withdrawal from these drugs will be followed by unchanged or increased sensitivity of the BIS. By contrast, behavioural treatments based on exposure are seen to increase input to the BIS, which under appropriate circumstances will become 'toughened up' and require a greater input of the same type in order to respond. By implication, combinations of tranquillizers and behavioural treatment should be less effective than behavioural treatment alone, since the drug effects will tend to block this toughening up process.

CONDITIONING MODELS OF FEAR

While Gray's approach does provide a plausible account of the brain mechanisms which may mediate the experience of anxiety, relatively little attempt has been made to integrate it with earlier models based on conditioning or other forms of learning. Attempts to construct learning models of anxiety began with Watson and Rayner's (1920) successful attempt to condition fear of a white rat in an 11-month-old child by pairing presentation of the animal with loud noise. On the basis of this observation it was argued that any neutral stimulus would come to elicit fear via classical conditioning if it were paired with a threatening stimulus.

This rather simplistic model encountered a number of difficulties almost immediately, among which was the fragility of the original demonstration. Several subsequent researchers (e.g. English 1929, Bregman 1934) failed to establish fear responses to neutral household objects in young infants, using a similar conditioning procedure. Furthermore, Watson's account is inconsistent with the observed characteristics of naturally occurring phobias. A central requirement of the model is that phobics must have experienced some past traumatic event associated with their feared stimulus. However, this does not appear to be a ubiquitous feature of all phobias. Although Öst & Hugdahl (1981) found that over 50% of severe phobics can recall such trauma, other studies have reported very much lower percentages (e.g. Goorny & O'Connor 1971, Rimm et al 1977). While it may of course be the case that relevant conditioning experiences actually occurred but were then subsequently forgotten, it then becomes difficult to see how the theory could be tested.

An even more embarrassing difficulty is the well-known tendency for classically conditioned responses to extinguish if they are no longer paired with an unconditioned stimulus (UCS). To maintain the conditioning model of anxiety it is therefore necessary to explain how conditioned response (CR) can be produced which grows in strength over time rather than extinguishing.

Two-factor learning theory

Mowrer has attempted to deal with such problems by introducing a two-factor learning model of fear acquisition, incorporating both classical and instrumental conditioning (Mowrer 1960). According to this account, the first stage in the acquisition of fear is the establishment of a CR to a particular conditioned stimulus (CS) paired with a noxious UCS. When this CS is next encountered the consequent elevation in anxiety will motivate an avoidance response, and the resulting decrease in anxiety will reinforce the occurrence of this avoidance.

While the two-factor theory does overcome some of the problems associated with Watson's account, it is not entirely compatible with laboratory evidence. Avoidance behaviour can indeed be conditioned in an analogous manner using laboratory animals. However, it is now believed that such behaviour is not causally mediated by an underlying drive state of autonomic arousal (Mineka 1979). Indeed, animals subjected to a prolonged avoidance learning schedule actually show a decline in their fear of the CS when the avoidance behaviour itself is not used as an index of such fear. Therefore, although the two-factor model may explain increases in avoidance behaviour, it has considerable difficulty accounting for the commonly observed growth of subjective distress which occurs as a phobia develops.

Mowrer's model is also incapable of accounting for various features of naturally occurring phobias. According to a simple learning model, any neutral CS paired with an aversive UCS may, perhaps through the mediating mechanism of avoidance learning, be capable of developing into a phobic stimulus. Phobias should therefore be fairly evenly distributed across a whole range of neutral stimuli, and inequalities of distribution should reflect the degree to which any stimulus has a probable history of traumatic association for a particular individual. As Seligman (1971) points out, however, phobic stimuli are not evenly distributed. Rather, they tend to consist of limited and non-arbitrary sets of situations: small animals, heights, crowded places, and so on. Indeed, stimuli with more probable genuine traumatic associations, such as motor cars or electrical sockets, hardly ever appear as phobic stimuli. Agras et al (1969) observed that the frequency of snake phobias was approximately double that of dental phobias in a small Vermont city, despite the fact that contact with a dentist was almost certainly a more frequent and a more painful event.

Related to this problem is the observation that exposure to genuinely traumatic events in real life may not lead to the development of phobias. Rachman (1977) reviews evidence demonstrating that remarkably few lasting anxiety reactions followed exposure to such a naturally occurring traumatic UCS as air-raids.

Seligman and 'preparedness'

How then can a conditioning model of anxiety account for the observed distribution of fears, the common failure to observe conditioning in the presence of a genuinely traumatic UCS, and the extreme resistance of phobias to normal extinction? In an attempt to cope with these problems, Seligman (1970) has challenged what he terms the 'equipotentiality assumption' — the notion that one CS is as good as any other in a conditioning paradigm. Seligman replaces this assumption with the concept of 'preparedness'. His basic argument is that, as a consequence of past evolutionary history, an organism will be innately prepared to learn certain CS–UCS associations. Furthermore, since the traditional laws of conditioning and extinction have been derived from experimental studies involving the pairing of arbitrary CSs and UCSs, these laws may not be directly applicable to instances of prepared learning. Seligman cites a considerable body of animal research to support the notion of preparedness. One of the most striking examples involves acquired taste aversion. In a series of studies, Garcia (cf. Garcia et al 1972) found that rats could easily learn to associate a particular taste with nausea, leading to subsequent avoidance, but failed to make the same association with an alternative CS such as a light. This association between taste and nausea could be learned on a single trial even with a delay of several hours, and proved highly resistant to subsequent extinction. On the basis of such observations, Seligman argues that the laws of prepared learning may differ from those derived from arbitrary associations, and proposes that phobias represent examples of prepared classical conditioning.

Although most of Seligman's examples have involved animal research, Öhman and his colleagues have found evidence with human subjects that the learning of prepared and unprepared associations show rather different characteristics (Öhman et al 1978). Using mild shock as a UCS and electrodermal response as an index of fear, Öhman conditioned CRs to both prepared and unprepared slides (e.g. snakes or spiders versus flowers or geometric shapes). He found robust conditioning with a single CS–UCS pairing for prepared but not for unprepared stimuli. Furthermore the CR extinguished very much more slowly for the prepared than for the unprepared slides. Taken together, such studies appear to confirm the importance of particular CS–UCS associations (in this case between snake or spider image and aversive tactile stimulation) in producing rapid conditioning which is highly resistant to extinction.

The incorporation of preparedness into classical conditioning accounts of fear acquisition overcomes a number of problems, such as the selectivity of phobias, rapidity of acquisition, and resistance to extinction. One problem with the concept of preparedness, however, is its potential circularity. That is, we can argue that only prepared stimuli are likely to be conditioned to phobic responses, yet researchers have typically defined stimuli as being prepared solely on the basis of whether or not they represent common phobias. Attempts to classify preparedness according to independent raters' judgements of 'evolutionary relevance' (De Silva et al 1977) failed to predict severity of phobia, suddenness of onset or treatment outcome.

Eysenck and the incubation of fear

Even if we accept Seligman's argument, and Öhman's finding that prepared associations extinguish slowly, conditioning models still have difficulty explaining how fear often tends to *increase* during the development of phobias, even when any original aversive UCS is no longer paired with the CS. This 'incubation' phenomenon cannot readily be accommodated by traditional models of conditioning. Accordingly, Eysenck (1979) has attempted to develop the theory of classical conditioning in a manner which overcomes this potential problem. His argument is that following the pairing of an aversive UCS with a neutral CS, the resulting CR will itself involve a noxious component (i.e. fear). Subsequent presentation of the CS alone will therefore, because it elicits the noxious CR, still be paired with an aversive stimulus. This pairing will tend to produce an increment in the CR strength. In other words, having conditioned the fear CR, presentations of the CS alone will result in two opposing tendencies: extinction and incubation. The observed consequences of subsequent CS presentation will therefore depend upon the relative strength of extinction and incubation, which in turn depends upon three crucial parameters. First, a strong original UCS will elicit a more intensely aversive CR, and hence increase the probability of incubation being the dominant tendency. Second, short subsequent exposures to the CS alone will ensure that the strength of the CR has little chance to decline (e.g. Nunes & Marks 1975, Mathews et al 1974), and, since its aversive properties will therefore be more intense, incubation will be the more likely consequence. Finally, personality variables are likely to play a role. For neurotic introverts, subsequent presentation of the CS alone will evoke a strong aversive CR and produce relatively little extinction — conditions favouring the occurrence of incubation. Thus, according to Eysenck, the risk of phobic development will be greatest in neurotic introverted subjects experiencing a relatively intense initial aversive UCS (paired with a prepared CS), and subsequently encountering frequent short exposures to the CS alone.

Problems with conditioning models

While conditioning models have an attractive elegant simplicity, they nevertheless fail to account fully for the onset and maintenance of all anxiety disorders. Two specific shortcomings will be considered here. The first criticism is that, although conditioning models may explain the development of some phobias, they have rather more difficulty accounting for generalized anxiety states. The concept of stimulus generalization has sometimes been invoked in the attempt to characterize such disorders as over-generalized phobias, but this frequently stands at odds with patients' reports concerning the development of their anxiety. An alternative approach has been to attribute generalized anxiety to interoceptive classical conditioning (Wolpe 1958, Razran 1961), in which the CS is some internal physiological event. According to this argument the anxiety only appears to be generalized, or free-floating, because the CSs (and possibly the UCSs) may be common every day internal events which are probably largely unconscious. Another related possibility which has been considered is that generalized anxiety arises from anxiety or arousal becoming conditioned to some aspect of relaxation itself. Some limited support for this idea is available from animal experiments (Denny 1976) and from reports of 'relaxation-induced anxiety' in some anxious clients (Heide & Borkovec 1984).

A second criticism of traditional conditioning models is that they attribute the genesis of phobias solely to an individual's past personal experience with the phobic stimulus. While this may be valid on some occasions, it is clearly inadequate in a great many cases. The high frequency of snake phobia, for instance, is inconsistent with the small proportion of the population having any direct contact with snakes whatsoever — traumatic or otherwise. A further possibility, which is considered in the next section, is that fears may be transmitted indirectly, by modelling or some other type of symbolic learning (Bandura 1971).

SYMBOLIC LEARNING AND FEAR

Extreme anticipatory fear can sometimes arise concerning a situation never actually encountered. Such fears may be attributable to the verbal transmission of information by others (as with a child fearful of the first visit to the dentist or hospital), or to modelling. There is a considerable correspondence between the fears of mother and child, and between children in the same family, with correlations of approximately 0.6 and 0.7 respectively (May 1950). The extent to which children are fearful of illness, or became anxious during air attack (Rachman 1977) correlates significantly with the fear displayed by their parents. While such correlational observations cannot be interpreted unequivocally, recent animal evidence shows beyond doubt that modelling can play a causal role.

Laboratory-reared rhesus monkeys, unlike their wild-reared counterparts, are not consistently afraid of snakes. Fear can be acquired quite rapidly in such infants if they watch their parents display terror in the presence of a snake. After a total of only eight minutes' exposure, most infants reach the same level of fear as that modelled by their parents (Mineka et al 1984). Furthermore, this close match in modelled fear is not specific to the parent–child context, since it has been replicated using unrelated pairs (Cook et al 1985). Conversely, prior observation of non-fearful behaviour in the presence of a snake prevents later fear acquisition.

Such data make it apparent that physical encounters with the fear-evoking object are not necessary for the acquisition of anxiety or phobias. More research is needed, however, before it becomes clear whether powerful effects in humans occur across all situations, or are limited to those involving particularly influential models, specific stages of development, or biologically 'prepared' stimuli.

Bandura and self-efficacy

Following a series of related studies demonstrating the power of participant modelling in the reduction of human phobias, Bandura (1977) formulated what has proved to be an influential social learning theory of anxiety. In the current form of this theory, Bandura discounts the role of conditioning on the grounds that cognitive factors such as expectancy tend to over-ride conditioning effects in humans (cf. Brewer 1974). Expectations related to phobic anxiety are likely to arise, or be modified, on the basis of verbally transmitted information, watching the behaviour of others and (most powerfully) observations of one's own behaviour and capabilities in phobic situations. These differences in the power of various types of information to alter expectations are said to explain why treatments involving real-life interaction with phobic situations (e.g. participant modelling or in vivo exposure) are generally more powerful than less direct forms (observational modelling or imaginal desensitization).

Relevant expectations are of two kinds: self-efficacy and outcome expectations. Outcome expectancy refers to beliefs held by the individual concerning the likelihood of aversive (or other) consequences, while self-efficacy refers to beliefs having to do with that individual's capacity to control these potential outcomes. Thus snake phobics are afraid because they envisage aversive outcomes (e.g. the snake attacking them) which they perceive themselves as powerless to control. Treatments which increase a sense of mastery over the situation (typically by enhancing self-efficacy) lead to increased approach behaviour as a result. Anxiety is seen as the outcome of these conscious evaluations, and as having no necessary relation to conditioning. Although Bandura's theory avoids the problems encountered by previous conditioning accounts, it is not without its own difficulties Testing the theory requires a valid index of expectations, which must be obtained independently from measures of behavioural change. Self-efficacy expectations are in fact obtained from answers to questions such as 'Could you pick the snake up?', so that the high correlations with behaviour typically obtained may show only that subjects are able to predict their own behavioural intentions, or that public endorsement tends to be a self-fulfilling prophecy. It is true that effective treatments are those which change self-efficacy ratings most, but this may not necessarily reveal the mechanism of such treatments. Conceivably, treatments such as desensitization are effective because they reduce conditioned fear reactions, or modify some cognitive process which is not directly accessible to self-report. If so, then the treated subject will be aware of less anticipatory anxiety and greater willingness to approach when thinking of the phobic object, without necessarily understanding why or how this change has occurred. Self-efficacy ratings may also reflect the same change and thus be highly accurate predictors of behaviour, without themselves being causally related to that behaviour.

That awareness of self-efficacy is not the *only* cause of behaviour change is suggested by the effect of offering large rewards for performance: incentives can change behaviour without altering self-efficacy. Equally, it is possible to change self-efficacy ratings by altering general mood state (Kavanagh & Bower 1985) or by providing positive expectations of change (Lane & Borkovec 1984) without necessarily changing behaviour. In the study by Lane & Borkovec (1984), self-efficacy ratings were more successful in predicting self-reported improvement than in predicting changes in either behavioural (e.g. dysfluency) or autonomic (e.g. heart rate) measures of speech anxiety. Even if self-efficacy ratings are highly correlated with some other aspects of behaviour (e.g. approach), this leaves open the question of whether behavioural changes are in fact caused by changes in self-efficacy, or whether both efficacy judgements and behaviour are both related to another causal factor or factors.

Eastman & Marzillier (1984), in a lengthy exchange with Bandura, argue that outcome expectations cannot be entirely excluded from judgements of efficacy. Such a separation appears to be possible in some cases, as when one may report low efficacy ratings concerning ability to run in a marathon despite high outcome expectancy concerning the likelihood of praise if one actually succeeds. However, it is not difficult to construct examples where the distinction is much more problematic. Is the agoraphobic's belief that going out will lead to a panic attack and possible collapse an efficacy or an outcome expectation? Eastman & Marzillier would seem to treat such a belief as a perceived outcome, while Bandura (1984) appears to regard it as 'inefficacy in exercising adequate control over her behaviour'. In practice, when subjects are asked to rate their confidence in being able to perform a fear-provoking task, we believe that they are likely to base their assessment on both ability and outcome expectations, in varying amounts depending on the individuals and the specific circumstances involved.

In sum, efficacy and outcome expectation ratings clearly correlate highly with approach behaviour in feared situations, but self-efficacy theory may be more an exercise in labelling than in explaining. Bandura has rightly drawn our attention to the fact that phobic subjects make decisions to approach or to avoid frightening situations, and decisions are surely cognitive events. However, it may require more than a simple self-report on whether one is able to perform an action to understand fully the processes influencing that action.

COGNITIVE MODELS OF ANXIETY

Bandura's approach attaches more importance to the role of thought than do the more traditional conditioning models. The relationship between thinking and emotion is, however, most strongly embodied in the cognitive model of anxiety proposed by Aaron Beck (1976, Beck & Emery 1985). According to this account, anxiety — whether normal or abnormal — is seen as an appropriate emotional reaction to the occurrence of highly threatening thoughts, usually concerning potential future dangers. Anxiety disorders are therefore conceptualized primarily as thinking disorders.

Beck and cognitive schemata

There is some evidence that generalized anxiety disorder is indeed associated with particularly threatening patterns of thinking (e.g. Beck et al 1974, Mathews & Shaw 1977, Hibbert 1984). For example, Beck et al (1974) employed a standardized interview schedule and self-completed records to investigate the occurrence of danger-related thoughts in 32 anxious patients. Every patient reported experiencing thoughts involving the anticipation of some physical or social danger, either in visual or verbal form, during episodes of anxiety. Furthermore, most subjects reported that these thoughts preceded the onset or exacerbation of the anxiety, and that the intensity of this emotion was moderated by the degree of belief in the thought. Similar results were reported by Hibbert (1984) using three standardized questions, who also demonstrated that those patients who experienced panic attacks had thoughts centring on physical dangers, whereas those without panic attacks had thoughts primarily concerned with psychosocial dangers. In the absence of appropriate control data, however, it is difficult to evaluate the degree to which such thinking patterns have a causal role, or differentiate clinical from normal anxiety.

Beck attributes the inappropriate occurrence of such thoughts to the operation of certain mental structures, or cognitive schemata, which systematically distort experience. The concept of schemata has been employed by cognitive scientists to accommodate a variety of phenomena, primarily involving the comprehension of complex information (eg Neisser 1976, Mandler 1984). A schema is conceptualized as a modular cognitive structure developed from past experience, which when active serves to select relevant details from a complex environment, and to provide a particular interpretation of the overall situation. Long-term memory is assumed to contain a vast range of such schemata and at any time only a small subset will be active. The same external situation may thus be represented internally in radically different ways, depending upon the nature of the schemata which are employed. Beck (1976) suggests that clinical anxiety reflects the overactivation of schemata which are predominantly concerned with the encoding and elaboration of threat-related information. The activity of these cognitive structures gives rise to processing biases, which ultimately lead to the presence of danger-related thoughts in anxious subjects. For example, Beck argues that anxious patients will show evidence of 'catastrophizing', or exaggerating the probability of negative events actually occurring; 'selective abstraction', or resolving ambiguity to produce the most threatening interpretation; and 'hypervigilance', or selective allocation of attention to the more threatening elements in any environment.

Processing biases in anxiety

Recent laboratory research has in general supported the hypothesis that anxious subjects have characteristic biases in the way they process emotionally relevant information. Butler & Mathews (1983 and in press) have confirmed that anxiety is associated with inflated subjective risk judgements specifically concerning the probability of personally experiencing aversive events in the future. For those events alone anxious patients were shown to produce higher risk estimates than did matched control subjects. Furthermore, as state anxiety increased in a normal group of subjects approaching an examination, so too did the perceived risk for negative events, especially in high-trait subjects. The interpretation of ambiguity has likewise been shown to be biased in anxious subjects. For example, Eysenck et al (1987) identified 28 homophones having one meaning related to threat, such as GUILT/GILT, or PAIN/PANE, and presented these on tape, mixed randomly with non-ambiguous filler material, in what subjects perceived as a spelling task. Their resulting spellings indicated the degree to which their favoured interpretation was biased towards the more threatening meaning, and the extent of this bias correlated 0.6 with a measure of trait anxiety. We are currently finding similar results with more complex ambiguous sentences.

A range of paradigms have also confirmed the presence of an attentional bias towards threat-related stimuli in anxious subjects. Mathews & MacLeod (1985) found clinically anxious, but not control, subjects to be differentially disrupted on a colour-naming task, when they were required to ignore threat-related rather than neutral distractor words. Similar findings were produced on a dichotic listening task, even when the distractor information was presented outside conscious awareness, suggesting that this bias may be relatively automatic (Mathews & MacLeod 1986). Using a rather different visual attention paradigm, MacLeod et al (1986) demonstrated that following the simultaneous presentation of a word pair, including one threatening and one neutral item, anxious patients moved attention towards the threat item, whereas control subjects moved attention away from it. Thus detection latencies for dot probes occurring in the area of the threat word were disproportionately fast compared with those appearing in the other area for the anxious subjects, but were disproportionately slow for the control subjects.

Bower's network model of mood and memory

Beck's notion of modular danger schemata does not represent the only means of explaining such biases. Bower (1981) has recently extended his network model of long-term memory (Anderson & Bower 1973) to accommodate similar observed relationships between mood and cognition. According to this model information is stored in nodes, with related nodes being connected through associative links. Accessing any information involves activating the relevant node, and this activation spreads to related information, which is thus rendered more easily accessible for future operations.

Bower's extension to this model involved the introduction of mood nodes into the network. Every emotion is represented by such a node, which is linked to all the others which have been commonly associated with this mood in the past. Thus an anxiety node will share associative links with nodes corresponding to a wide range of threat-related information. Entering a particular emotion state is assumed to activate its corresponding mood node, and this activation then spreads through the network to partially activate related nodes. In consequence, mood-congruent information is, in general, more accessible than mood-incongruent information, for a wide range of processing operations. According to this account, therefore, the processing biases observed in anxiety would reflect the disproportionate ease with which threat-related information can be accessed while in this mood.

Bower's original network model is a rather more passive system than is Beck's notion of active schemata which direct attention and impose structure on experience. However, more recent extensions to Bower's account (e.g. Bower & Cohen 1982), largely concerning the way in which the cognitive system operates upon this network data base, make the distinction between the two models less clear-cut. In any case, both accounts agree that anxiety is indeed associated with cognitive biases which yield a more dangerous subjective representation of the world. It therefore seems possible that the elevated levels of anxiety experienced by clinical patients may, at least on occasions, represent a 'realistic' emotional response to a distorted representation of the environment.

Finally, it is important to consider whether the cognitive processing biases which characterize anxiety represent a transient feature of mood (i.e. state anxiety), or reflect more stable personality variables (i.e. trait anxiety). One possibility, which we favour and which is compatible with both Beck's and Bower's formulations, is that both trait and state anxiety may contribute to such processing biases in rather different ways. Trait anxiety may be associated with certain structural aspects of the cognitive system. In Beck's terms, high trait anxiety may represent the existence of highly integrated danger schemata, while in Bower's account it may reflect an extremely rich network of associations linking the anxiety node to related threatening information. State anxiety, on the other hand, may reflect the current degree of activity within such cognitive structures. If so, then the degree to which cognitive biases are actually manifest will be an interactive function of both trait and state anxiety levels. This interactive view is consistent with much of our own current data, which indicate that the relationship between state anxiety and threat-related cognitive biases is commonly only significant in high-trait-anxiety subjects. For example, in a study to be reported elsewhere, we employed the previously described visual attention paradigm to investigate the influence of increasing state anxiety in high- and low-trait-anxious students approaching an important examination. As state anxiety increased, the high-trait students showed an enhanced tendency to shift attention towards threatening examination-related words, such as 'failure' or 'humiliated', resembling the pattern shown by clinical patients. In contrast, however, increases in state anxiety for the low-trait students resulted in an enhanced tendency to shift attention *away* from such material. This result suggests that stressful situations may elicit different biases, which in high-trait-anxiety subjects will highlight potential threats, but in low-trait subjects will tend to block out such information.

INTEGRATED THEORIES OF ANXIETY

As indicated in the introduction to this chapter, theoretical models of anxiety have tended to utilize either physiological, behavioural or verbal responses as their primary source of data. Such models tend to be particularly successful in accounting for data within their chosen domain, but typically have less to say about other aspects. In this final section, we shall consider to what extent these single-system models can be replaced with more integrated theories, drawing on data from more than one primary source.

Lang's cognitive psychophysiology

The growing consensus that opposition between pathophysiological and psychological views of anxiety has proved unproductive, suggests that models involving interactions between different systems may be more useful. In developing a theory of emotional imagery, Lang took as his starting point the serendipitous finding that clients showing large physiological reactions during imaginal desensitization appeared to have a better treatment outcome (Lang et al 1970). Such individuals also showed a higher degree of concordance between subjective and physiological reactions to phobic imagery. Lang concluded that the ability to generate a more complete response to imagery was responsible for the better therapeutic outcome.

In his current elaboration of this finding, Lang (1985) proposes that emotional images arise from the activation of a hierarchical cognitive structure, containing stimulus, response and meaning propositions. The base level of this hierarchical structure consists of information concerning efferent responses and motor programmes. Activation of such propositions by instructed imagery may result in detectable autonomic and motor activity, due to efferent 'leakage'. In the second hierarchical level are propositions concerned with attributes of emotional stimuli, such as the writhing movements of a snake. The highest level is a true semantic network containing meaning propositions such as 'I am frightened' or 'snakes are dangerous'. Phobic anxiety corresponds to the activation of this entire hierarchical structure, which tends to be all-or-none. That is, although some aspects may be accessed alone, strong associative links among the various components make it very probable that the structure is activated as a complete unit. This is said to be particularly true in a highly anxious individual, whereas in a less anxious individual the reduced coherence of the entire structure makes such total activation less likely.

Lang's theoretical approach to emotional imagery clearly owes something to Bower's (1981) network theory of emotion on the one hand, and Pylyshyn's (1973) propositional theory of imagery on the other. However, unlike Bower he does not postulate the existence of a central emotional node linking all congruent events, but instead assumes that emotional states arise directly from the activation of propositions within the emotional representation. It is further assumed that propositions within the structure can be changed only if they are currently activated, thus explaining why desensitization appears to be more successful in the presence of large reactions to phobic imagery instructions. Much of Lang's experimental work has been concerned with varying the type of phobic imagery, in terms of whether both stimulus and response propositions are included, or only stimulus information (Lang 1985). Those who are given instructions or training that emphasize response propositions (for example 'your heart is racing') consistently show larger physiological reactions to phobic imagery, and which are more highly correlated with verbal report. Thus, although Lang's theory is predominantly cognitive, it makes clear predictions concerning psychophysiological data, which have generally been strongly confirmed.

One of the most important clinical predictions that arises from Lang's theory is that a good response to those treatments which involve anxiety-evoking imagery depends on the extent to which the entire emotional representation is accessed. Since training in attention to response propositions apparently results in greater overall activation, it would seem to follow that this form of training should produce better treatment outcome. However, comparisons of systematic desensitization with or without response training have not in fact been carried out, so that this crucial question remains unanswered. While the lack of critical testing leaves the validity of Lang's theory in considerable doubt, there is less doubt about its heuristic usefulness. Unlike other models, it clearly embodies the idea that the cognitive and psychophysiological systems must be systematically related to one another, and in some respects may be interdependent.

Panic attacks: a somatic-cognitive loop?

While Lang's theory has been useful in its attempt to bridge cognitive theorizing and psychophysiological experimentation, it has little to say on the subject of how individuals interpret and react to their own physiological responses. More recently, a number of clinical researchers have focused on precisely this issue, and in this section we shall consider the possibility of a cognitive-somatic loop in panic attacks (Clark 1986). It is well known that panic attacks can be provoked in certain anxious individuals by a range of physical agents, such as lactate infusions, caffeine, voluntary overbreathing, and inhalation of carbon dioxide. While this has previously been interpreted as evidence of biological vulnerability, recent studies (e.g. Clark & Hemsley 1982, Van den Hout & Griez 1984) suggest that different individuals may experience the same physiological sensations either as extremely frightening, or as mildly pleasurable, depending upon their expectations and interpretations of their own reactions. Thus it appears likely that these physical agents do not promote panic directly, but rather induce a physiological state which may or may not lead to panic, depending upon how it is subjectively interpreted. If the further assumption is made that certain individuals are prone to misinterpret common physiological reactions in a catastrophic way, the scene is set for a vicious circle that may spiral into panic. For example, when an individual perceives some stimulus (whether internal or external) as threatening, both subjective apprehension and characteristic physiological reactions will occur. If the physiological reactions result in perceptible bodily sensations, such as overbreathing leading to dizziness, a catastrophic misinterpretation of these sensations as dangerous will lead to increased anxiety levels, and so on. Methods of treatment for panic based on this model have been developed recently by Griez & Van den Hout (1986) and Salkovskis et al (1985).

Both the idea of a cognitive-somatic loop and the emotional imagery model of Lang represent steps towards integrating data gathered from different perspectives within a single theory of anxiety states. Their range is limited, however, in that only some clinical phenomena are addressed (phobic imagery and panic attacks), and they do not clearly accommodate data generated from neuropsychological and information-processing research. While a fully integrated theory is almost certainly premature, we will close the chapter with a discussion of this possibility.

An integrated model of anxiety states

A major problem in attempting an integrated theory is that different explanations seem to work best with different clinical phenomena. For example, prepared learning explanations apply more naturally to phobias than they do to generalized anxiety states. Biological or information-processing approaches seem more applicable to generalized anxiety than they do to phobias. By combining learning, neurophysiological and information-processing approaches into one theoretical framework, perhaps it will be possible to give a coherent account of all abnormal anxiety phenomena.

In our integrated account we first assume that emotional responses (including anxiety) normally begin with the evaluation of incoming information as having relevance to the goals or expectations of that individual. We suppose that language-based semantic processing is not essential for such an evaluation, since comparable emotional states appear to exist in species other than man. We further assume that this evaluative system is innately prepared to react to some biologically important stimuli. Finally, we assume that emotional responses to stimuli can be acquired or modified involuntarily, without any awareness that such a change has taken place. This last assumption is based on information-processing experiments which suggest that liking for stimuli may be increased, or autonomic responses to conditioned stimuli may be extinguished, following subliminal exposure to them (Seamon et al 1984, Öhman 1985).

Incoming information may thus trigger evaluative/emotional responses as a result of innate preparation, learning, or after being selectively processed for threat-related associative meaning at a higher level in the cognitive system. As an example of these routes, consider whether or not the discovery of a small lump on one's body is likely to produce anxiety. Conceivably, anxiety could be a prepared response to certain alterations in one's bodily appearance. More plausibly, earlier experiences of similar events may have resulted in physical blemishes being a conditioned stimulus for embarrassment and social anxiety. Finally, anxiety may result from higher-level processing to the extent that the lump is interpreted as a sign of a serious illness, such as cancer. Activation via this final route would of course depend on abstract knowledge of the disease and its consequences, combined with any relevant personal experiences related to cancer.

Although anxiety may thus be provoked via several different routes, it would be parsimonious to suppose that all routes converge into a final common pathway. The behavioural inhibition system described by Gray (1982) provides an example of such a final common pathway. Clearly, the BIS must have associated with it some pre-programmed representations of situations like heights, to explain why freezing and avoidance occur in infants faced with a visual cliff for the first time. Since other situations can later come to evoke identical reactions, either as a result of conditioning or symbolic learning, it is clear that the same neurophysiological mechanisms can be recruited by newly formed cognitive representations at a higher level. We would further propose that conditioning experiences with biologically prepared stimuli result in representations capable of activating the behavioural inhibition system in the presence of such stimuli (specific phobias), while symbolic learning may give rise to more extensive representations of personal danger capable of evoking similar reactions to a wider range of stimuli (generalized anxiety).

In the absence of direct conditioning experiences, we assume that such widespread representations of danger may arise out of a combination of biological predisposition, threatening life events and acquired processing style. Consider an emotionally labile individual, who is exposed to a life event possibly denoting danger, such as a serious illness in a close family member. The perceived threat, in this case the possible death of a loved one, will give rise to a marked emotional response, together with elaborations in the cognitive representations of disease, to incorporate strengthened associations with danger. Later on, the same individual may perceive cues such as their own physiological reactions, and interpret them in the light of the stored representations of danger through illness.

Why should some individuals react in this way, and perhaps develop an anxiety disorder, while others cope more effectively and remain healthy? Our speculation is that this depends on the type and extent of selective processing bias used when exposed to ambiguously threatening situations. An attentional bias favouring the pick-up of threat-related information, and an interpretative bias to construe the situation in its most dangerous form, are likely to result in progressively greater elaborations to the stored representations of personal danger. Such elaboration would thus explain the otherwise mysterious growth of anxiety as the disorder develops. These perceptual and inferential biases may be relatively automatic, in the sense that they are effortless, involuntary and may not be consciously accessible. Nonetheless, the result will be the awareness of increased anxiety in the presence of various internal or external cues, such as those related to illness, which have now acquired the capacity to activate the neurophysiological anxiety system. Because these cues may be relatively ubiquitous and unavoidable, the resulting experience is of persistent and generalized anxiety, which may occasionally develop into panic attacks.

Although vague and incomplete, this integrated model avoids unproductive conflict between opposed views of anxiety, yet at the same time has some clinical implications. Among other things it suggests that there may be a role for exposure to anxiety cues in generalized anxiety states, even when clients are unaware of the existence of such cues. It suggests that cognitive therapy will be effective to the extent that the relevant danger cues are represented semantically, which is perhaps more likely to be true in generalized anxiety states than in specific phobias. In all anxiety conditions, it suggests that treatment manipulations which never arouse anxiety will be relatively ineffective, since they do not involve accessing the relevant representations. While these detailed proposals may well turn out to be incorrect, we are convinced that the goal of a more integrated view of anxiety is a worthwhile one to pursue, both for scientific and clinical reasons.

REFERENCES

Agras S, Sylvester D, Oliveau D 1969 The epidemiology of common fears and phobias. Comprehensive Psychiatry 10: 151–156

Anderson J R, Bower G H 1973 Human associative memory. Winston, Washington, DC

Bandura A (ed) 1971 Psychological modelling. Atherton Press, Chicago

Bandura A 1977 Self efficacy: toward a unifying theory of behavioral change. Psychological Review 84: 191–215

Bandura A 1984 Recycling misconceptions of perceived self-efficacy. Cognitive Therapy and Research 8: 231–255

Barrett E S 1972 Anxiety and impulsiveness: towards a neuropsychological model. In: Spielberger C D (ed) Anxiety: current trends in theory and research, Vol 1. Academic Press, New York

Beck A T 1976 Cognitive therapy and the emotional disorders. International Universities Press, New York

Beck A T, Emery G 1985 Anxiety disorders and phobias: a cognitive perspective. Basic Books, New York

Beck A T, Laude R, Bohnert M 1974 Ideational components of anxiety neurosis. Archives of General Psychiatry 31: 319–325

Bower G H 1981 Mood and memory. American Psychologist 36: 129–148

Bower G H, Cohen P R 1982 Emotional influences in memory and thinking: data and theory. In: Clark M S, Fisk S T (eds) Affect and Cognition. Lawrence Erlbaum, New Jersey

Bregman E 1934 An attempt to modify the emotional attitudes of infants by the conditioned response technique. Journal of Genetic Psychology 45: 169–198

Brewer W F 1974 There is no convincing evidence for operant or classical conditioning in adult humans. In: Weinman W B, Palermo D S (eds) Cognition and Symbolic Processes. Lawrence Erlbaum, New Jersey

Buss A H 1962 Two anxiety factors in psychiatric patients. Journal of Abnormal Psychology 65: 426–427

Butler G, Mathews A 1983 Cognitive processes in anxiety. Advances in Behaviour Research and Therapy 5: 51–62

Butler G, Mathews A Anticipatory anxiety and risk perception. Cognitive Therapy and Research (in press)

Cannon W B 1929 Bodily changes in pain, hunger, fear and rage: An account of recent researchers into the function of emotional excitement. 2nd edn. Appleton-Century-Crofts, New York
Carr D B, Sheehan D V 1984 Panic anxiety: a new biological model. Journal of Clinical Psychiatry 45: 323–330
Clark D M 1986 A cognitive approach to panic. Behaviour Research and Therapy 24: 461–470
Clark D M, Hemsley D R 1982 The effects of hyperventilation and its relation to personality. Journal of Behaviour Therapy and Experimental Psychiatry 13: 41–47
Cook M, Mineka S, Wolkenstein B, Laitsch K 1985 Observational conditioning of snake fear in unrelated rhesus monkeys. Journal of Abnormal Psychology 94: 591–610
Denny R 1976 Post-aversive relief and relaxation and their implications for behavior therapy. Journal of Behavior Therapy and Experimental Psychiatry 7: 315–322
De Silva P, Rachman S, Seligman M E P 1977 Prepared phobias and obsessions: therapeutic outcomes. Behaviour Research and Therapy 15: 65–78
Eastman C, Marzillier J S 1984 Theoretical and methodological difficulties in Bandura's self-efficacy theory. Cognitive Therapy and Research 8: 213–229
English H B 1929 Three cases of the 'conditioned fear response'. Journal of Abnormal Psychology 34: 221–225
Eysenck H J 1979 The conditioning model of neurosis. Behavioral and Brain Sciences 2: 155–166
Eysenck H 1967 The biological basis of personality. In: C Thomas, Springfield, Ill
Eysenck M, MacLeod C, Mathews A 1987 Cognitive functioning in anxiety. Psychological Research 49: 189–195
Finlay-Jones R A, Brown G W 1981 Types of stressful life-event and the onset of anxiety and depressive disorders. Psychological Medicine 11: 803–815
Garcia J, McGowan B K, Green K F 1972 Biological constraints on conditioning. In: Black A H, Prokasy W F (eds) Classical conditioning II: current research and theory. Appleton-Century-Crofts, New York
Goorny A B, O'Connor P J 1971 Anxiety associated with flying. British Journal of Psychiatry 119: 159–166
Gray J A 1982 The neuropsychology of anxiety. Clarendon Press, Oxford
Griez E, Van den Hout M A 1986 CO_2 inhalation in the treatment of panic attacks. Behaviour Research and Therapy 24: 145–150
Heide F, Borkovec T D 1984 Relaxation-induced anxiety: mechanism and theoretical implications. Behaviour Research and Therapy 2: 1–12
Hibbert G A 1984 Ideational components of anxiety: their origin and content. British Journal of Psychiatry 144: 618–624
Hodgson R I, Rachman S J 1974 Desynchrony in measures of fear. Behaviour Research and Therapy 12: 319–326
Jerremalm A, Jansson L, Öst L-G 1986 Individual response patterns and the effects of different behavioural methods in the treatment of dental phobia. Behaviour Research and Therapy 24: 587–596
Kavanagh D J, Bower G H 1985 Mood and self-efficacy: impact of joy and sadness on perceived capabilities. Cognitive Therapy and Research 9: 507–525
Kiser R S, Brown C A, Sanghera M K, German D C 1980 Dorsal raphe nucleus stimulation reduces centrally-elicited fearlike behaviour. Brain Research 191: 265–272
Lader M, Marks I 1971 Clinical anxiety. Heinemann, London
Lader M H, Wing L 1966 Physiological measures, sedative drugs, and morbid anxiety. Oxford University Press, London
Lane T W, Borkovec T D 1984 The influence of therapeutic expectancy/demand on self-efficacy ratings. Cognitive Therapy and Research 8: 95–106
Lang P J 1968 Fear reduction and fear behavior: Problems in treating a construct. In: Shlien J M (ed) Research in psychotherapy, Vol III, pp 90–103. American Psychological Association, Washington, DC
Lang P J 1985 The cognitive psychophysiology of emotion: fear and anxiety. In: Tuma A H, Maser J D (eds) Anxiety and the anxiety disorders. Lawrence Erlbaum, New Jersey
Lang P J, Melamed B G, Hart J D, 1970 Psychophysiological analysis of fear modification using an automated desensitization procedure. Journal of Abnormal Psychology 76: 220–234

Lehrer P M, Woolfolk R L 1982 Self-report assessment of anxiety: somatic, cognitive, and behavioural modalities. Behavioral Assessment 4: 167–177
McKeon J, Roa B, Mann A 1984 Life events and personality trait in obsessive-compulsive neurosis. British Journal of Psychiatry 144: 185–189
MacLeod C, Mathews A, Tata P 1986 Attentional bias in emotional disorders. Journal of Abnormal Psychology 95: 15–20
Mandler G 1984 Mind and Body. Wiley, New York
Marks I 1969 Fears and Phobias. Heinemann, London
Marks I, Lader M 1973 Anxiety states (anxiety neurosis): a review. Journal of Nervous and Mental Disease 156: 3–18
Mathews A, MacLeod C 1985 Selective processing of threat cues in anxiety states. Behaviour Research and Therapy 23: 563–569
Mathews A, MacLeod C 1986 Discrimination of threat cues without awareness in anxiety states. Journal of Abnormal Psychology 95: 131–138
Mathews A, Shaw P 1977 Cognitions related to anxiety, a pilot study of treatment. Behaviour Research and Therapy 15: 503–505
Mathews A, Johnston D W, Shaw P M, Gelder M G 1974 Process variables and the prediction of outcome in behaviour therapy. British Journal of Psychiatry 125: 256–264
May R 1950 The Meaning of anxiety. Ronald Press, New York
Mineka S 1979 The role of fear in theories of avoidance learning, flooding, and extinction. Psychological Bulletin 86: 985–1010
Mineka S, Davidson M, Cook M, Keir R 1984 Observational learning of snake fear in rhesus monkeys. Journal of Abnormal Psychology 93: 355–372
Mowrer O H 1960 Learning theory and behavior. Wiley, New York
Neisser U 1976 Cognition and reality: principles and implications of cognitive psychology. Freeman, San Francisco
Nunes J S, Marks I M 1975 Feedback of true heart rate during exposure in vivo. Archives of General Psychiatry 32: 933–936
Öhman A 1985 Face the beast and fear the face: animal and social fears as prototypes for evolutionary analysis of emotion. Psychophysiology 23: 123–145
Öhman A, Fredrikson M, Hugdahl K 1978 Towards an experimental model for simple phobic reactions. Behaviour Analysis and Modification 2: 97–114
Öst L-G, Hugdahl K 1981 Acquisition of phobias and anxiety response patterns in clinical patients. Behaviour Research and Therapy 19: 439–447
Öst L-G, Jerremalm A, Janssen L, 1981 Individual response patterns and the effects of different behavioural methods in the treatment of social phobia. Behaviour Research and Therapy 19: 1–16
Pitts F N, McClure J N 1967 Lactate metabolism in anxiety neurosis. New England Journal of Medicine 277: 1329–1336
Pylyshyn Z W 1973 What the mind's eye tells the brain: a critique of mental imagery. Psychological Bulletin 80: 1–22
Rachman S 1977 The conditioning theory of fear acquisition: a critical examination. Behaviour Research and Therapy 15: 375–388
Rachman S J, De Silva P 1978 Normal and abnormal obsessions. Behaviour Research and Therapy 16: 233–248
Rachman S J, Hodgson R I 1974 Synchrony and desynchrony in fear and avoidance. Behaviour Research and Therapy 12: 311–318
Rachman S, Seligman M E P 1976 Unprepared phobias: 'Be prepared'. Behaviour Research and Therapy 14: 333–338
Razran G 1961 The observable unconscious and the inferable conscious in current Soviet psychophysiology: Interoceptive conditioning, semantic conditioning, and the orienting reflex. Psychological Review 68: 81–150
Redmond D E, Huang Y H 1979 New evidence for a locus coeruleus–norepinephrine connection with anxiety. Life Sciences 25: 2149–2162
Reiman E M, Raichle M E, Butler F K, Herscovitch P, Robins E 1984 A focal brain abnormality in panic disorders, a severe form of anxiety. Nature 310: 683–685
Rimm D, Janda L, Lancaster D, Nahl M, Dittman K 1977 An exploratory investigation of the origin and maintenance of phobias. Behaviour Research and Therapy 15: 231–238
Salkovskis P M, Jones D R O, Clark D M 1985 Respiration control in the treatment of

panic attacks: a replication and extension with concurrent measurement of behaviour and pCO_2. British Journal of Psychiatry 148: 256

Schwartz G E, Davidson R J, Goleman D J 1978 Patterning of cognitive and somatic processes in the self-regulation of anxiety: effects of meditation versus exercise. Psychosomatic Medicine 40: 32–328

Seamon J G, Marsh R L, Brody N 1984 Critical importance of exposure duration for affective discrimination of stimuli that are not recognised. Journal of Experimental Psychology: Learning, Memory and Cognition 10: 465–469

Seligman M E P 1970 On the generality of the laws of learning. Psychological Review 77: 406–418

Seligman M E P 1971 Phobias and preparedness. Behaviour Therapy 2: 307–320

Taylor L, Chave S 1964 Mental health and environment. Longman, London

Van den Hout M A, Griez E 1984 Panic symptoms after inhalation of carbon dioxide. British Journal of Psychiatry 144: 503–507

Watson J B, Rayner R 1920 Conditioned emotional reactions. Journal of Experimental Psychology 3: 1–14

Wolpe J 1958 Psychotherapy by reciprocal inhibition. Stanford University Press, Stanford

9

Padmal de Silva

Obsessive-compulsive disorder

INTRODUCTION

Obsessive-compulsive disorder is one of the conditions traditionally regarded as neurotic illnesses. Although it takes many forms, the main features of the clinical condition are well recognized. It is relatively rare, the prevalence of the disorder among psychiatric out-patients being estimated between 0.3% and 0.6%. Among in-patients the prevalence is higher, but definitely under 5% (Black 1974, Hare et al 1972, Rachman & Hodgson 1980). The exact figures must be treated with some caution since differences in survey methodology, diagnostic criteria and clinical practices and policy considerably influence these. Whilst the prevalence in the general population has been estimated to be about 0.5%, more recent data from the USA suggest a higher rate. Initial data from the National Epidemiology Catchment Area survey show a 6-month prevalence of 1.3–2.0%, and a life-time risk of 1.9–3.0% (Myers et al 1984, Robins et al 1984). Despite some claims of a female preponderance, there is no conclusive evidence of a sex bias. The onset of the disorder is usually in adolescence or early adulthood, with an onset after the age of 45 being quite rare (Black 1974, Rachman & Hodgson 1980, Rasmussen & Tsuang 1986). Obsessive-compulsive disorders can often be handicapping, with a considerable impact on the patient's life.

THE PHENOMENA

Definitions and descriptions

The phenomena that constitute obsessive-compulsive disorder have been detailed by various authorities including classical writers such as Janet (1903), Jaspers (1923) and Lewis (1936), as well as more recent investigators like Akhtar et al (1975), Emmelkamp (1982) and Rachman & Hodgson (1980). The current position with regard to obsessive-compulsive phenomenology is reflected in the American Psychiatric Association's *Diagnostic and Statistical Manual* (DSM III, APA 1980), which describes the phenomena as follows:

The essential features are recurrent obsessions or compulsions. *Obsessions* are recurrent, persistent ideas, thoughts, images, or impulses that are ego-dystonic, that is, they are not experienced as voluntarily produced, but rather as thoughts that invade consciousness and are experienced as senseless or repugnant. Attempts are made to ignore or suppress them. *Compulsions* are repetitive and seemingly purposeful behaviors that are performed according to certain rules or in a stereotyped fashion. The behavior is not an end in itself, but is designed to produce or to prevent some future event or situation. However, the activity is not connected in a realistic way with what it is designed to produce or prevent, or may be clearly excessive. The act is performed with a sense of subjective compulsion coupled with a desire to resist the compulsion (at least initially). The individual generally recognises the senselessness of the behavior (this may not be true for young children) and does not derive pleasure from carrying out the activity, although it provides a release of tension. The most common obsessions are repetitive thoughts of violence (e.g. killing one's child), contamination (e.g. becoming infected by shaking hands), and doubt (e.g. repeatedly wondering whether one has performed some action, such as having hurt someone in a traffic accident). The most common compulsions are handwashing, counting, checking and touching. (p. 238)

It is stressed that these features should not be secondary to another mental disorder since similar phenomena can sometimes result from certain other disorders.

Diversity of the phenomena

What is clear from this and other descriptions (e.g. Rachman & Hodgson 1980, Rasmussen & Tsuang 1986) is that there is more than one type of phenomenon that may manifest itself in an obsessive-compulsive disorder. The traditionally held view among clinicians that it is essentially a singular or unitary condition, while correct at one level, can be misleading as the clinical manifestations may be markedly diverse. It has recently been pointed out that the limited progress that has been made in our understanding of these problems may partly be due to the tendency to regard them as unitary. It is important, therefore, to recognize the diversity of the phenomena and of the ways in which they present clinically (cf. de Silva 1986, Rachman 1982, Sturgis 1984).

First and foremost, it needs to be stressed that, while related, obsessions and compulsions are not the same phenomenon. This is clearly recognized in the DSM III definition but not in many others, including the World Health Organization's International Classification of Diseases (ICD 9, WHO 1978). Indeed, some authors have maintained that there is no essential difference between compulsions and obsessions (Cooper 1983, Reed 1985). Others have argued that the cardinal phenomenon, regardless of the manifestation, is essentially one of compulsion (Carr 1974). Related to this, it has also been argued that the inconsistent and confusing uses of the two terms 'obsession' and 'compulsion' in the terminology of English psychiatric writing is due to the faulty way in which the original German and French terms were translated (Reed 1985).

The clearing of this inconsistency and confusion is in fact not too difficult and can be accomplished by a close analysis of the clinical phenomena. The DSM III account comes close to achieving this and the research of contemporary investigators, particularly Rachman and his associates, provides the necessary empirical and experimental basis for a full analysis (Rachman & Hodgson 1980). The two main factors that are considered in the DSM III account as essential, either alone or together, are obsessions and compulsions and these are quite distinct phenomena. An *obsession* is an unwanted intrusive cognition; it intrudes into consciousness, and the person normally resists this and attempts to dismiss it. It is persistent, repetitious, generally uncomfortable although not attributed to an external source, and is experienced as senseless or repugnant. The experience is essentially a *passive* one, with the person being the passive recipient or victim of it. A not uncommon clinical example which is typical of this phenomenon is the repeated intrusion of a thought such as 'I must have killed someone' or 'I may strangle or stab someone'. A *compulsion*, on the other hand, is an active phenomenon. It is brought about actively by the person. Consider someone touching the door handle three times on every occasion he closes a door. This is not, in contrast to an obsession, a passive occurrence and is something in which the person engages actively. It is caused by a strongly felt subjective urge, usually referred to as a 'compulsive urge', and in this is unlike a muscle spasm or a tic. This urge is often resisted and the person may fight hard not to carry out the act. It is thus very different from the obsession, which is a passive experience.

It is important to recognize that both obsessions and compulsions can take a variety of forms. An obsession can be a thought, image, or an impulse and is often a combination of two, or even all three of these (de Silva 1986, Rachman & Hodgson 1980). Some clinical examples are given below:

1. Thought that he had cancer (male, 46 years)
2. Thought plus visual image that he may have knocked someone down with his car (male, 29 years)
3. Impulse, with associated doubting thought, to shout obscenities during prayer or a church service (female, 19 years)
4. Image of corpses rotting away (female, 27 years)
5. Thoughts of serious accident or harm occurring to his family (male, 38 years)

A compulsion can be an overt form of motor behaviour, like washing hands repeatedly, or covert and cognitive in nature as in the silent utterance of words in a certain fixed sequence. The DSM III makes no explicit recognition of the fact that a compulsion can be, and not infrequently is, cognitive in nature, and most of the literature assumes that compulsions are

expressed as motor behaviour. This is a serious error. Examples of compulsions are:
1. Repeated and extensive washing of hands to get rid of contamination by germs (female, 26 years)
2. Checking gas taps, door handles, and electric switches three times each time he went past them (male, 28 years)
3. Imagining in sequence the photographs of members of his family, his parents, pictures of Jesus Christ and the Virgin Mary, and then photographs of two other persons (male, 38 years)
4. Cleaning and washing around bed and nearby wall to get rid of germs and dirt (female, 15 years)

Constituent elements of obsessive-compulsive experiences

In clinical cases an obsession may occur without an associated compulsion, as when a young woman had intrusive thoughts and images of her wedding reception which she found distressing, but which led to no active compulsion. More often obsessions lead to related compulsive behaviour, as when an obsessional thought of contamination by germs or dirt leads to extensive washing of hands and body each time the obsession is experienced. In such cases the individual feels a strong need to wash and an inability to relax until this has been done. Compulsions without obsessions are very rare but can occur. An example is a man who had a compulsion to imagine each number plate he saw with the numbers transformed in a certain way (e.g. multiplied by two or squared). The relationship between the obsession and the compulsion is perhaps best understood in the context of all the key variables which are associated with an obsessive-compulsive experience. These are presented schematically in Table 9.1.

Table 9.1 Elements of an obsessional-compulsive experience

A	(i) Trigger	External/internal/none
	(ii) Obsession	Thought/image/impulse/none
	(iii) Discomfort	+
	(iv) Compulsive urge	+/−
	(v) Compulsive behaviour	Motor/cognitive/none
	(vi) Discomfort reduction	+/?
B	(i) Fears of disaster	+/−
	(ii) Reassurance seeking	+/−
	(iii) Avoidance	+/−

This scheme will fit most obsessive-compulsive episodes if these are taken as discrete events, which most of them are. This is not to say that all the elements given in the table are found in every single obsessional experience; nor is there always an invariant sequence of them, although most would follow the order given under A (i to vi). A patient's main problem may be the recurrent intrusion (A-ii) of the thought and associated visual image that he may have killed someone. This thought might be triggered (A-i) by the hearing or reading of news of murders and other violent acts (external trigger) and, less frequently, whenever he remembers a dead relation (internal trigger). The cognition is hard to dismiss and results in a strong feeling of discomfort, or even anxiety (A-iii). Associated with this may be a sharply felt urge (A-iv) to look at his hands. More often than not he will yield to this urge and so indulge in this compulsive behaviour (A-v). The compulsion may well follow a set pattern with his looking first at the left hand and then at the right with the whole sequence being followed three times. Completion of the compulsion markedly reduces the feeling of discomfort (A-vi). This marks the end of the obsessive-compulsive episode and the victim may then be relatively free of this experience for several hours until the whole thing becomes triggered off once more.

Is other examples a trigger may lead to an intrusive image, and to discomfort, with a compulsive urge which is translated into cognitive compulsive behaviour. A woman complained of being assailed by images (A-ii) of asymmetrical patterns or objects. In her case the compulsive behaviour (A-v) was to imagine or visualize the offending patterns or objects in a perfect symmetrical form. Doing so brought relief (A-vi). Other instances may only involve the distressing intrusive cognition without any compulsive act or urge. Mention was made above of the young woman who had thoughts and images of her wedding (A-ii). The cognitions particularly centred on the flower arrangements at the reception which she felt were not right. These thoughts assailed her repetitively, they were hard to dismiss and caused distress (A-iii). She had no associated compulsive behaviour, either overt or covert. As also mentioned above, a small number of cases have a compulsive urge with resultant compulsive behaviour with no preceding obsession. This is the case for a young woman who always had to look at the four corners (A-v) of any room she entered. Entering a room was the trigger (A-i) for this urge (A-iv) but there was no intrusive cognition (obsession). Finally, there are a small number of cases where the carrying out of the compulsive behaviour does not bring about a reduction of the discomfort/anxiety and may even increase it (Beech 1971).

This account and examples do not illustrate the factors under B in Table 9.1, although these may be present in a good number of cases. Fears of disaster (B-i) are common and can be manifest at the occurrence of the obsession (A-ii), or even upon exposure to the trigger (A-i). They contribute to the discomfort felt by the person (A-iii) and thus to the strength of the compulsive urge (A-iv). Many patients resort to reassurance seeking (B-ii) which they usually receive from their family members. Often an obsessional thought (A-ii) in the form of a doubt (e.g. 'Did I do it correctly?', or 'Was it done the right way') leads to this externally elicited form of relief. Avoidance (B-iii) is found in many cases where there is a clear external trigger to set off the whole experience. Thus a woman who gets the thought that she might attack her own children with knives or other sharp objects (A-ii) and mainly in the presence of such items (A-i), may avoid knives, scissors, etc. when she is on her own (B-iii). Patients who have obsessions about contamination by dirt or germs, usually leading to extensive cleaning and washing rituals if exposed to stimuli that they believe are contaminating, tend to avoid such situations as far as possible. In extreme cases a patient may have only a small safe area in the home where he/she can move about freely. A patient may not wash in the morning, for example, because this behaviour requires a long, complicated ritual. Another may go to bed in his day clothes to avoid prolonged and exhausting compulsions involved in changing.

Resistance

It has already been mentioned that both the obsession and the compulsion may be resisted by the sufferer. In his much quoted paper, Sir Aubrey Lewis (1936) argued that the central and indeed essential feature of obsessive-compulsive disorder was the strong resistance that the patient had. More recent studies (e.g. Rachman & Hodgson 1980, Stern & Cobb 1978) have shown that whilst resistance is very common it is not found invariably. It is possible that in the early stages a patient may resist his obsessions and/or compulsive urges strenuously, but after repeated failures over a period of time may begin to show much less resistance. There are chronic obsessive-compulsive patients where resistance to symptoms is quite low (Rasmussen & Tsuang 1986).

Other key terms

Other terms used to describe aspects of obsessive-compulsive disorders need to be mentioned. A *ritual* in the present context is a compulsive behaviour, either overt or covert, which has a rigid set pattern or sequence of steps with a clear-cut beginning and end. An example is a checking ritual where a system of checks is carried out in an invariant sequence. Most compulsive behaviours have a ritualistic quality to them. A *rumination* is a train of thoughts, usually unproductive and prolonged, on a particular topic. A young man had complicated and time-consuming ruminations on the question 'Am I genetically flawed?'. He would ruminate on this for long periods, going over various considerations and arguments and contemplating what superficially appeared as evidence. A rumination has no satisfactory conclusion, nor is there a set sequence of steps with a clear-cut end point, so it is different from a cognitive ritual. Not surprisingly, ruminations are hard to classify as either obsessions or compulsions. The decisive issue is whether they come as an intrusive experience, in which case they would fall into the category of obsessions, or whether there is a compulsive urge to think through a topic, in which case they would be compulsions. Clinically, it seems to be the case that most ruminations are compulsions and that they are usually preceded by an obsession. To illustrate this, the intrusive cognition 'Am I mad' or 'Am I going mad' would lead to the compulsive urge to think through the subject. The muddled 'thinking through' that follows is the rumination.

Primary slowness

Another category of obsessive-compulsive disorder which may present difficulties in terms of analysis is what has been described as 'primary obsessional slowness'. Rachman (1974) identified a small group of obsessive-compulsive patients whose behaviour was characterized by extreme slowness and which was not secondary to other rituals or ruminations. The behaviours most affected in this way seem to be in relation to self-care, such as washing, shaving, bathing and dressing (Rachman & Hodgson 1980). The patient takes a long time to accomplish these activities, often dwelling at each stage and moving in small, slow steps. The available data indicate that this slowness may best be seen as the result of a compulsive urge to engage in the behaviours in question in certain specific ways, making sure that each step is properly carried out.

Content of obsessions and compulsions

The main defining features of obsessive-compulsive disorders are the formal characteristics of the phenomena rather than their content (see also Reed 1985). However, it is clear that there are certain common themes that form the subject of these experiences. The data from empirical studies (Akhtar et al 1975, Dowson 1977, Rachman & Hodgson 1980, Rasmussen & Tsuang 1986, Reed 1985) show that contamination and dirt, disease and illness, violence and aggression, and moral and religious topics are amongst the most common. There are also symptoms related to order involving symmetry, numbers and sequence. Also found are sexually related themes. An investigation of the 'preparedness' (Seligman 1970, 1971) of the content of the obsessions in clinical series in London (de Silva et al 1977) showed that most of these were highly 'prepared' in the sense that they could be considered to be biologically relevant for humans in terms of their evolutionary significance. In this they are like most phobias. Thus, while obsessive-compulsive disorders are defined by their formal properties, it has to be recognized that their content is neither random nor widely diverse. Indeed, the commonality of content across different cultures is remarkable (Akhtar et al 1975).

The question of normality

An important issue is whether obsessive-compulsive disorders are a clinical entity entirely discontinuous from normal behaviour and experience or whether they are only quantitatively different from the normal. The apparent bizarreness of many obsessive-compulsive symptoms has encouraged some writers to consider the disorder as very different from normal behaviour and experience. Some have even maintained that obsessive-compulsive symptoms are a defence against a psychotic breakdown, and that many obsessive-compulsives may end up being schizophrenic (e.g. Bleuler 1955). There is no clear evidence that this is the case (for a review see Black 1974, Rachman & Hodgson 1980). Yet some features of the disorder certainly lend themselves to being seen as very abnormal and bizarre. Recent findings on the strength with which some of these patients hold certain beliefs associated with their obsessions and compulsions leading to these being described as 'overvalued ideas' and even 'delusional', serve to emphasize this point (Foa 1979). While the behaviour and feelings of a phobic patient can be seen as an extreme manifestation of normal behaviour, at least some obsessive-compulsive symptoms seem qualitatively different from what is usually regarded as normal.

However, much of obsessive-compulsive symptomatology is not unique to the small number of persons who come for help and get labelled as having 'obsessive-compulsive neurosis'. The two main characteristics of the disorder, the obsession and the compulsion, are not infrequently found in normal persons. In a study designed to assess the prevalence and characteristics of obsessions in a non-clinical population, Rachman & de Silva (1978) found that a very large proportion of normals did have obsessions remarkably similar to their clinical counterparts. The figure was around 80%. Both in form and content, these obsessions were very similar to, and indeed indistinguishable from, those reported by obsessive-compulsive patients. The main differences were those of degree of severity. These findings have been replicated by Salkovskis & Harrison (1984). This is not a surprising finding when one considers the essential nature of an obsession. An obsession is an unwanted cognition that intrudes into consciousness, and there are many studies showing that certain experiences, usually stressful, tend to cause intrusive cognitions. A case in point is the impressive series of studies by Horowitz (1969, 1975), and comparable data come from the more recent literature on post-traumatic stress disorder (e.g. Laufer et al 1984). The main differences between these phenomena and clinical obsessions are that the latter are more persistent, more repetitive, may cause more discomfort, and are harder to remove. In addition, in the clinical cases there is often no clear experience that can be recalled as having led directly to the particular cognition in question. The content of some obsessions is also impersonal and a direct link with any previous stress experience cannot then be assumed (de Silva 1986).

As for compulsions, it is clear that many people do have superstitious and stereotyped behaviours that resemble clinical compulsive behaviour. More importantly, a number of people who never come to clinics or hospitals do have compulsive behaviours very much like those of their clinical counterparts, although not as disabling (Rachman & Hodgson 1980, Lewis 1965). A recent report by Frost et al (1986) provides clear evidence of this. Nearly 10% of a sample of 384 people scored 5 or more (range of possible scores 0–9) on the checking subscale of the Maudsley Obsessional-Compulsive Inventory (MOCI). Only 34% were completely free of 'symptoms' (i.e. scored 0). In a second study of 148 female students the proportion of checkers, as determined by the same criterion, was 12%, with only 19% being complete non-checkers. The typical checking behaviours that these non-clinical subjects engaged in were very similar to those of compulsive patients; e.g. checking to make sure that doors are looked, checking that appliances are turned off, and checking clothing for dirt. A recent Italian study (Sanavio & Vidotto 1985) using the MOCI showed checking, contamination and cleaning, doubts and intrusive thoughts and, in males, slowness in a large ($N = 868$) non-clinical sample.

Obsessional personality

A further issue is the relationship of obsessive-compulsive disorders to what has been described as the obsessional or compulsive personality. There have been different views expressed by writers and clinicians on this issue. One view is that the obsessive-compulsive disorder is an exaggeration of the obsessive-compulsive personality. In Freudian terms this is the 'anal-erotic' personality. A second view is that those with the disorder have an obsessional premorbid personality. The obsessional (or anankastic) personality is considered to be characterized by orderliness, meticulousness, parsimony. neatness and perfectionism. The evidence for the presumed relationship between the disorder and personality is not strong. The problems involved in assessing personality reliably, not to mention premorbid personality, make the relationship difficult to evaluate satisfactorily (Rachman & Hodgson 1980). In a detailed review, Pollak (1979) concluded that as a cluster of traits, obsessive-compulsive personality appears to have empirical validity and that it can be statistically differentiated from the symptoms of obsessive-compulsive disorder through factor analysis. On the whole clinical data indicate that a proportion of obsessive-compulsive patients do have the personality traits premorbidly but that there are many who do not (Cooper 1983, Lewis 1965, Rack 1977, Rosenberg 1967a). Equally important is the fact that a large majority of those with the obsessional personality do not develop the disorder at all.

THEORETICAL APPROACHES

The literature offers many theories and models aimed at explaining obsessive-compulsive disorders. For the most part, the tendency has been to assume that the disorders represent a unitary phenomenon with each theoretical model being offered to account for a diversity of symptoms and presentations. More recent reviews (e.g. de Silva 1986, Rachman 1982, 1985, Sturgis 1984) suggest that such a unitary view may be mistaken. Apart from the fact that obsessions and compulsions are distinct phenomena there are also differences between subgroups of patients with compulsive rituals. Rachman & Hodgson (1980) and Foa and her team (Foa et al 1980, Steketee et al 1982), amongst others, have documented important differences between those whose main compulsions are checking behaviours and those whose main problem consists of washing and cleaning rituals. It is important to recognize this diversity in proffering and evaluating theories for explaining these disorders. It must also be noted that the accounts offered for the aetiology of the disorders may not be adequate to account for their maintenance, and vice versa.

Aetiological factors

Before discussing the various theories it is necessary to take a brief look at what is known about factors influencing the aetiology of obsessive-compulsive disorders. The data on aetiology are often weak and mostly obtained retrospectively. In many cases no specific time of onset can be established. In cases with a reported acute onset a single, clear precipitating event is often not found, although stresses of various sorts in the period of time leading up to onset are often reported. These stresses are of a general kind such as overwork, sexual and marital problems, and the illness/death of a close relative (Emmelkamp 1982, Rachman & Hodgson 1980).

The role of social learning processes in the aetiology of these disorders has also been discussed (e.g. Rachman & Hodgson 1980). There does not seem to be much strong evidence for direct vicarious conditioning or for observational learning, although the latter may be a factor in some cases. Where social learning may have a role in aetiology it has been suggested that the learning is more likely to be that of general behaviour patterns such as overdependence and timidity, usually fostered by parental attitudes, rather than of any specific compulsive behaviours. These general patterns are thought to make the individual more vulnerable to the development of obsessive-compulsive problems.

The possible role of genetic factors has also been explored. Firstly, there are reports of familial aggregation. There is an increased rate of psychiatric disorder among the parents and siblings of obsessive-compulsive patients (Kringlen 1965, Rosenberg 1967b, Slater & Cowie 1971). Whilst there is an increased rate of phobias and anxiety states, there is not a particularly strong specific association with obsessive-compulsive disorders. On the other hand, Carey & Gottesman (1981) examined relatives of obsessive-compulsive patients and found raised rates of both obsessive-compulsive neurosis and obsessional personality features among the parents, siblings and children of the patient group. These findings need to be interpreted with caution since social learning and other psychological factors cannot be ruled out as contributing to these higher than average rates. Secondly, there are some twin studies. The relative rarity of the disorder makes large twin studies difficult and so firm conclusions are not warranted on the basis of the available data. However, there are interesting findings. Carey & Gottesman (1981) have shown a higher concordance rate among monozygotic than dizygotic twins as far as obsessive-compulsive neurosis is concerned. Similarly, Murray et al (1981) have reported a considerable genetic contribution to 'obsessionality' (both traits and symptoms) in a large series of normal twins. Crucial studies of monozygotic twins reared apart would give a more definite estimate of the genetic contribution to the disorder but are lacking. At the moment it appears that there may be a genetic contribution which is probably in the form of a general emotional oversensitivity or neuroticism, and which predisposes the individual to develop the disorder.

It appears then that the genesis of obsessive-compulsive disorders is influenced by a multiplicity of factors, possibly including a genetic predisposition, social learning as mediated by parental modelling and parental control in childhood, and various life stresses and learning experiences. With these in mind let us now turn to the theories.

The psychoanalytic approach

Historically the oldest and best-known theoretical account of obsessive-compulsive disorders is the psychoanalytic one. Freud's writings on obsessive-compulsive problems display different and changing views over time (e.g. 1895, 1913). What is loosely described as the psychoanalytic view is in fact a version of these as developed by later writers such as Fenichel (1945). Repressed memories, desires and conflicts are held to be the source of neurotic anxiety which manifests itself as various symptoms. Fixation at a particular stage of psychosexual development, caused by various factors during the formative years, determines the nature of the manifest problem when the neurosis appears in later life. Obsessive-compulsive disorders are assumed to be linked to the anal-sadistic stage of development in which toilet training is a major feature and with which anger and aggression are also associated. Those who do not successfully negotiate this phase of psychosexual development are vulnerable to obsessive-compulsive problems in later years.

Although interesting the psychoanalytic theory does not lend itself to empirical testing and the available literature offers little in the way of convincing evidence in its support.

The learning approach

The behavioural/learning view has been more widely held and discussed in recent years and derives from Mowrer's two-factor theory of learning (1939,

1960). Certain stimuli and situations may acquire anxiety-producing properties by a process of classical conditioning. On later occasions the anxiety (conditioned emotional response) which results from exposure to the conditioned stimulus is terminated by an escape or avoidance response. This produces anxiety relief, thus reinforcing the response. This is a case of instrumental conditioning. Extending these views to obsessive-compulsive behaviour it is assumed that the compulsive acts are performed in response to anxiety generated by certain stimuli, which may include the individual's own obsessions, and are strengthened as a result of the anxiety reduction that follows (Dollard & Miller 1950). The model is essentially one of learned anxiety reduction.

Rachman & Hodgson (1980) have suggested that in these patients the critical negative emotion should be considered as discomfort rather than anxiety since in many cases patients report feelings other than those of anxiety. The view is then that discomfort reduction is the crucial element in the maintenance of obsessive-compulsive behaviour.

There is considerable evidence in general support of this position. The studies of Rachman and his associates carried out in London in the 1970s provide appreciable corroboration (Hodgson & Rachman 1972, Rachman et al 1976, Rachman & Hodgson 1980, Roper & Rachman 1975, Roper et al 1973). In these experiments it was found that both checkers and cleaners show heightened anxiety/discomfort when exposed to certain situations and/or stimuli (cues) which normally generated their ritualistic behaviours. For example, a cleaner made to touch an item which he believed to be contaminated would typically report a marked heightening of anxiety or discomfort. When the compulsive behaviour, e.g. hand-washing, was carried out there was considerable reduction in discomfort. Associated with the discomfort, and following the same course, was the compulsive urge subjectively felt by the patient. In a small number of cases the execution of the compulsive behaviour actually led to an increase in discomfort. Nevertheless, despite the exceptions, the model appears to be robust.

Further evidence supporting the model comes from two sources. Likierman & Rachman (1980) showed that repeated trials of exposure to cues in the same patient led to progressively lower levels of both discomfort and felt compulsive urge, and to progressively quicker dissipation of this under conditions of response prevention (i.e. the patient not being allowed to carry out his compulsive behaviour). This shows that there is a cumulative effect in repeated exposure to discomfort cues or, in other words, a habituation process. This fits well into the discomfort reduction model. If the compulsive behaviours were maintained by the reduction of anxiety/discomfort achieved by carrying out the behaviour, then the prevention of these behaviours in the presence of the relevant cues should have certain effects. With repeated exposures the urge to engage in the compulsive behaviours, and the behaviours themselves, should gradually reduce. This is exactly what the Likierman & Rachman (1980) experiment demonstrated. The second line of supporting evidence comes from the numerous treatment studies of obsessive-compulsive patients using the exposure–response prevention paradigm which generally fit in with the discomfort reduction model. These studies are summarized in detail elsewhere (e.g. Emmelkamp 1982, Foa et al 1985, Marks 1981, Rachman 1982, 1985) and will not be further covered here.

Difficulties for the learning approach

The discomfort reduction aspect of this approach is thus supported by both experimental and treatment studies, although the exceptions in which the ritual actually increases anxiety must be acknowledged to be a problem. On the other hand, the theory is on less sure grounds with regard to the aetiology of the disorder. Why is it that only certain types of stimuli tend to lead to these behaviours, as shown by de Silva et al (1977)? Why is it that many patients do not have a traumatic (conditioning) experience as the starting point for their problem behaviours? The criticisms of the Mowrer two-factor theory as a model for neurosis are well known and need not be repeated here (Eysenck 1976, Rachman 1977). Dollard & Miller (1950) proposed that certain behaviour patterns which previously led to anxiety reduction, such as hand-washing or checking, become exaggerated and take the form of compulsions. For example, washing in childhood is often associated with avoidance of, or escape from, parental criticism. However, how and why some behaviours turn into adult compulsions, or why only some individuals are subject to them, is not explained. Also the learning model does not offer much help in understanding obsessions that are not accompanied by compulsive behaviours. Finally the elaborate, repetitive, and even bizarre nature of compulsive behaviour which is best seen as active avoidance, unlike the passive avoidance found in phobias (cf. Gray 1982, Rachman & Hodgson 1980), needs to be explained more fully than the conditioning theory would allow.

Data from animal avoidance learning

Some writers have examined the animal-learning literature as a possible source of understanding of obessive-compulsive disorders. In a key paper, Teasdale (1974) suggested that compulsive behaviours may be considered as avoidance behaviours which are under poor stimulus control. They are reminiscent of the unnecessarily high frequency of responses shown by animals in experiments using the Sidman avoidance paradigm, where the delivery of the shock is unsignalled (Sidman 1955). Compulsive rituals can also be seen as not having good feedback or safety-signal properties and hence their inefficiently high rate of occurrence (Rachman & Hodgson 1980, Teasdale 1974). For example, a patient will not know easily whether the germs he is trying to wash off have been effectively removed since there is no safety signal or feedback to indicate that this has happened. The same applies to many checking rituals intended to ward off future disasters.

Another aspect of the avoidance literature which has been cited as possibly relevant comes from the findings of Fonberg (1956), as cited by Wolpe (1958). In this study, she first trained dogs to make a response (e.g. leg-lifting) to avoid an aversive stimulus. They were then subjected to a second conditioning procedure aimed at inducing an experimental 'neurosis' by making the required discrimination increasingly difficult. As the animals' behaviour became more and more 'neurotic', it was observed that they began to show the previously learned avoidance response (leg-lifting) at a high frequency, although no more discriminative stimuli for this particular response were presented. What seemed to be happening was that a response learned to avoid aversive stimulation re-emerged in a different setting when anxiety was induced in a different way. The relevance of this to the present topic is that it appears to provide a parallel for the wide variety of situations in which compulsive behaviours are performed by the patient.

Other examples from animal-learning studies that have been cited as possibly throwing light on these disorders include the much quoted Solomon et al (1953) study of traumatic avoidance in dogs, and Maier's (1949) work on fixation in rats. In the former a well-learned avoidance response became stereotyped in nature. These stereotyped responses persisted for hundreds of trials, despite the absence of further exposures to the aversive stimulus. In the Maier experiment, animals developed extremely strong fixations after being repeatedly forced to jump from a Lashley jumping stand in an insoluble problem situation. Maier reported that the behaviour showed a clearly compulsive quality in that the rats went on making the fixated response even after the problem had been made soluble. Even more interesting were behavioural signs that they 'knew' the correct response; as when the rat with a right position fixation would orient itself to the left (which was now the correct side) but still jump to the right.

Thus there are several findings from animal avoidance learning which have been considered as possibly relevant to the understanding of obsessive-compulsive disorders. None of these provides a full, or even closely approximate, analogy. However, they throw some light on the possible ways in which obsessive-compulsive behaviours may be acquired, why they occur in different settings, why some of them appear unrelated to the situation in which they are manifest, and why they are strongly persistent.

Other approaches

Beech and Perigault

It was noted that there are exceptional cases in whom the carrying out of the compulsive ritual does not reduce discomfort but actually increases it.

The theory offered by Beech & Perigault (1974) assumes that this is in fact the case with most rituals. They consider that rituals are behaviours that cause a deterioration in mood. They also propose that moods are central to the generation of obsessional thoughts and thus these patients are particularly vulnerable to mood disturbances. According to them the thoughts are the result of the patient's attempt to explain the negative mood. Although mood disturbance does have an association with obsessive-compulsive disorder the overall evidence for the Beech–Perigault position is not particularly strong. In any case its applicability is restricted to a small proportion of patients. Most patients do show discomfort reduction upon completion of the ritual and thus would not fit into this model.

Beech & Perigault (1974) have also suggested that those who develop obsessive-compulsive disorders may be prone to a high level of arousal. This in turn could lead them to be particularly vulnerable not only to classical or avoidance learning, but also to pseudo-conditioning, one-trial learning and poor habituation. There is some tentative evidence that these patients may be subject to chronic overarousal (Turner et al 1985). This is also consistent with their high level of neuroticism (Turner & Michelson 1984).

Cognitive deficit approaches

It has been suggested that these patients have a major difficulty in decision making which may explain their symptoms (e.g. Beech & Liddell 1974, Milner et al 1971). Reed (1976, 1985) has also emphasized this aspect of obsessive-compulsive problems. There is some evidence of this (Volans 1976) but it is not clear that it can be taken as an explanation of obsessive-compulsive phenomena. Emmelkamp (1982) has argued that the decision-making difficulty could equally well be a consequence of the symptoms. The proper evaluation of decision-making difficulties in these disorders must await further investigation.

Adopting a somewhat different approach, Carr (1974) has argued that obsessive-compulsive patients make very high subjective estimates of the probability of aversive outcomes. Compulsive behaviours develop to reduce the threat of these outcomes. The behaviours lead to the relief of anxiety and reduce the subjective threat. Further arguments along these lines are presented by McFall & Wollersheim (1979).

A more general cognitive theory has been offered by Reed (summarized by Reed 1985). According to Reed the main problem is 'that the obsessional finds difficulty in the spontaneous structuring of experience and attempts to compensate for this by imposing artificial, rigidly defined boundaries, category limits, and time markers. The rigidity and specificity of definition themselves lead to further uncertainty as to the "appropriate" allocation of category items, schematization, completion times, etc.' (ibid., p. 220). Reed attempts to explain all the major phenomena of the disorder in terms of this central concept. For example, checking may be seen as a failure in 'terminating response', coupled with uncertainty in categorical-limit attributions. Rituals are an example of the imposition of artificial structure geared to the arbitrary definition of tasks and situations. A study by Persons & Foa (1984) provides some independent evidence of certain features of the thought patterns of ritualizers consistent with Reed's views. Ritualizers appeared to use 'complex concepts', i.e. concepts that are excessively complex and over-specific. There are further data on the possible role of cognitive deficits in obsessive-compulsive problems. Sher et al (1983) found that non-clinical compulsive checkers had poorer memories for prior actions than non-checkers. They were also found to underestimate their ability to distinguish memories of real and imagined events ('reality monitoring'). Both these factors were considered to contribute to checking rituals. A subsequent study by Sher et al (1984) confirmed the previous findings and also showed that compulsive checkers had a particular memory deficit for meaningfully linked sequences. Despite this work it is not yet possible to make a proper evaluation of Reed's position or of any other cognitive-deficit model. The postulated central deficit appears to assume too much uniformity in the phenomena. Both clinical and other data show too great a diversity. Such models also fail to take into account the selective nature of the content of obsessive-compulsive problems.

The use of a model derived from Beck

Another recent contribution (Salkovskis 1985) proposes an analysis in terms of Beck's concept of negative automatic thoughts (e.g. Beck 1967, 1976). Salkovskis takes the position of Rachman (1971, 1976) that intrusive cognitions are best regarded as internal stimuli. He argues that these provoke cognitive responses in the form of negative automatic thoughts concerning responsibility or blame for harm to self or others. This leads to such behaviours as overt rituals, asking for reassurance or cognitive compulsions. Salkovskis (1985) has offered a detailed analysis of the problems in question along these lines, also taking mood disturbance into account. Whilst this is an interesting approach it needs to be subjected to empirical test to substantiate the role of automatic thoughts in these experiences. Also the intrusive cognition is by itself quite anxiety arousing in many clinical cases and there is no need to assume mediation by a further link. In any case this model does not contradict the discomfort-reduction model, nor does it challenge the overall treatment strategy based on the latter.

New theories of anxiety

Foa and Kozak

Two new approaches to the understanding of all anxiety disorders have been proposed recently and deserve mention. The first is that of Foa &

Kozak (1985, 1986). Briefly, the theory takes as its starting point Lang's (1979) bio-informational theory, which states that fear exists as an information network in memory. This consists of information about the stimuli concerned, the fear responses and their meanings. This network or prototype is a programme for the fear behaviour itself which takes place when the affective memory is activated. Foa & Kozak (1985, 1986) have proposed that neurotic fears differ structurally from normal fears in that they are marked by the presence of erroneous estimates of threat, unusually high negative valence for the threatening event, and exaggerated response elements. They are also very resistant to modification. They argue that the persistence may be because of failure to access the fear network, either due to active avoidance or the fact that the content of the network is such that it precludes spontaneous encounters that evoke anxiety. In addition, there may be some impairment in the change mechanism itself, such as excessive arousal with failure to habituate, cognitive defences, faulty premises and erroneous rules of inference. Foa & Kozak (1985) give examples of different types of fear stimuli that may exist in obsessive-compulsive patients. Some would be characterized by excessive associations between the stimuli concerned and the anxiety response, and mistaken evaluations of possible harm from the stimuli. For others the fear responses may be associated with mistaken meaning rather than with a particular stimulus. An example of the former is a patient who fears catching venereal disease from public toilets and washes excessively to prevent this. The latter is exemplified by, say, someone who is disturbed by perceived asymmetry and has to rearrange objects to reduce anxiety. It is not the object that is feared in this case: the individual is disturbed by the view that certain arrangements are improper. It is suggested that whilst there is no one fear structure in obsessive-compulsive patients, they all seem to have an impairment in the rules for making inferences about harm. It is this that leads to persisting unnecessary and repetitious behaviours.

This is a promising view which has the advantage of avoiding the oversimplicity of some other learning-based models. The incorporation of cognitive factors into a learning/habituation model is an impressive feature and seems able to explain certain treatment failures (e.g. Foa 1979) more easily than other theories. These are patients whose beliefs about their compulsions are so strong that they are not easily modified by disconfirmation. It is plausible to assume that their inferential rules with regard to harm and related matters are impaired. The Foa and Kozak theory does not, however, take account of obsessions per se and this is a problem with several theories. It must be noted that it is not offered as an alternative to the learning view but as an elaboration of it.

Gray

The second view of anxiety is that of Gray (1982), which is based on the concept of the 'behavioural inhibition system' and with activity in this system constituting anxiety. The system responds to certain kinds of input (stimuli that warn of punishment and non-reward, novel stimuli and innate fear stimuli) with its outputs, which are inhibition of ongoing motor behaviour, increased arousal and increased attention to environmental stimuli. The main function of the system is to act as a monitor comparing actual with expected stimuli. Under conditions of mismatch between predicted and actual events, or in those where the predicted event is aversive, the system assumes a controlling function over behaviour. It then acts in various ways which include trying out new motor programmes. There are certain tasks which require the system to participate constantly in controlling behaviour. These are tasks containing multiple sources of interference which can be overcome only by the maximum use of the system's capacity for multidimensional comparison of stimuli and response patterns.

Gray (1982) states that the very occurrence of obsessions and the repetitiveness of most compulsions are both hard to explain by the learning-anxiety reduction model. He argues that his theory offers a more natural model. The behavioural inhibition system, which continually engages in a monitoring function, searches with particular care for those stimuli that are unexpected or threatening. If the system becomes hyperactive it will end up tagging too many stimuli as important and/or searching for them too persistently. The obsessive-compulsive patient thus scans his environment to an excessive degree for potential threats in the form of checking rituals. Certain rituals function both in a checking role and as active avoidance responses. Thus hand-washing is both an effective way of checking for dirt and a way to remove it, and this is why it is repetitive. If it were merely an active avoidance behaviour the repetition would not occur. Also the scanning for potential threats can extend to internal repositories of information concerning such threats. An illustration of such a scan may be when a patient, anxious about cutting himself, checks his memory to verify where he disposed of a razor blade. Secondly, there are some threats which are of purely internal origin (e.g. fear of one's own impulses). The checking of the system that produces the feared behaviour may in fact prime the system to produce it. Thus the obsessional impulses may come intrusively and repeatedly, arising from the very checking process that attempts to ensure their absence. A similar analysis can be applied to obsessive thoughts and images.

Gray attempts to explain the selectivity of obsessions and compulsions in a number of ways. For example, the concern with dirt and the related checking for dirt and cleaning behaviours may be of evolutionary significance and a parallel to grooming behaviour seen in certain animal species. This reflects the considerable danger dirt presents for survival. To cite another example, the concern for orderliness may arise from the fact that any disorder produces novel arrays of stimuli. This is a situation that, according to the theory, necessarily activates the behavioural inhibition system.

It is not possible to evaluate Gray's theory fully in the present context but some comments can be made. A model to account for both obsessions and compulsions is both ambitious and attractive but the evidence does not really favour a unitary mechanism. Also the view of something like cleaning rituals as checking-cum-cleaning behaviours does not fit in well with clinical observations. The model seems to be particularly strong in relation to checking compulsions but not so plausible in relation to other aspects of obsessive compulsive problems. In any case, even as a theory of anxiety Gray's model has yet to be fully evaluated in terms of the predictions that can be derived from it.

The explanation of obsessions

It is necessary at this point to discuss obsessions briefly. Many of the theoretical models address themselves to the origins and maintenance of compulsions, especially overt rituals. In theory they could apply equally well to cognitive rituals. If cognitive compulsive behaviour reduces discomfort then it is likely that it will be manifest to avoid impending discomfort. But what of the obsession, the intrusive cognition that in some cases occurs on its own and in others leads to a compulsion? In both these instances what is primarily needed is an explanation as to why the cognition occurs in the first place. This relatively neglected aspect of obsessive-compulsive disorder has only recently received systematic study. Following Rachman's (1971) view that such experiences may not be uncommon in the normal population, research has confirmed that normal people do have similar unwanted intrusive cognitions, or 'normal obsessions' (Parkinson & Rachman 1980, Rachman & de Silva 1978, Salkovskis & Harrison 1984). The amount of disturbance that they cause seems to determine how difficult they are to control (Rachman 1985). The discomfort they generate may lead to anxiety-reducing compulsions. It appears that their genesis may be related to stress, both contrived and uncontrived. Studies by Horowitz have shown that experimentally delivered traumatic input causes intrusions of related cognitions later on (e.g. Horowitz 1975). Similar intrusions are found in those undergoing uncontrived stress experiences (Rachman & Parkinson 1981). These common, normal experiences seem to be short-lived and removal of the stress dramatically reduces them. On the other hand, unresolved stress may cause them to become chronic. This would be especially so in cases where the initial stress is not clear-cut or where there are multiple stresses. Further, Sutherland et al (1982) have shown experimentally that depression helps to evoke unwanted intrusive cognitions and also makes these difficult to remove. In the light of present knowledge, perhaps the best explanation for the persistence of obsessions, and of how normal intrusions become more chronic and achieve clinically significant levels of severity, lies within the broad concept of emotional processing as proposed by Rachman (1980). Elements of stressful material which have not been successfully processed emotionally, may appear in an intrusive way from time to time and cause distress. This can, and indeed does, happen to most people. The individual is more vulnerable to these when mood is low and when affected by fresh stresses. In those who are predisposed in certain ways (whether genetic, due to early social experiences, or whatever), such experiences are likely to become more persistent, more intense, more distressing, and more difficult to control. While in some cases the intrusion directly reflects the stress, in others it may do so only indirectly or in a fragmented form. In numerous cases where the obsession is associated with a compulsion, the explanation of the compulsion is still plausible along the lines of discomfort reduction. It is interesting that Foa & Kozak (1986) also make use of the concept of emotional processing as a major part of their theory.

Concluding comments

When all is considered where do the different theoretical positions stand? It is clear that none of the existing theoretical accounts provides a fully satisfactory explanation of obsessive-compulsive disorders. The discomfort reduction aspect of the learning approach is, on the whole, broadly plausible for explaining the maintenance or persistence of compulsive behaviours. However, the aetiology, selectivity and nature of these behaviours cannot be easily accommodated within a simple learning model, although some of the phenomena resemble certain experimentally produced instances of avoidance learning. Clinical investigations point to a multiply determined aetiology with influences from inheritance, social learning, stress and mood disturbance. There also seems to be a preparedness factor determining content. Specific traumatic conditioning experiences are not widespread. Obsessions seem most likely to be stress linked and their persistence is best explained in terms of poor emotional processing. If a unitary explanation is sought for both obsessions and compulsions, the lack of satisfactory processing may still be seen as the major explanatory concept. This would still need to incorporate discomfort reduction to account for the maintenance of compulsions. Models based on information processing and other cognitive deficits provide interesting insights into some aspects of the disorder, but evidence for their validity as general explanations is weak. Gray's theory, which attempts a single account of both obsessions and compulsions within his model of anxiety, has yet to be tested. As it stands at present it has to depend upon various assertions about the phenomena which are not well supported by clinical observations. The Foa–Kozak theory has many promising features and awaits evaluation.

There is still some way to go before a really satisfactory account of the phenomena associated with obsessive-compulsive disorders can be achieved. It is entirely possible that several explanations will be needed in order to cope with the different phenomena that can appear. The existing accounts provide an impetus for further investigation in offering specific predictions that can be tested. The newer theories are particularly welcome in that they offer new lines for research.

ACKNOWLEDGEMENT

The author wishes to thank David R. Hemsley for his comments on an earlier draft of this chapter.

REFERENCES

Akhtar S, Wig N N, Varma V K, Pershad L, Verma S K 1975 A phenomenological analysis of symptoms in obsessive-compulsive neurosis. British Journal of Psychiatry 127: 342–348
American Psychiatric Association 1980 Diagnostic and statistical manual of mental disorders, 3rd edn. APA, Washington
Beck A T 1967 Depression: clinical, experimental, and theoretical aspects. University of Pennsylvania Press, Philadelphia
Beck A T 1976 Cognitive therapy and the emotional disorders. International Universities Press, New York
Beech H R 1971 Ritualistic activity in obsessional patients. Journal of Psychosomatic Research 15: 417–422
Beech H R, Liddell A 1974 Decision-making, mood states and ritualistic behaviour among obsessional patients. In: Beech H R (ed) Obsessional states. Methuen, London
Beech H R, Perigault J 1974 Toward a theory of obsessional disorder. In: Beech H R (ed) Obsessional states. Methuen, London
Black A 1974 The natural history of obsessional neurosis. In: Beech H R (ed) Obsessional states. Methuen, London
Bleuler E 1955 Dementia praecox or group of schizophrenias. International Universities Press, New York
Carey G, Gottesman I I 1981 Twin and family studies of anxiety, phobic and obsessive disorders. In: Klein D F, Rabkin J (eds) Anxiety: new research and changing concepts. Raven, New York
Carr A 1974 Compulsive neurosis: a review of the literature. Psychological Bulletin 81: 311–318
Cooper J E 1983 Obsessional illness and personality. In: Russell G F M, Hersov L A (eds) The neuroses and personality disorders. Cambridge University Press, Cambridge
de Silva P 1986 Obsessional-compulsive imagery. Behaviour Research and Therapy 24: 333–350
de Silva P, Rachman S J, Seligman M E P 1977 Prepared phobias and obsessions: therapeutic outcome. Behaviour Research and Therapy 15: 65–78
Dollard J, Miller N E 1950 Personality and psychotherapy: an analysis in terms of learning, thinking, and culture. McGraw-Hill, New York
Dowson J H 1977 The phenomenology of severe obsessive-compulsive disorders. British Journal of Psychiatry 131: 75–78
Emmelkamp P M G 1982 Phobic and obsessive-compulsive disorders: theory, research and practice. Plenum, New York
Eysenck H J 1976 The learning model of neurosis: a new approach. Behaviour Research and Therapy 14: 251–268
Fenichel 0 1945 The psychoanalytic theory of neurosis. Norton, New York
Foa E B 1979 Failure in treating obsessive-compulsives. Behaviour Research and Therapy 16: 391–399
Foa E B, Kozak M J 1985 Treatment of anxiety disorders: implications for psychopathology. In: Tuma A H, Maser J D (eds) Anxiety and the anxiety disorders. Erlbaum: Hillside, NJ
Foa E B, Kozak M J 1986 Emotional processing of fear: exposure to corrective information. Psychological Bulletin 99: 20–25
Foa E B, Steketee G, Turner R M, Fischer S C 1980 Effects of imaginal exposure to feared

disasters in obsessive-compulsive checkers. Behaviour Research and Therapy 18: 449–455
Foa E B, Steketee G, Ozarow B J 1985 Behavior therapy with obsessive-compulsives: from theory to treatment. In: Mavissakahian M, Turner S M, Michelson L (eds) Obsessive-compulsive disorders: psychological and pharmacological treatments. Plenum, New York
Freud S 1895 Obsessions and phobias. In: Strachey J (ed) Standard edition of the complete psychological works of Sigmund Freud. Hogarth, London, 3: 45–61
Freud S 1913 The disposition to obsessional neurosis. In: Strachey J (ed) Standard edition of the complete psychological works of Sigmund Freud. Hogarth, London, 12: 317–326
Frost R O, Sher K J, Geen T 1986 Psychopathology and personality characteristics of nonclinical compulsive checkers. Behaviour Research and Therapy 24: 133–143
Gray J A 1982 The neuropsychology of anxiety. Clarendon, Oxford
Hare E, Price J, Slater E 1972 Fertility in obsessional neurosis. British Journal of Psychiatry 121: 197–205
Hodgson R J, Rachman S J 1972 The effects of contamination and washing in obsessional patients. Behaviour Research and Therapy 10: 111–117
Horowitz M 1969 Psychic trauma: return of images after a stress film. Archives of General Psychiatry 20: 552–559
Horowitz M 1975 Intrusive and repetitive thoughts after experimental stress. Archives of General Psychiatry 32: 1457–1463
Janet P 1903 Les obsessions et la psychasthénie. Alcan, Paris
Jaspers K 1923 General psychopathology (translated by Hoenig J, Hamilton M W 1963). University of Chicago Press, Chicago
Kringlen E 1965 Obsessional neurotics: a long-term follow-up. British Journal of Psychiatry 111: 709–722
Lang P 1979 A bio-informational theory of emotional imagery. Psychophysiology 16: 405–512
Laufer R S, Brett E A, Gallops M 1984 Post-traumatic stress disorder (PTSD) reconsidered: PTSD among Vietnam veterans. In: Van der Kolk B A (ed) Post-traumatic stress disorder: psychological and biological sequelae. American Psychiatric Press, Washington
Lewis A 1936 Problems of obsessional illness. Proceedings of the Royal Society of Medicine 29: 325–336
Lewis A 1965 A note of personality and obsessional illness. Psychiatria et Neurologia 150: 299–305
Likierman H, Rachman S J 1980 Spontaneous decay of compulsive urges: cumulative effects. Behaviour Research and Therapy 18: 387–394
McFall M G, Wollersheim J P 1979 Obsessive-compulsive neurosis: a cognitive-behavioral formulation and approach to treatment. Cognitive Therapy and Research 3: 333–348
Maier N R F 1949 Frustration: the study of behavior without a goal. McGraw-Hill, New York
Marks I M 1981 Cure and care of neuroses. Wiley, New York
Milner A D, Beech H R, Walker V J 1971 Decision processes and obsessional behaviour. British Journal of Social and Clinical Psychology 10: 88–89
Mowrer O H 1939 A stimulus–response theory of anxiety. Psychological Review 46: 553–565
Mowrer O H 1960 Learning theory and behavior. Wiley, New York
Murray R M, Clifford C, Fulker D W, Smith A 1981 Does heredity contribute to obsessional traits and symptoms? In: Tsuang M T (ed) Genetic issues. Academic, New York
Myers J K, Weissman M M, Tischler G L et al 1984 Six-month prevalence of psychiatric disorders in three communities. Archives of General Psychiatry 41: 959–962
Parkinson L, Rachman S J 1980 Are intrusive thoughts subject to habituation? Behaviour Research and Therapy 18: 409–418
Persons J B, Foa E B 1984 Processing of fearful and neutral information by obsessive-compulsives. Behaviour Research and Therapy 22: 259–265
Pollak J M 1979 Obsessive-compulsive personality: a review. Psychological Bulletin 86: 225–241
Rachman S J 1971 Obsessional ruminations. Behaviour Research and Therapy 9: 229–235
Rachman S J 1974 Primary obsessional slowness. Behaviour Research and Therapy 12: 463–471

Rachman S J 1976 The modification of obsessions: a new formulation. Behaviour Research and Therapy 14: 437-449
Rachman S 1977 The conditioning theory of fear acquisition: a critical examination. Behaviour Research and Therapy 15: 375-385
Rachman S J 1980 Emotional processing. Behaviour Research and Therapy 18: 51-60
Rachman S J 1982 Obsessional-compulsive disorders. In: Bellack A S, Hersen M, Kazdin A E (eds) International handbook of behavior modification and therapy. Plenum, New York
Rachman S J 1985 Obsessional-compulsive disorders. In: Bradley B P, Thompson C (eds) Psychological applications in psychiatry. Wiley, Chichester
Rachman S J, de Silva P 1978 Abnormal and normal obsessions. Behaviour Research and Therapy, 16: 233-248
Rachman S J, Hodgson R J 1980 Obsessions and compulsions. Prentice Hall, Englewood Cliffs
Rachman S J, Parkinson L 1981 Unwanted intrusive cognitions. Advances in Behaviour Research and Therapy 3: 89-123
Rachman S J, de Silva P, Roper G 1976 The spontaneous decay of compulsive urges. Behaviour Research and Therapy 14: 445-453
Rack P 1977 Clinical experience in the treatment of obsessional states. Journal of International Medical Research 5: 81-91
Rasmussen S A, Tsuang M T 1986 Clinical characteristics and family history in DSM-III obsessive-compulsive disorders. American Journal of Psychiatry 143: 317-322
Reed G F 1976 Indecisiveness in obsessional-compulsive disorder. British Journal of Social and Clinical Psychology 15: 443-445
Reed G F 1985 Obsessional experience and compulsive behaviour: a cognitive-structural approach. Academic, London
Robins L N, Helzer J L, Weissman M M et al 1984 Life time prevalence of specific psychiatric disorder in three sites. Archives of General Psychiatry 41: 949-958
Roper G, Rachman S J 1975 Obsessional-compulsive checking: replication and development. Behaviour Research and Therapy 14: 25-32
Roper G, Rachman S J, Hodgson R J 1973 An experiment on obsessional checking. Behaviour Research and Therapy 11: 271-277
Rosenberg C 1967a Personality and obsessional neurosis. British Journal of Psychiatry 113: 471-477
Rosenberg C 1967b Familial aspects of obsessional neurosis. British Journal of Psychiatry 114: 477-478
Salkovskis P M 1985 Obsessional-compulsive problems: a cognitive behavioural analysis. Behaviour Research and Therapy 23: 571-583
Salkovskis P M, Harrison J 1984 Abnormal and normal obsessions: a replication. Behaviour Research and Therapy 22: 549-552
Sanavio E, Vidotto G 1985 The components of the Maudsley Obsessional-Compulsive Questionnaire. Behaviour Research and Therapy 23: 659-662
Seligman M E P 1970 On the generality of the laws of learning. Psychological Review 77: 406-418
Seligman M E P 1971 Phobias and preparedness. Behavior Therapy 2: 307-320
Sher K J, Mann B, Frost R O, Otto R 1983 Cognitive deficits in compulsive checkers: an exploratory study. Behaviour Research and Therapy 21: 357-363
Sher K J, Frost R O 1984 Cognitive dysfunction in compulsive checkers: further exlorations. Behaviour Research and Therapy 22: 493-502
Sidman M 1955 Some properties of warning stimulus in avoidance behavior. Journal of Comparative and Physiological Psychology 48: 444-450
Slater E, Cowie V 1971 The genetics of mental disorders. Oxford University Press, London
Solomon R, Kamin L, Wynne L 1953 Traumatic avoidance learning: the outcomes of several extinction procedures with dogs. Journal of Abnormal and Social Psychology 48: 291-302
Steketee G, Foa E B, Grayson J B 1982 Recent advances in the behavioral treatment of obsessive-compulsives. Archives of General Psychiatry 39: 1365-1371
Stern R S, Cobb J P 1978 Phenomenology of obsessive-compulsive neurosis. British Journal of Psychiatry 132: 233-239

Sturgis E 1984 Obsessional and compulsive disorder. In Adams H E, Sutker P B (eds) Comprehensive handbook of psychopathology. Plenum, New York
Sutherland G, Newman B, Rachman S J 1982 Experimental investigations of the relation between mood and intrusive unwanted cognitions. British Journal of Medical Psychology 55: 127–138
Teasdale J 1974 Learning models of obsessional-compulsive disorder. In: Beech H R (ed) Obsessional states. Methuen, London
Turner S M, Michelson L 1984 Obsessive-compulsive disorders. In: Turner S M (ed) Behavioral theories and treatment of anxiety. Plenum, New York
Turner S M, Beidel D C, Nathan R S 1985 Biological factors in obsessive-compulsive disorders. Psychological Bulletin 97: 430–450
Volans P J 1976 Styles of decision-making and probability appraisal in selected obsessional and phobic patients. British Journal of Social and Clinical Psychololgy 15: 305–317
Wolpe J 1958 Psychotherapy by reciprocal inhibition. Stanford University Press, Stanford
World Health Organization 1978 Mental disorders: glossary and guide to their classification in accordance with the ninth revision of the International Classification of Diseases. WHO, Geneva

10   *Ronald Blackburn*

Psychopathy and personality disorder

PERSONALITY DISORDER AND PERSONALITY THEORY

Psychiatric conceptions

The identification of personality disorder represents an attempt to distinguish psychological abnormalities which are attributable to regularities in a person's behaviour from those which signal a discontinuity of function. In the most recent edition of the *International Classification of Diseases* (ICD 9: World Health Organization 1978), personality disorders are defined as: 'Deeply ingrained maladaptive patterns of behaviour generally recognizable by the time of adolescence or earlier and continuing throughout most of adult life, although often becoming less obvious in middle or old age. The personality is abnormal either in the balance of its components, their quality and expression, or in its total aspects'. The third edition of the *Diagnostic and Statistical Manual* (DSM III: American Psychiatric Association 1980) confines attention to personality traits, which are: '. . . enduring patterns of perceiving, relating to, and thinking about the environment and oneself, and are exhibited in a wide range of important social contexts. It is only when *personality traits* are inflexible and maladaptive and cause either significant impairment in social or occupational functioning or subjective distress that they constitute *Personality Disorders.*' ICD 9 identifies eight categories of disorder and DSM III eleven. The categories are listed in Table 10.1, and it will be seen that although there is substantial overlap, DSM III omits affective and explosive disorders, which are dealt with under other headings, and also includes several additional categories which are of relatively recent origin. This chapter will pay particular attention to the DSM III classification, which has generated more interest in this class of disorders than previous classifications.

It will be noted that the widely used category of psychopathic personality does not appear in Table 10.1. During the early part of the century, this term was a generic one covering all forms of personality disorder, and etymologically psychopathic means nothing more specific than 'psychic abnormality'. In ICD 9, abnormal personality is still referred to as 'this deviation or psychopathy'. However, since its introduction by Kraepelin in 1904, the

Table 10.1 Categories of Personality Disorder in DSM III and ICD 9 equivalents

DSM III	ICD 9
Paranoid	— Paranoid
Schizoid	— Schizoid
Schizotypal	
Histrionic	— Hysterical
Narcissistic	
Antisocial	— Personality disorder with predominantly asocial or sociopathic manifestations
Borderline	
Avoidant	
Dependent	— Asthenic
Compulsive	— Anankastic
Passive-aggressive	
	Affective
	Explosive

concept of psychopathic personality has undergone considerable transformation, and in more recent decades has been used in a narrower sense to denote deviations of an antisocial kind. The current equivalents are to be found in the 'sociopathic' category of ICD 9, and the antisocial personality disorder of DSM III.

Among the novel features of DSM III are the provision of operational criteria for the identification of each disorder, the affirmation that diagnostic labels describe *behaviours* rather than people, and the requirement that the clinician make diagnoses on both Axis I (Clinical Syndromes) and Axis II (Personality Disorders). This differentiation of two subsets of mental disorder does not imply any causal independence, and instances of more serious psychiatric disorder may commonly be extensions of coping strategies which characterize particular personality disorders (Millon 1981). The distinction is nevertheless consistent with the argument of Foulds (1971) that personality deviation and 'personal symptomatology' belong in different universes of discourse, and that a person may therefore exhibit either, neither or both. Clinicians and researchers have frequently failed to recognize this distinction, and the disjunctive use of an 'either–or' categorization is still not uncommon. In the past, this may have been reflected in observations that between 5% and 17% of the psychiatric population exhibited personality disorders (Lion 1981). Field trials of DSM III, however, indicated that the diagnosis was applicable to 50–60% of the adult psychiatric population sampled. Yet only a small amount of the research literature on psychopathology has been devoted to this subject.

Traits, consistency, and personality theory

Within psychology, personality refers to a field of investigation rather than a process or entity, but personality theories share the premise that there are stable attributes of the person which contribute to behaviour, and whose organization accounts for individual distinctiveness. The definition of personality disorders as inflexible and maladaptive traits reflects the traditional assumption that people are characterized by consistencies in their behaviour which manifest themselves in varying situations. However, the validity of this assumption has been challenged in recent years in the course of the 'person–situation' debate. If, as was earlier argued by Mischel (1968), social behaviour does not show appreciable cross-situational consistency, and trait ascriptions are largely illusions imposed by the conceptual categories of our 'implicit personality theories' (Shweder 1975), then the theoretical or practical value of identifying personality disorders must be doubted. While the controversy has abated in the wake of 'interactionist' solutions (Magnusson & Endler 1977), it has contributed to a decline of interest among clinicians in personality theory and assessment. It is also perhaps one reason why less than 4% of the space in recent textbooks of abnormal psychology has been devoted to personality disorders (Turkat & Alpher 1983). It is therefore appropriate to consider the current status of the trait concept in psychological theory.

One of the main objections to trait description appears to have been the implication that traits represent primary *causes* of behaviour. However, this assumption has been seriously entertained by only a few theorists, and the argument has centred less on *whether* attributes of the person are determinants of behaviour than on *what* it is that the person contributes. For example, reference to dispositions or tendencies is indispensable to any account of behaviour, whether they are 'generalized' (e.g. X is phobic), or 'situationally specific' (e.g. X panics in supermarkets). Both of these are dispositional statements, since the interest of psychologists is in behavioural *tendencies*, not unrepeated occurrences. Moreover, each of these examples refers to a property of the person, in the very real sense that it is the person who possesses the energy which produces action (Allport 1966). While it may be more useful to describe a person's behaviour in terms of specific rather than generalized dispositions for many purposes, this simply entails a narrowing of trait descriptions rather than their elimination (Alston 1975). Furthermore, the argument that generalized traits do not 'exist' in the form of cross-situational consistencies can no longer be sustained, since ample evidence is now available that individual differences in a number of socially relevant variables show substantial stability over time and setting (Block 1977, Hogan et al 1977, Olweus 1979, 1981, Epstein 1979, Epstein & O'Brien 1985).

There is, then, sufficient stability in behaviour to make useful probability statements about an individual's proclivities on the basis of trait measures which do not specify situations (Epstein & O'Brien 1985). This view does not deny the role of situations in constraining behaviour, nor does it imply a unidirectional causality from the person to behaviour. What traits refer to is behaviour *in the aggregate*, and they do not reliably predict single behavioural occurrences in specific situations. Similarly, a trait cannot be inferred from a single observation of behaviour. As they are summary descriptions of average behaviour, rather than statements about behavioural invariance, traits cannot provide a fundamental account of behaviour (Alston 1975), and a more complete explanation is provided by reference to cognitive-motivational variables, or what Alston calls 'the desire–belief structure'. With the exception of some radical behaviourists, most contemporary theorists appeal to such variables in accounting for behaviour. These include proponents of trait description (Olweus 1981, Epstein & O'Brien 1985) as well as social learning theorists (Mischel 1973, Bandura 1978) and psychodynamic writers (Erdelyi 1985). In this respect, there seems to be some agreement that traits provide a first step in describing the prominent features of a person's behavioural repertoire, but that reference to 'latent' dispositions in the form of cognitive structures and their interaction with environmental events is required to explain both consistency and variability.

Social learning theorists, such as Mischel, now appear to accept that people display cross-situationally consistent behaviour, but argue that this may be the exception rather than the rule. They reject mechanistic versions of interactionism in which people are seen to 'react' or 'emit behaviours' in different situational contexts on the basis of prior conditioning history, and instead argue for a reciprocal interaction between person, situation and behaviour (Bandura 1978). Thus, people *create* their environment by enacting behaviours, on the basis of goals and outcome and efficacy expectations. Environmental consequences in turn influence behaviour and expectations. In these terms, adaptive behaviour implies flexibility and situational discriminativeness. Inflexible behaviour is likely to reflect the influence of cognitive structures which override environmental consequences, or levels of 'construction competence' which do not match situational requirements. Personal consistency may therefore be particularly pronounced in maladjusted populations. Observations of aggressive children and adults support this view (Raush 1965, Blackburn 1984, Mischel 1984).

Current psychological approaches to personality disorder

Given that as much as a half of the psychiatric population may exhibit personality disorders, their neglect in the literature suggests that clinicians are reluctant to identify them, or that they call them something else (Turkat & Levin 1984). One likely reason is that people who might meet the criteria for a personality disorder often seek help only in the face of a personal crisis, and their problems may be identified as relatively focal emotional or relationship difficulties. However, even when a presenting problem is clearly long-standing, it may be identified in terms other than personality disorder. Social skills training is commonly directed towards behavioural difficulties related to the criteria for personality disorders, such as social avoidance, lack of assertiveness or anger control, but only rarely is reference made to personality disorder in this context. A major reason for this is the behaviourist model of social skill, which sees such behaviour in molecular terms and as 'highly situation specific' (Bellak 1983). Social skills training, however, has not been conspicuously successful, and Trower (1984) attributes this to the 'passive organism' model of behaviourism and to the neglect of person variables such as goals and expectations which are entailed in the active generation of a person's environment.

Some behaviourally oriented clinicians, however, seem prepared to accept a more molar concept of socially skilled behaviour. Turner & Hersen (1981) note that the syndromes of personality disorder amount to a classification of social problem behaviours, the common features being an inability to maintain satisfactory interpersonal relationships and to obtain gratification from the environment. They propose that these syndromes can be conceptualized as the outcome of an intricate reinforcement history characterized by complex reinforcement schedules which result in particular behaviours becoming dominant in several habit hierarchies. Inflexible traits, in these terms, reduce to classes of operant behaviours.

Marshall & Barbaree (1984) similarly conceptualize personality disorders as unskilful behaviours governed by discriminative cues and reinforcing consequences in particular social environments, but also draw on social learning analyses to include cognitive person variables. They propose that the traits held to characterize the different categories of personality disorder can be formulated in terms of consistent dysfunctional or maladaptive perceptions, cognitions or overt responses in an interpersonal context, and suggest that the various diagnostic criteria can be sorted into non-overlapping behavioural categories or dimensions describing different kinds of dysfunction.

A cognitive orientation to personality disorder is found in the work of interpersonal theorists such as Carson (1970, 1979) and McLemore & Benjamin (1979), who also see such disorders primarily as disturbances in social behaviour. Carson presents an analysis which explicitly relates interpersonal traits to cognitive-environment interactions. He suggests that most people develop a preferred 'style' of relating to others in the context of a differentiated repertoire. Preferred interpersonal style relates to beliefs and expectancies about self and others and entails the relatively persistent enactment of behaviours which elicit a complementary reaction from others. In turn, this yields information relevant to beliefs and expectations. Inflexible styles may result from aversive experiences, and are self-perpetuating. A hostile-dominant person, for example, anticipates hostility from others and behaves in a way which is likely to confirm this expectation. Snyder (1981) provides evidence for the pervasiveness of such self-fulfilling prophecies or 'self-confirmatory biases' in everyday activities. McLemore & Benjamin (1979) describe a more detailed form of this analysis which permits an examination of specific interpersonal behaviours as they occur in particular relationships or situational contexts.

In summary, then, psychiatric conceptions of personality disorder are congruent with several current psychological models, and may be construed in terms of stable and rigid interpersonal behavioural repertoires which fail to engender desirable outcomes for the person or others. Trait descriptions provide the first step in identifying such repertoires.

CLASSIFICATION OF PERSONALITY DISORDERS

Historical perspective

The relationship between the concepts of personality disorder and psychopathic personality continues to be a source of confusion in the clinical and research literature. The nature of this has been discussed by Pichot (1978) and Millon (1981), who identify both conceptual and terminological differences between English-speaking and German psychiatrists. At issue is the confounding of two universes of discourse, on the one hand the psychological universe of personality and personality deviation, and on the other the socio-cultural universe of society's rules and their violation. From both a scientific and clinical viewpoint it is of interest to know whether socially undesirable behaviour, such as criminal activity, substance abuse, or sexual deviation, is a *consequence* of particular personality dispositions, or whether particular dispositions make rule-violation more likely. However, a recurring theme in psychiatry has been the identification of a syndrome of psychopathic or antisocial *personality* on criteria of socially deviant activity alone. This not only pre-judges the question of the contribution of the person to undesirable forms of activity, but also contaminates the identification of a clinical syndrome with moral value judgement (Mowbray 1960, Millon 1981). Detailed and scholarly historical analyses are provided by Maughs (1941), as well as by Pichot and Millon. Here, an attempt is made to identify the significant punctuations in what was described by Cameron & Margaret (1951) as 'this tortuous and perplexing historical development'.

In 1837, Pritchard introduced the concept of 'moral insanity' to account for socially damaging or irresponsible behaviour which was not associated with known forms of mental disorder. Behaviour identified as morally objectionable was thereby attributed to a diseased 'moral faculty'. Despite resistance from many British psychiatrists, the influence of this concept persisted and was seen in the English Mental Deficiency Act of 1913, which described a class of 'moral imbeciles' as 'persons who from an early age display some permanent moral defect coupled with strong vicious or criminal propensities'. Pichot sees the persistence of this tradition in the legal category of Psychopathic Disorder of the English 1959 Mental Health

Act, which was defined as 'a persistent disorder or disability of mind ... which results in abnormally aggressive or seriously irresponsible conduct on the part of the patient, and requires or is susceptible to medical treatment'. The wording originally proposed was actually 'a persistent disorder of *personality*' (see Department of Health and Social Security 1975), but this was objected to on the quite logical grounds that personality disorder should not be inferred from antisocial conduct. However, the final wording merely ensures that 'a persistent disorder of mind' is also inferred, in entirely circular fashion from the antisocial conduct it supposedly 'results in', in precisely the same way as the earlier 'moral insanity' or 'moral defect'. It will be noted that 'persistent disorder of mind' does not fall within either the ICD 9 or DSM III definitions of personality disorder. Psychopathic Disorder, then, means little more than a proclivity to engage in morally objectionable behaviour.

Nineteenth-century German psychiatry avoided the moral value implications of Pritchard's concept by introducing the term 'psychopathic inferiority'. This also related to a wide range of social deviants, but attributed their deviation to biological 'inferiority' rather than moral defect. The description was favoured for a time in America but replaced by the adjective 'sociopathic' to denote revised assumptions that the origins were social (Partridge 1930). While in recent years, sociopathic and psychopathic have been used interchangeably to refer to antisocial personality, it should be noted that 'sociopathic personality disturbance' in DSM I was a generic term covering antisocial reaction, dyssocial reaction, sexual deviation and addictions. The 'sociopathic' rubric was dropped in 1968 when 'antisocial personality' became one of several distinct personality disorders in DSM II.

In Germany, Schneider (1923: first English edition 1950) developed the ideas of Kraepelin, who had suggested several varieties of 'psychopathic personality'. However, Schneider's particular contribution was to reject antisocial behaviour as a criterion of *personality* disorder. He proposed a concept of personality as continuous variation of traits in the population at large, and suggested that psychopathic personalities are not ill, but rather are distinguished by the statistical abnormality of their personality. Of the ten varieties he identified, seven are represented in the ICD 9 class of Personality Disorders. The eighth, the 'asocial or sociopathic' category, violates Schneider's original concept in introducing antisocial behaviour as a criterion, although it also bears some resemblance to his 'affectionless' category.

Although Schneider's psychopathic personalities became the personality disorders of ICD and also DSM II, some American psychiatrists, notably Karpman (1941) and Cleckley (1976: first edition 1941) objected to this equation. They preferred to narrow the meaning of 'psychopathic' and to dispense with the category of personality disorders, most of which they believed belonged with the neurotic or psychotic disorders. Karpman proposed that psychopaths were either *primary*, in being characterized by egoistic, uninhibited instinctual expression unmodified by conscience or guilt, or *secondary*, in that antisocial behaviour was an outcome of dynamic disturbance of a neurotic or psychotic kind. This classification by inferred aetiology has little value in the absence of adequate descriptive criteria, but the distinction between primary and secondary psychopaths has been used by several researchers to distinguish antisocial personalities who are guilt-free or non-anxious from those who exhibit emotional difficulties. Cleckley also suggested relegating most categories of personality disorder to the neuroses or psychoses, but identified psychopathic personality as 'a distinct clinical entity' characterized not simply by socially deviant behaviour, but by a number of dispositions. His 16 criteria of psychopathic personality are: (1) superficial charm; (2) absence of psychotic signs; (3) absence of nervousness; (4) unreliability; (5) untruthfulness and insincerity; (6) lack of remorse or shame; (7) inadequately motivated antisocial behaviour; (8) failure to learn from experience; (9) egocentricity and incapacity for love; (10) emotional poverty; (11) lack of insight; (12) unresponsiveness in interpersonal relations; (13) uninviting behaviour, sometimes with alcohol; (14) empty suicide threats; (15) impersonal sex life; (16) failure to follow a life plan. Factor analyses of ratings of these criteria show that most of them contribute to a general factor of hostility versus lack of warmth or affection (Hare 1980, Blackburn & Maybury 1985). They partially overlap with the criteria of psychopathic personality offered by McCord & McCord (1964), i.e. 'an asocial, aggressive, highly impulsive person, who feels little or no guilt and is unable to form lasting bonds of affection with other human beings'.

The latter descriptions emphasize personality dispositions, and Cleckley's concept in particular has provided the basis for operational definitions of psychopathic personality in much psychological research. Cleckley's concept is also congruent with the DSM II description of antisocial personality and with the similar criteria for the ICD 9 'asocial or sociopathic' category (. . . disregard for social obligations, lack of feeling for others, and impetuous violence or callous unconcern . . . often affectively cold and may be abnormally aggressive or irresponsible . . . tolerance for frustration is low . . . blame others).

In DSM III, however, history of antisocial behaviour again becomes the essential criterion for antisocial personality disorder, and the only personality traits among the criteria are irritability and aggressiveness, impulsivity and recklessness, none of which is in fact necessary to the diagnosis. Moreover, many of Cleckley's criteria relate to other disorders such as histrionic or narcissistic personality. In Millon's view this is a return to the value-laden notion originating with Pritchard. DSM III appears to reflect a general acceptance of Schneider's view of personality disorders, and a rejection of Karpman's and Cleckley's claim that most belong with the neuroses or psychoses. But it confounds the classification of these disorders by introducing an additional principle of classification in the form of chronic social deviation or rule-breaking. Given that personality traits and acts of social rule-breaking belong in different universes of discourse, there is no a priori reason to suppose that rule-breakers are confined to a single personality type. In other words, it is unlikely that psychopathic or antisocial personalities defined in terms of *socially* deviant behaviour are homogeneous with respect to *personality* deviation, and the evidence indicates that they are not. Many of those who meet the DSM III criteria for antisocial personality also meet the criteria for other personality disorders, such as narcissistic or borderline (Kosten et al 1982, McManus et al 1984). Similarly, at least four distinct personality types can be detected among those identified as having psychopathic disorders by the English Mental Health Act (Blackburn 1975). Chronic rule violation, then, is not sufficient to identify a unitary personality disorder or 'a distinct clinical entity'.

What has been missing from attempts to classify personality disorders and to define psychopathic personality is empirical research on classification guided by a comprehensive theoretical model of personality. As Hempel (1961) noted, the syndromes of psychiatry have the status of scientific terms which must be subject to empirical validation. At the present time, all of the categories of personality disorder represent hypotheses of trait covariation and their validity as homogeneous classes of dispositions remains to be established. As has been observed on several occasions, adequate classification must precede aetiological explanation.

Categories of personality disorder

In this section, the DSM III categories of personality disorder are briefly described, and evidence as to their validity as distinct types considered. The DSM III categorization was influenced by Millon's dimensional system of personality classification, although the final version departs from it in several respects (Millon 1981). In particular, Millon dissents from the identification of schizotypal, borderline and paranoid disorders as separate types, preferring to see them as more pathological variants of basic patterns. Millon's three dimensions are active–passive, self–other orientation, and pleasure–pain motivation. Eight 'coping patterns' are derived from combining activity or passivity with four levels of self–other orientation (dependent, independent, ambivalent, detached), pleasure–pain differences being confined to schizoid and avoidant disorders. This categorization provides a coherent (although as yet untested) theoretical framework for understanding some of the proposed attributes of the different personality disorders, and the disorders are therefore discussed in terms of Millon's scheme.

Dependent and histrionic disorders

Dependent disorders are defined in DSM III by the following criteria: passively allows others to assume responsibility for major areas of life, subordinates own needs to those on whom he or she depends, lacks self-confidence. *Histrionic* disorders are defined by: overly dramatic and intensely expressed behaviour as seen in self-dramatization, drawing attention to self, craving for excitement, over-reaction to minor events or irrational tantrums, and interpersonal disturbance in the form of shallowness of response, egocentricity, vanity, dependent and helpless behaviour and proneness to manipulative suicidal threats. In Millon's scheme, both categories are characterized by strong dependence on others in the form of need for approval and affection, but adopt passive or active strategies to achieve it. Thus the dependent personality is submissive and manipulable, the histrionic more actively soliciting approval through attracting the attention of others.

Histrionic replaces the older 'hysterical' category, which is retained in ICD 9. Lazare et al (1970) found evidence for a 'hysterical' factor in a factor analysis of self-report scales, but contrary to prediction found that aggression, oral aggression and obstinacy had loadings on this factor. Additional support for the existence of such a factor is provided by Presly & Walton (1973). Of four factors extracted from psychiatrists' ratings of personality-disordered patients, one was defined by ingratiation, need for attention, excessive emotional display, unlikeability and insincerity, and was accordingly labelled 'hysterical'. They also noted that the diagnosis was applied more frequently to females, whereas males more often attracted the diagnosis of sociopathic personality. This sex bias persists in DSM III, the most frequent personality disorder diagnoses for females being dependent and histrionic, while for males they are antisocial and compulsive (Kass et al 1983).

Dependent personality has been related to the 'oral character' of psychoanalytic theory, and Lazare et al (1970) provide some support for this in the form of a corresponding self-report factor. Kline & Storey (1977), however, distinguish 'oral optimist' and 'oral pessimist' factors, the former being related to extroversion, the latter to neurotic suspicion. A factor of 'submissiveness' was identified by Presly & Walton (1973), this being made up of ratings of timidity, meekness, and intropunitiveness. However, these traits would also be applicable to the avoidant pattern.

Narcissistic, antisocial and paranoid disorders

DSM III criteria for *narcissistic* disorders are: grandiose sense of self-importance, preoccupied with fantasies of unlimited success or power, exhibitionism, indifference or rage in response to criticism, and disturbances in interpersonal relationships such as assumptions of entitlement, exploitativeness, alternation between over-idealization and devaluation in relationships, and lack of empathy. *Paranoid* disorders are characterized by: pervasive suspiciousness and mistrust, as shown by expectations of trickery, guardedness, concern with hidden motives or pathological jealousy, hypersensitivity as shown by easily feeling slighted, exaggeration of difficulties, and restricted affectivity in the form of taking pride in rationality, lacking humour and lacking sentimentality. *Antisocial* disorders are defined by detailed criteria of delinquent and socially irresponsible behaviour beginning before the age of 15, and involving violation of the rights of others. As noted earlier, reference to traits is limited to irritability and aggressiveness, impulsivity and recklessness. Millon considers that this category is more appropriately designated as 'aggressive', and suggests that the major criteria are hostile affectivity, social rebelliousness, vindictiveness and disregard for danger. In Millon's scheme, narcissistic and aggressive personalities share a need for independence and self-reliance, but the former passively relies on an image of extreme self-worth, while the latter actively maintains autonomy as a result of extreme mistrust and hostility. Narcissistic personalities are therefore arrogant and take others for granted, whereas aggressive personalities seek to dominate others in the face of anticipated hostility. According to Millon, paranoid personalities show characteristics of these two in the form of more extreme mistrust, self-importance, and externalized hostility, although they have some features in common with compulsive personalities.

The inclusion of narcissistic disorder in DSM III is largely a reflection of the interest in this category among psychoanalysts such as Kernberg (1970), although there is not in fact an agreed description or formulation of the disorder in the psychodynamic literature. A 'competitive-narcissistic' interpersonal style was identified by Leary & Coffey (1955), who, however, noted that few patients exhibited it, perhaps because of the incompatability of the patient role with the need to maintain autonomy. Similarly, paranoid personalities are likely to be found in clinical settings only when delusional ideas become florid. Perhaps for these reasons, empirical research on these categories is lacking.

In view of the extensive literature on psychopathic or antisocial personality, this subject is dealt with separately later in the chapter.

Compulsive, passive-aggressive and borderline disorders

DSM III criteria for *compulsive* disorders are: restricted ability to express warm emotions, as shown in conventionality, perfectionism, insistence that others submit to his or her way of doing things, excessive devotion to work to the exclusion of pleasure, and indecisiveness. *Passive-aggressive* personalities are characterized by: resistance to demands for adequate performance, resistance being expressed, for example, in procrastination, stubbornness, intentional inefficiency, ineffectiveness in social and occupational roles and persistence of the above when effective behaviour is possible. *Borderline* personalities are defined by at least five of: impulsivity, unstable and intense relationships, intense anger, identity disturbance, affective instability, self-damaging acts, and chronic feelings of emptiness and boredom. According to Millon, compulsive and passive-aggressive personalities are both ambivalent over reliance on self or on external demands. The former opt for a conforming, over-controlled style, characterized by recourse to rules and authority, stubbornness and stinginess, and an ingratiating, obsequious manner. The latter are irritable and moody, and vacillate between despondency and spite. Millon follows Kernberg (1970) in seeing borderline disorders as a level of organization representing extreme forms of several disorders (compulsive, passive-aggressive, histrionic, dependent), rather than as a distinct type of personality disorder.

Compulsive disorders are synonymous with obsessive-compulsive or obsessional personality, and with the anankastic category of ICD 9. The category has often been linked with the 'anal character' of psychoanalytic theory, and several factor analytic studies have provided evidence for an 'obsessional' or 'anal' factor, defined by traits such as obstinacy, orderliness or parsimony. One reviewer regards the evidence for an 'anal' factor to be inconclusive (Hill 1976), and Stone & Gottheil (1975) found that it contributes relatively little to inter-individual variation and is unrelated to bowel habits. Pollak (1979), however, concluded that empirical studies have validated the broader construct of obsessive-compulsive personality, and that it is distinct from the similarly named symptom disorder.

Passive-aggressive disorders have not generally been recognized outside American psychiatry, and they are among the least reliably identified personality disorders. In one of the few studies of this category, Small et al (1970) described an 11-year follow-up of 100 such patients given this label, and considered that they differed from matched controls in terms of history of interpersonal strife, verbal aggression, anger outbursts, impulsivity and manipulation. Diagnostic reliability was not reported.

From a review of clinical descriptions of borderline patients, Gunderson & Singer (1975) concluded that six characteristics had been described with sufficient frequency to warrant a basis for a rational diagnosis, these being intense hostile or depressive affect, impulsive acts such as self-mutilation, addiction or promiscuity, relatively well-maintained social adaptation, brief psychotic experiences, bizarre responses to projective tests, and oscillation between superficial and intense relationships. A few recent studies have examined MMPI profiles of borderline personalities as defined by DSM III criteria. Evans et al (1984), for example, found that borderlines produced high-ranging or 'floating' profiles, and scored significantly higher than chronic schizophrenic or acute psychotic patients on several scales. While their sample showed a number of test differences from other samples of borderline patients, they nevertheless suggest that the validity of the category is supported. However, in view of the disagreements regarding the construct, more critical evidence for validity would be separation from other categories of personality disorder. Many borderlines meet the criteria for other disorders, notably schizotypal, dependent and antisocial (Kosten et al 1982, Clarkin et al 1983), and hence the independence of this category must be doubted.

Schizoid, avoidant and schizotypal disorders

DSM III criteria for *schizoid* disorders are: emotionally cold and aloof, indifferent to the feelings of others, few friendships, absence of eccentricities of speech, thought or behaviour. The latter are shown by *schizotypal* disorders, which are characterized by combinations of magical thinking, ideas of reference, social isolation, recurrent illusions, odd speech, inadequate interpersonal rapport, suspiciousness, and social anxiety. *Avoidant* disorders are defined by: hypersensitivity to rejection, unwillingness to enter into relationships without strong guarantees of acceptance, social withdrawal, desire for affection and acceptance, and low self-esteem. In Millon's scheme, both schizoid and avoidant disorders represent detachment from others, the former taking a passive form, the latter active. They also differ in capacity to experience pleasure and pain. Where the schizoid personality has a limited capacity for emotional and social involvement with others, and is socially isolated by preference, the avoidant personality has a conflict between mistrust and fear of humiliation and the need for affection. Either set of characteristics may be exhibited in schizotypal disorders in which cognitive eccentricities are the most significant feature.

The schizoid personality has antecedents in early psychiatric classifications, and is discussed in the psychoanalytic literature. Schizotypal personality, however, is of relatively recent origin in the literature, and was introduced into DSM III to distinguish 'borderline schizophrenia' from borderline personality (Spitzer et al 1979), although Millon considers it to represent a more pathological form of his two detached types. A genetic link between schizotypal disorder and schizophrenia is assumed, but undemonstrated, although Golden & Meehl (1979) claim to have isolated a corresponding 'latent taxon' in the MMPI responses of non-schizophrenic patients. There is no demonstrable link between schizoid disorder and predisposition to schizophrenia (Bower et al 1960). On the other hand, the long-term stability of schizoid traits has been demonstrated (Wolff & Chick 1980), and there may be some relation of these to social introversion. Scarr (1969) reports that twin studies suggest a high heritability for social introversion, and that traits of withdrawal and social anxiety are highly stable from birth to adolescence. A 30-year retest correlation of 0.74 for the MMPI Social Introversion scale in normal adults (Leon et al 1979) seems consistent with Scarr's findings. Scarr hypothesized that there is a genotype predisposing the individual to react in relatively outgoing or withdrawn ways to interactions with cues and contingencies in the environment.

Patients who present with problems of social interactions may commonly meet the criteria for avoidant disorders. Nichols (1974) noted the common features of 'social phobics', and his observations parallel the DSM III criteria for avoidant personality. He suggests that socially 'phobic' individuals are more appropriately construed as being extreme with respect to a personality variable of social anxiety. This may well be equivalent to social introversion as discussed by Scarr, since personality measures of shyness, social anxiety and social introversion are usually highly intercorrelated.

The utility of current classification systems

Classification within abnormal psychology serves a number of communication and predictive purposes (Blashfield & Draguns 1976), and the diagnosis of personality disorder should indicate the nature of a person's behavioural difficulties as well as the difference between these and the problems of other patients. It should also predict the kind of intervention procedures which are likely to be beneficial, and should provide a basis for the formulation of explanatory principles and a guide to the conduct of research. At the present time, none of these functions is adequately realized, due to limitations in the reliability with which personality disorders are identified, and the lack of firm evidence that the concepts represent clinically and scientifically valid distinctions among classes of deviant social behaviour.

Although DSM III attempts to improve on the reliability of psychiatric diagnosis, field trials indicated that overall reliability (kappa) for personality disorders as a class was 0.5, with kappas for specific categories ranging from 0.26 to 0.75 (American Psychiatric Association 1980). Only a few categories, such as antisocial personality disorder, achieve inter-rater reliabilities above the acceptable kappa level of 0.70. Several factors contribute to this low level of reliability. First, the criteria of category membership are typically attributes which require a subjective decision as to their presence or absence. Further, they range from the visible (e.g. physically self-damaging acts, frequent displays of temper) to the inferential (e.g. identity disturbance, preoccupation with fantasies of unlimited success). There are also practical difficulties in determining whether or not a particular attribute represents an 'enduring' trait, since both self-descriptions obtained in interview and psychological test responses may be contaminated by associated symptom disorders or temporary mood states (Bianchi & Fergusson 1977). Reliability of classification can be improved by the use of structured and multi-method measurement procedures. Promising candidates include a rating schedule associated with ICD 9 criteria (Tyrer & Alexander 1979), the MCMI (Millon 1983), which purports to measure both DSM III personality disorders and symptom disorders, and a structured interview for the assessment of DSM III personality disorders (Stangl et al 1985).

As indicated earlier, there is research evidence for the validity of some individual categories of personality disorder, but the validity of the class as a whole has not been established. In particular, it remains to be demonstrated that the current categories represent an optimal partition of the universe of inflexible personality traits. The recognition of categories and their criteria has not been guided by a uniform theoretical scheme, and the current classifications do not conform with the requirements of 'classical' taxonomy that categories should be defined by singly necessary and conjointly sufficient criteria which yield homogeneous and mutually exclusive classes (Hempel 1961, Blashfield & Draguns 1976). In fact, DSM III does not assume homogeneity within categories and several are defined by a multiple choice of criteria. Also, multiple classification is recommended, and in practice there is significant overlap between categories, in particular histrionic, narcissistic, borderline and antisocial (Kosten et al 1982, Stangl et al 1985, Blashfield et al 1985).

In research on categorization, Rosch (1978) has demonstrated that the classical requirements of homogeneity are rarely met in either everyday or scientific classifications. Rather is it the case that people categorize objects in terms of a few salient or *prototypical* features, only some of which are shared by all members of a category. Cantor et al (1980) propose that psychiatric diagnosis follows prototypical categorization, and that heterogeneity of category membership is not unreasonable. Several categories of personality disorder have been shown to comply with the prototype model (Clarkin et al 1983, Blashfield et al 1985). However, prototypic classification raises serious difficulties in attempting to validate a category, since 'pure' instances will be rare, and abandonment of the 'classical' approach is likely to impede the process of validation (Adams & Haber 1984). These and other issues related to the application of DSM III criteria of personality disorder are discussed by Widiger & Kelso (1983).

A similar problem is the separation of personality disorder from normality implied by discrete categorical classification, and the meaning of *disorder* in this context. Both the ICD 9 and DSM III classifications follow Schneider in assuming continuity between normal and abnormal behaviour, but inflexible traits become personality disorder only when subjective distress or social impairment is also present. This clearly implies that inflexible traits themselves are not sufficient for the identification of disorder. Foulds (1971) recognized this, and suggested that personality disorder be distinguished from 'discordant personality' in which inflexible traits are 'manageable' by the person. He also recognized that not all inflexible traits are equally likely to produce impairment or distress, and suggested that certain traits are themselves 'deviant', possible criteria being differential distribution in samples of personality-disordered and normal individuals. Extrapunitive hostility, suspicion, lack of control, and expediency meet these criteria (Foulds 1971, McIver & Presly 1974). Nevertheless, there is a significantly arbitrary element in the distinction between extremes of normal behavioural variation and personality disorder, and some clinicians have objected to the implication that personality disorders are diseases or illnesses (Schwartz & Schwartz 1976). The argument centres on the definition of disease or illness, which is not agreed (Blackburn 1983a).

However, there seems to be increasing acceptance that personality disorders reflect learned behaviour patterns and not bodily diseases (Millon 1981).

Categorical versus dimensional classification

The problems of reliability and validity surrounding the classification of personality disorders arise largely from the use of a categorical system, and it has long been argued that a dimensional system of classification is inherently more reliable, avoids problems of overlapping categories or borderline cases, and is more powerful in the evaluation of empirical relationships (Eysenck 1960, Strauss 1973). Further, a dimensional system can be converted into a category scheme on theoretical or empirical bases, while at the same time the arbitrariness of the dichotomy between deviant and normal is made explicit. The advantages of a dimensional approach to personality disorders are discussed by Frances (1982) and Widiger & Kelso (1983), and research has indicated the possible forms this might take.

Three related strategies can be discerned in the efforts to date. The first is to look for dimensionality among the traits describing personality disorder, most typically through the use of factor analysis. A comprehensive study of this kind is described by Presly & Walton (1973), who had psychiatrists rate 87 patients on 46 traits of personality disorder. The four factors extracted from the data were labelled social deviance (in preference to psychopathy), submissiveness, obsessional-schizoid, and hysterical. A cluster analysis of scores on these dimensions generated several patterns or types, which, however, showed little resemblance to conventional categories of personality disorder. A similar study is described by Tyrer & Alexander (1979), who obtained trait ratings on 130 psychiatric outpatients. Three factors accounted for most of the variance, these being described as sociopathy, passive dependence and dysthymia. A hierarchical cluster analysis of scores on the three dimensions yielded four groups (sociopathic, passive-dependent, schizoid and anankastic), which cut across ICD personality disorder categories. Although there are differences in these two studies, the first factor obtained in each of them is very similar, being defined in particular by several items related to Cleckley's criteria of psychopathy (egocentricity, callousness, irresponsibility). A similar general factor has been found in analyses of Cleckley's criteria (Hare 1980, Blackburn & Maybury 1985), and given that these criteria relate to several DSM III categories of personality disorder, it would seem that the traits distinguishing personality disorders are reducible to a few dimensions, one of which resembles Cleckley's concept of psychopathy. It would also seem likely that the current categories could be replaced by a smaller number representing patterns of variation along these dimensions.

A second strategy entails translating the current categories into established or theoretical dimensional systems of personality description, such as that of Eysenck. Eysenck's interest in personality disorders has been largely confined to psychopathic personality, which he construes broadly in terms of antisocial behaviour. He has suggested that primary psychopaths are relatively extreme with respect to psychoticism, secondary psychopaths being neurotic extroverts (Eysenck & Eysenck 1978). Little support has been forthcoming for this proposal (Blackburn 1975, Hare 1982). While interest in other categories has been limited, Paykel & Prusoff (1973) provide some evidence that the oral (dependent) personality is a neurotic introvert, the hysterical a neurotic extrovert, and the obsessional a stable ambivert.

In contrast, considerable interest has been shown in identifying personality disorders in terms of the dimensional system of classifying interpersonal behaviours originating in the work of Leary (Carson 1970, McLemore & Benjamin 1979, Wiggins 1982, Blackburn 1983a). In this model, a two-dimensional space is defined by orthogonal axes of power (dominance versus submission) and affiliation (love versus hate). Interpersonal behaviours represent differing blends of these two, and are arrayed around the space in the form of a circle, or Guttman circumplex. Categories of interpersonal style are formed by combining behaviours at a molar level (e.g. quadrants of the circle corresponding to hostile-dominant or friendly-submissive styles) or by a more detailed differentiation of behaviours around the circle (McLemore & Benjamin 1979). In an early study, Leary & Coffey (1955) worked with the octants of the interpersonal circle, and demonstrated from self-ratings and clinical ratings that six categories of personality disorder could be defined in terms of rigidity of interpersonal style. For example, obsessives were characterized by a self-effacing style, schizoids by a distrustful style, and psychopaths by an aggressive style. Wiggins (1982) and Blackburn (1983a) have suggested ways in which DSM III categories might be related to the interpersonal circle. While this remains to be tested empirically, a study of psychiatrists' concepts (i.e. prototypes) of the characteristics of DSM II categories of personality disorder by Plutchik & Platman (1977) showed that they were systematically related to each other in a circular ordering around a two-dimensional space. Further evidence on the relevance of the interpersonal circle to the classification of personality disorder is provided by Blackburn & Maybury (1985), who showed that Cleckley's criteria of psychopathy fall at the hostility pole of the affiliation axis.

Marshall & Barbaree (1984) have also suggested that the categories of personality disorder can be translated into a dimensional system, but their dimensions are for the most part classes of behavioural dysfunction suggested by the social skills literature rather than by a theoretical model of personal dispositions. They propose nine dimensions, which are not regarded as entirely independent: inappropriate assertive responses, interpersonal aversiveness, dominance-submission, dysfunctional social cognitions, social anxiety, dysfunctional affiliation, inappropriate or restricted emotion, compulsions, and antisocial behaviour. Within this scheme, for example, avoidant disorders are characterized by extreme social anxiety, dysfunctional affiliation and dysfunctional social cognitions. The scheme has a pragmatic appeal insofar as it focuses on targets of treatment intervention.

One further strategy is to generate an alternative empirical taxonomy from established personality dimensions, cluster analysis being the common method of choice. Lorr et al (1965) obtained therapist ratings of interpersonal style in non-psychotic patients, and identified four clusters which essentially represent the extremes of the power and affiliation axes of the interpersonal circle. The defining characteristics of the groups were: (a) exhibitionistic, dominant, competitive; (b) hostile, mistrusting, detached; (c) agreeable, nurturant, sociable; and (d) inhibited, submissive, abasive. No marked agreement was found with diagnostic categories, but some correspondence with DSM III categories is suggested by these characteristics. Histrionic and narcissistic traits are suggested by (a), for example, while (d) suggests features of avoidant and dependent disorders.

Studies of self-report personality characteristics in forensic psychiatric and prison samples have yielded an apparently similar taxonomy (Blackburn 1975, Henderson 1982). The four groups distinguished in these studies were described by Blackburn as: (1) primary psychopath (impulsive, aggressive, hostile, extraverted); (2) secondary psychopath (impulsive, aggressive, hostile, withdrawn); (3) controlled or conforming (unaggressive, defensive, sociable); (4) inhibited (unaggressive, withdrawn, introverted). Blackburn (1983a) suggested that these types represent preferred styles falling at different points of the interpersonal circle. This hypothesis was supported by Willner & Blackburn (1986), who found significant differences between the groups in their anticipated reactions to interpersonal situations involving threat or friendly interactions, differences being maintained across situations.

PSYCHOPATHIC PERSONALITY

Assessment and the validity of the construct

It was argued above that a history of antisocial behaviour is inappropriate as a criterion of a personality disorder, and the utility of the construct of psychopathic or antisocial personality lies in the extent to which it tells us how attributes of the person contribute to undesirable behaviour. Attempts to identify the personality traits distinguishing the psychopath are to be found in the descriptions offered by McCord & McCord (1964), Cleckley (1976) and Millon (1981), who broadly refer to two sets of attributes. On the one hand, Cleckley and the McCords give weight to a lack of warmth or affection in relationships (e.g. egocentricity, insincerity, lack of remorse, callousness, lack of empathy), while on the other the McCords and Millon also emphasize aggressive impulsivity (aggressiveness, irritability, irresponsibility, vindictiveness, recklessness). These correspond to identifiable behavioural dimensions (Blackburn 1979a, Hare 1980), which are correlated rather than identical (Blackburn & Maybury 1985). However, several investigators distinguish between primary and secondary psychopaths on the basis of differences in level of anxiety (Lykken 1957, Schmauk 1970). Empirical justification for this distinction is provided by the finding of two groups of impulsive, hostile offenders who occupy opposite extremes of a dimension of social anxiety and withdrawal (Blackburn 1975, 1979a).

As employed in research during the past three decades, the concept of the psychopath is broader than that implied by the current categories of antisocial or sociopathic personality, and it probably embraces other categories of personality disorder. Traits associated with psychopathy in the literature are among the DSM III criteria for histrionic (superficial charm, insincerity, egocentricity), narcissistic (lack of empathy, exploitativeness), schizoid, paranoid, compulsive (lack of warmth) and borderline disorders (impulsivity, lack of anger control). Research on psychopathy has usually ignored the differentiation of personality disorders, and it must be assumed that the need for the primary–secondary distinction arises from the association of other disorders with the sociopathic category. Primary psychopaths may therefore include histrionic and narcissistic personalities, while borderline and other disorders may make up secondary psychopaths.

The bulk of recent research has employed one of the following to identify psychopaths: (a) *Cleckley's Criteria* in the form of ratings or global assessments; Hare (1980) has developed a *Research Checklist* from earlier work with Cleckley's criteria, although he includes several items relating to past history of antisocial behaviour; (b) combined elevations of the *Pd* (Psychopathic Deviate) and *Ma* (Hypomania) scales of the MMPI; Blackburn (1979a) developed the SHAPS (Special Hospitals Assessment of Personality and Socialization) largely from MMPI items, and distinguished primary and secondary psychopaths by means of orthogonal factors of Psychopathy and Social Withdrawal; (c) the *So* (Socialization) scale of the California Psychological Inventory (Gough 1965); (d) a factor dimension of *psychopathy* identified by Quay (1978) in case history data, behaviour ratings and self-report questionnaires.

These procedures emphasize different personality characteristics and do not produce identical subject groups. MMPI-derived criteria and Quay's factor emphasize impulsivity, Cleckley's criteria lack of affection. Hare (1985) examined inter-relationships of Cleckley ratings, the Research Checklist, *Pd*, *So*, and DSM III diagnosis of antisocial personality disorder. Most intercorrelations were significant, but the majority were in the range between 0.3 and 0.5. Somewhat surprisingly, DSM III diagnosis correlated significantly with Cleckley ratings (0.57), *Pd* (0.29) and *So* (−0.37). Diagnoses of other personality disorders were not, however, included in the study.

Theories and research on psychopathy

Explanatory models of psychopathy are concerned with elucidating the characteristics of the individual which mediate socially undesirable behaviours, and much of the work in this area reflects a continuation of the assumption that the disorder is due to hereditary weakness. While evidence from twin and adoptive studies indicates a genetic or congenital constitutional contribution to *criminality* (Mednick & Hutchings 1978), insufficient attention is given in the literature to distinguishing this from psychopathic *personality*. However, Schulsinger (1972) employed a clinical criterion of psychopathy, and found a significantly greater incidence of psychopathy in the biological relatives, particularly fathers, of adoptees who became psychopaths than in their adoptive relatives or the relatives of non-psychopathic adoptees. On the other hand, comparable evidence has been found for the role of familial factors in the generation of psychopathy. Oltman & Friedman (1967), for example, demonstrated significantly more frequent loss of a parent in childhood among 'personality disorders', the loss being mainly by separation. They suggest that this is likely to reflect prior parental discord. McCord & McCord (1964) also observed greater instability in the families of psychopaths and noted that erratic discipline and parental rejection were common. These biological and environmental contributions are not incompatible, and Quay (1977) suggests that a child who is constitutionally hyperactive, aggressive and insensitive to punishment is more likely to generate parental rejection, with the result being failure of socialization.

Most psychological research on psychopathy has been oriented towards the search for a *deficiency* which would account for a failure of socialized learning and the inhibition of behaviour which attracts societal disapproval and punishment. Cleckley (1976) proposed that psychopaths are characterized by 'semantic dementia', a defect in the ability to become aware of what emotional experiences mean to others. Along similar lines, Gough (1948) suggested that psychopaths are deficient in the ability to assume the role of 'the generalized other'. Widom (1976) obtained evidence consistent with these notions in the repertory grids of psychopaths. She found that they did not differ from controls in their use of emotional constructs, but tended to construe more situations as 'dull'. Further, they failed to distinguish their own constructs as any different from those of other people. Schalling (1978) has speculated that this apparent lack of empathic awareness might reflect a weak vividness of imagery consequent on low levels of cortical arousal.

Rather more research attention has been given to the possibility of a defect in psychophysiological functioning, particularly in mechanisms governing the acquisition of classically conditioned responses of anxiety. Influential in this context has been the use of the Miller–Mowrer two-process learning theory to account for socialization (Trasler 1973). The model assumes that socialized restraints develop through the acquisition of conditioned fear (anxiety) responses which function as an aversive drive state. This drive state is reduced by passive avoidance learning, i.e. the inhibition of responses which have punishing consequences. Unsocialized behaviour will therefore result from either inadequate exposure to appropriate conditioning schedules involving punishment of unacceptable behaviour or from characteristics of the individual which impair the acquisition of conditioned fear responses. The psychopath is held to represent the latter case, and low levels of autonomic arousal or reactivity have been postulated as central to this deficiency.

Seminal research by Lykken (1957) demonstrated poorer passive avoidance learning in primary and secondary psychopaths in response to shock, and also slower conditioning of electrodermal responses (EDRs) associated with punishment. Parenthetically, it may be noted that the inferior performance of secondary psychopaths, defined by high levels of trait anxiety, is an embarrassment to the model. The deficiency in passive avoidance of physical punishment was replicated by Schmauk (1970), but he found that this was not a generalized deficiency, since psychopaths were able to learn to avoid a material punishment, loss of money. This indicates that psychopaths are responsive to punishment when self-interest is involved. A study by Hare & Quinn (1971) also demonstrated that psychopaths do not have any general deficit in conditionability. Using a design which entailed conditioning of both EDRs and heart rate responses to aversive and non-aversive unconditioned stimuli, they found that impaired conditionability in psychopaths was restricted to EDRs associated with a physically noxious stimulus.

Subsequent research by Hare & Craigen (1974) and Hare et al (1978) has suggested that the smaller EDRs of psychopaths may reflect the activity of a defensive cortical-baroreceptor system, which enables them to 'tune out' the aversive effects of a noxious stimulus. Fowles (1980) has alternatively proposed that the smaller EDRs of psychopaths in these studies are consonant with a deficiency in the Behavioural Inhibition System described by Gray (1975). According to Gray, this system involves forebrain circuits which are activated by conditioned stimuli for punishment and frustrative non-reward, and mediates anxiety. A weakness or deficiency of this system could account for the psychopath's lack of anxiety and failure to inhibit punished behaviour.

The available evidence, however, indicates that psychopaths fail to respond to aversive stimulation or inhibit punished responses only under restricted conditions. Moreover, it is questionable whether low anxiety can account for the unsocialized behaviour of psychopaths (Blackburn 1983b). Psychopaths are heterogeneous with respect to anxiety, secondary psychopaths being distinguished by high anxiety levels. Further, there is no evidence that socialization is primarily mediated by punishment rather than by positive reinforcement, modelling or cognitive learning of moral principles. There are also alternative explanations for the failure of psychopaths to respond to punishment. Siegel (1978), for example, has shown that psychopaths avoid punishment when it is predictable, but not when it is uncertain. He suggests that cognitive factors, such as decision criteria based on assumptions of 'magical immunity', are involved.

A further limitation of the deficit approach is that it fails to consider the motivation for the unsocialized behaviour of psychopaths. One theory which does so is that of Quay (1977), who relates the impulsivity and rebelliousness of psychopaths to proneness to boredom and 'pathological stimulation seeking'. He hypothesized that the substrate for this is under-responsiveness to sensory input or rapid habituation. While there is little support for the proposal that psychopaths display these physiological characteristics, at least in peripheral autonomic activity, there is relatively consistent evidence that psychopaths are 'sensation-seekers' (Blackburn, 1978). It is possible that this can be attributed to low cortical arousal levels, and clinical data have long indicated that psychopaths are characterized by EEG abnormalities, predominantly in the form of excessive slow-wave activity associated with low arousal. However, Blackburn (1979b) and Howard (1984) found this to be most prominent in secondary psychopaths.

In recent investigations, the search for deficits in psychopaths has focused more on neuropsychological functioning and cognitive processing. Heilbrun (1982), for example, has found that the relationship of psychopathy to impulse control, empathy, and history of violence varies with the level of intelligence. A specific deficit in cognitive processing associated with frontal lobe functioning was demonstrated by Gorenstein (1982), but not confirmed by Hare (1984). However, Hare & McPherson (1984) provide evidence that lateralization of performance in a dichotic listening task was less in psychopaths, and propose that language processes are not strongly lateralized in psychopaths, a possible correlate of 'semantic dementia'.

An alternative approach has been to construe psychopathy less in terms of inherent defect than in terms of consequences of failures in the socializing environment which produce maladaptive but active coping styles. Marshall & Barbaree (1984) refer to the evidence for a history of erratic and punitive rearing in psychopaths, and suggest that this would be sufficient to lead to unresponsiveness to physical punishment or social disapproval, and responsiveness to tangible costs when these are immediate. They also note that punitive behaviour in the parents is likely to provide models for inappropriate behaviour, as well as generating an 'oppositional' approach in personal relations. Blackburn & Lee-Evans (1985) similarly argue that psychopaths are biased to perceive malevolent intent in others. They demonstrated that psychopaths anticipate stronger reactions of anger to interpersonal threat, and suggest that psychopaths are influenced by hostile expectations which lead to hypervigilance for threat and self-justification for harmful and exploitative behaviour. This proposal is consistent with

Millon's (1981) view of the aggressive coping pattern, and with Carson's (1979) model of the functions of hostility and dominance in interpersonal exchange.

CONCLUSIONS

The interest of clinicians and researchers in personality disorders has so far been limited by the inadequacy of available classifications and by the pervasive influence of the compelling but unenlightening concept of the psychopath. The greater prominence given to these disorders in DSM III indicates that they deserve greater attention, and the revised classification provides an impetus to the development of clinically relevant theories based on coherent models of personality and behaviour. When seen from the perspective of the variety of these disorders, psychopathic personality appears to be a redundant concept which may be more adequately represented by reference to several disorders apart from the regrettably named 'antisocial' category. While the explanation of antisocial behaviour remains of interest to psychopathology, the focus of attention in understanding personality disorders must be the psychological attributes of the person and their contribution to problems in social behaviour.

REFERENCES

Adams H E, Haber J D 1984 The classification of abnormal behaviour: an overview. In: Adams H E, Sutker P B (eds) Comprehensive handbook of psychopathology. Plenum, New York

Allport G W 1966 Traits revisited. American Psychologist 21: 1–10

Alston W P 1975 Traits, consistency, and conceptual alternatives for personality theory. Journal for the Theory of Social Behaviour 5: 17–48

American Psychiatric Association 1980 Diagnostic and statistical manual of mental disorders, 3rd edn. Washington, DC

Bandura A 1978 The self in reciprocal determinism. American Psychologist 33: 344–358

Bellak A S 1983 Recurrent problems in the behavioural assessment of social skill. Behaviour Research and Therapy 21: 29–41

Bianchi G N, Fergusson D M 1977 The effect of mental state on EPI scores. British Journal of Psychiatry 131: 306–309

Blackburn R 1975 An empirical classification of psychopathic personality. British Journal of Psychiatry 127: 456–460

Blackburn R 1978 Psychopathy, arousal and the need for stimulation. In: Hare R D, Schalling D (eds) Psychopathic behaviour: approaches to research. Wiley, Chichester

Blackburn R 1979a Psychopathy and personality: the dimensionality of self-report and behaviour rating data in abnormal offenders. British Journal of Social and Clinical Psychology 18: 111–119

Blackburn R 1979b Cortical and autonomic arousal in primary and secondary psychopaths. Psychophysiology 16: 143–150

Blackburn R 1983a Are personality disorders treatable? In: Shapland J, Williams T (eds) Mental disorder and the law: effects of the new legislation. Issues in Criminological and Legal Psychology No 4, British Psychological Society, Leicester

Blackburn R 1983b Psychopathy, delinquency and crime. In: Gale A, Edwards J (eds) Physiological correlates of human behaviour. Academic Press, London

Blackburn R 1984 The person and dangerousness. In: Müller D J, Blackman D E, Chapman A J (eds) Psychology and law. Wiley, Chichester

Blackburn R, Lee-Evans J M 1985 Reactions of primary and secondary psychopaths to anger evoking situations. British Journal of Clinical Psychology 24: 93–100

Blackburn R, Maybury C 1985 Identifying the psychopath: the relation of Cleckley's criteria to the interpersonal domain. Personality and Individual Differences 6: 375–386

Blashfield R K, Draguns J G 1976 Evaluative criteria for psychiatric classification. Journal of Abnormal Psychology 85: 140–150

Blashfield R, Sprock J, Pinkston K, Hodgin J 1985 Exemplar prototypes of personality disorder diagnoses. Comprehensive Psychiatry 26: 11–21

Block J 1977 Advancing the psychology of personality: paradigmatic shift or improving the quality of research? In: Magnusson D, Endler N S (eds) Personality at the crossroads. Erlbaum, Hillsdale, NJ

Bower E, Shellhammer T, Daily T M 1960 School characteristics of male adolescents who later become schizophrenic. American Journal of Orthopsychiatry 30: 712–729

Cameron N, Margaret A 1951 Behaviour pathology. Houghton Mifflin, Boston

Cantor N, Smith E E, French R, Mezzich J 1980 Psychiatric diagnosis as prototype categorisation. Journal of Abnormal Psychology 89: 181–193

Carson R C 1970 Interaction concepts of personality. Allen & Unwin, London

Carson R C 1979 Personality and exchange in developing relationships. In: Burgess R L, Huston T L (eds) Social exchange in developing relationships. Academic Press, New York

Clarkin J F, Widiger T A, Frances A, Hurt S W, Gilmore M 1983 Prototype typology and the borderline personality disorder. Journal of Abnormal Psychology 92: 263–275

Cleckley H 1976 The mask of sanity, 6th edn. Mosby, St Louis

Department of Health and Social Security 1975 Report of the committee on abnormal offenders. HMSO, London

Epstein S 1979 The stability of behaviour: I. On predicting most of the people much of the time. Journal of Personality and Social Psychology 37: 1097–1126

Epstein S, O'Brien E J 1985 The person–situation debate in historical and current perspective. Psychological Bulletin 98: 513–537

Erdelyi M 1985 Psychoanalysis: Freud's cognitive psychology. Freeman, San Francisco

Evans R W, Ruff R M, Braff D L, Ainsworth T L 1984 MMPI characteristics of borderline personality inpatients. Journal of Nervous and Mental Disease 172: 742–748

Eysenck H J 1960 Classification and the problem of diagnosis. In: Eysenck H J (ed) Handbook of abnormal psychology, 1st edn. Pitman, London

Eysenck H J, Eysenck S B G 1978 Psychopathy, personality and genetics. In: Hare R D, Schalling D (eds) Psychopathic behaviour: approaches to research. Wiley, Chichester

Foulds G A 1971 Personality deviance and personal symptomatology. Psychological Medicine 1: 222–233

Fowles D C 1980 The three arousal model: implications of Gray's two-factor learning theory for heart rate, electrodermal activity, and psychopathy. Psychophysiology 17: 87–104

Frances A 1982 Categorical and dimensional systems of personality diagnosis: a comparison. Comprehensive Psychiatry 23: 516–527

Golden R, Meehl P 1979 Detection of the schizoid taxon with MMPI indications. Journal of Abnormal Psychology 88: 217–233

Gorenstein E E 1982 Frontal lobe function in psychopaths. Journal of Abnormal Psychology 91: 368–379

Gough H G 1948 A sociological theory of psychopathy. American Journal of Sociology 53: 359–366

Gough H G 1965 Manual for the California psychological inventory. Consulting Psychologists Press, Palo Alto

Gray J A 1975 Elements of a two-process theory of learning. Academic Press, New York

Gunderson J, Singer M 1975 Defining borderline patients: an overview. American Journal of Psychiatry 132:1–10

Hare R D 1980 A research scale for the assessment of psychopathy in criminal populations. Personality and Individual Differences 1: 111–119

Hare R D 1982 Psychopathy and the personality dimensions of psychoticism, extraversion and neuroticism. Personality and Individual Differences 3: 35–42

Hare R D 1984 Performance of psychopaths on cognitive tasks related to frontal lobe function. Journal of Abnormal Psychology 93: 133–140

Hare R D 1985 A comparison of procedures for the assessment of psychopathy. Journal of Consulting and Clinical Psychology 53: 7–16

Hare R D, Craigen D 1974 Psychopathy and physiological activity in a mixed-motive game situation. Psychophysiology 11: 197–206

Hare R D, McPherson L M 1984 Psychopathy and perceptual asymmetry during verbal dichotic listening. Journal of Abnormal Psychology 93: 141–149

Hare R D, Quinn M 1971 Psychopathy and autonomic conditioning. Journal of Abnormal Psychology 77: 223–235

Hare R D, Frazelle J, Cox D N 1978 Psychopathy and physiological responses to threat of an aversive stimulus. Psychophysiology 15: 165–172

Heilbrun A B 1982 Cognitive models of criminal violence based on intelligence and psychopathy levels. Journal of Consulting and Clinical Psychology 50: 546–557

Hempel G C 1961 Fundamentals of taxonomy. In: Zubin J (ed) Field studies in the mental disorders. Grune & Stratton, New York

Henderson M 1982 An empirical classification of convicted violent offenders. British Journal of Criminology 22: 1–20

Hill A B 1976 Methodological problems in the use of factor analysis: a critical review of the evidence for the anal character. British Journal of Medical Psychology 49: 145–159

Hogan R, Desoto C B, Solano C 1977 Traits tests and personality research. American Psychologist 32: 255–264

Howard R C 1984 The clinical EEG and personality in mentally abnormal offenders. Psychological Medicine 14: 569–580

Karpman B 1941 On the need for separating psychopathy into two distinct clinical types: symptomatic and idiopathic. Journal of Criminology and Psychopathology 3: 112–137

Kass F, Spitzer R L, Williams J B W 1983 An empirical study of the issue of sex bias in the diagnostic criteria of DSM-III Axis II personality disorders. American Psychologist 38: 799–801

Kernberg O F 1970 A psychoanalytic classification of character pathology. Journal of the American Psychoanalytic Association 18: 800–822

Kline P, Storey R 1977 A factor analytic study of the oral character. British Journal of Social and Clinical Psychology 16: 317–328

Kosten T R, Rounsaville B J, Kleber H D 1982 DSM-III personality disorders in opiate addicts. Comprehensive Psychiatry 23: 572–581

Lazare A, Klerman G L, Armor D J 1970 Oral, obsessive and hysterical personality patterns: replication of factor analysis in an independent sample. Journal of Psychiatric Research 7: 275–290

Leary T, Coffey H S 1955 Interpersonal diagnosis: some problems of methodology and validation. Journal of Abnormal and Social Psychology 50: 110–124

Leon G R, Gillum B, Gillum R, Gouze M 1979 Personal stability and change over a 30-year period — middle age to old age. Journal of Consulting and Clinical Psychology 47: 517–524

Lion J R 1981 A comparison between DSM III and DSM II personality disorders. In: Lion J R (ed) Personality disorders: diagnosis and management, 2nd edn. Williams & Wilkins, Baltimore

Lorr M, Bishop P F, McNair D M 1965 Interpersonal types among psychiatric patients. Journal of Abnormal and Social Psychology 70: 468–472

Lykken D T 1957 A study of anxiety in the sociopathic personality. Journal of Abnormal and Social Psychology 55: 6–10

McCord W, McCord J 1964 The psychopath: an essay on the criminal mind. Van Nostrand, New York

McIver D, Presly A S 1974 Towards the investigation of personality deviance. British Journal of Social and Clinical Psychology 13: 397–404

McLemore C W, Benjamin L S 1979 Whatever happened to interpersonal diagnosis? A psychosocial alternative to DSM III. American Psychologist 34: 17–34

McManus M, Alessi N E, Grapentine W L, Brickman A 1984 Psychiatric disturbance in serious delinquents. Journal of the American Academy of Child Psychiatry 23: 602–615

Magnusson D, Endler N S 1977 Interactional psychology: present status and future prospects. In: Magnusson D, Endler N S (eds) Personality at the crossroads. Erlbaum, Hillsdale, NJ

Marshall W L, Barbaree H E 1984 Disorders of personality, impulse, and adjustment. In:

Turner S M, Hersen M (eds) Adult psychopathology and diagnosis. Wiley, New York
Maughs S 1941 A concept of psychopathy and psychopathic personality: its evolution and historical development. Journal of Criminal Psychopathology 2: 329–356
Mednick S A, Hutchings B 1978 Genetic and psychophysiological factors in asocial behaviour. In: Hare R D, Schalling D (eds) Psychopathic behaviour: approaches to research. Wiley, Chichester
Millon T 1981 Disorders of Personality: DSM-III, Axis II. Wiley, New York
Millon T 1983 Millon clinical multiaxial inventory manual, 3rd edn. Interpretive Scoring Systems, Minneapolis
Mischel W 1968 Personality and assessment. Wiley, New York
Mischel W 1973 Toward a cognitive social learning reconceptualisation of personality. Psychological Review 80: 252–283
Mischel W 1984 Convergences and challenges in the search for consistency. American Psychologist 39: 351–364
Mowbray R M 1960 The concept of the psychopath. Journal of Mental Science 106: 537–542
Nichols K A 1974 Severe social anxiety. British Journal of Medical Psychology 47: 301–306
Oltman J, Friedman S 1967 Parental deprivation in psychiatric conditions. Diseases of the Nervous System 28: 298–303
Olweus D 1979 Stability of aggressive reaction patterns in males: a review. Psychological Bulletin 86: 852–875
Olweus D 1981 Continuity in aggressive and withdrawn, inhibited patterns. Psychiatry and Social Science 1: 141–159
Partridge G E 1930 Current conceptions of psychopathic personality. American Journal of Psychiatry 10: 53–99
Paykel E S, Prusoff B A 1973 Relationships between personality dimensions: neuroticism and extraversion against obsessive, hysterical and oral personality. British Journal of Social and Clinical Psychology 12: 309–318
Pichot P 1978 Psychopathic behaviour: a historical overview In: Hare R D, Schalling D (eds) Psychopathic behaviour: approaches to research. Wiley, Chichester
Plutchik R, Platman S R 1977 Personality connotations of psychiatric diagnoses. Journal of Nervous and Mental Disease 165: 418–422
Pollak J M 1979 Obsessive-compulsive personality: a review. Psychological Bulletin 86: 225–241
Presly A S, Walton H J 1973 Dimensions of abnormal personality. British Journal of Psychiatry 122: 269–276
Quay H C 1977 Psychopathic behaviour: reflections on its nature, origins, and treatment. In: Weizmann F, Uzigiris I (eds) The structuring of experience. Plenum, New York
Quay H C 1978 Classification. In: Quay H C, Werry J S (eds) Psychopathological disorders of childhood, 2nd edn. John Wiley, New York
Raush H L 1965 Interaction sequences. Journal of Personality and Social Psychology 2: 487–499
Rosch E 1978 Principles of categorisation. In: Rosch E, Lloyd B B (eds) Cognition and categorisation. Erlbaum, Hillsdale, NJ
Scarr S 1969 Social introversion–extraversion as a heritable response. Child Development 40: 823–832
Schalling D 1978 Psychopathy-related personality variables and the psychophysiology of socialisation. In: Hare R D, Schalling D (eds) Psychopathic behaviour: approaches to research. Wiley, Chichester
Schmauk F J 1970 Punishment, arousal, and avoidance learning in sociopaths. Journal of Abnormal Psychology 76: 325–335
Schneider K 1923 Psychopathic personalities. Cassell, London
Schulsinger F 1972 Psychopathy, heredity and environment. International Journal of Mental Health 1: 190–206
Schwartz R A, Schwartz I K 1976 Are personality disorders diseases? Diseases of the Nervous System 86: 613–617
Shweder R A 1975 How relevant is an individual difference theory of personality? Journal of Personality 43: 455–484
Siegel R A 1978 Probability of punishment and suppression of behaviour in psychopathic and nonpsychopathic offenders. Journal of Abnormal Psychology 87: 514–522

Small I F, Small J G, Alig V B, Moore D F 1970 Passive-aggressive personality disorder: a search for a syndrome. American Journal of Psychiatry 126: 973–983

Snyder M 1981 Seek and ye shall find: testing hypotheses about other people. In: Higgins E, Herman C, Zanna M (eds) Social cognition: the Ontario symposium. Erlbaum, Hillsdale, NJ

Spitzer R L, Endicott J, Gibbon M 1979 Crossing the border into borderline personality and borderline schizophrenia. Archives of General Psychiatry 36: 17–24

Stangl D, Pfohl B, Zimmerman M, Bowers E, Corenthal C 1985 A structured interview for the DSM-III personality disorders, Archives of General Psychiatry 42: 591–596

Stone G C, Gottheil E 1975 Factor analysis of orality and anality in selected patient groups. Journal of Nervous and Mental Disease 160: 311–323

Strauss J S 1973 Diagnostic models and the nature of psychiatric disorder. Archives of General Psychiatry 29: 445–449

Trasler G B 1973 Criminal behaviour. In: Eysenck H J (ed) Handbook of abnormal psychology. 2nd edn. Pitman, London

Trower P 1984 A radical reformulation and critique: from organism to agent. In: Trower P (ed) Radical approaches to social skills training. Croom Helm, London

Turkat I D, Alpher V S 1983 An investigation of personality disorder descriptions. American Psychologist 38: 857–858

Turkat I D, Levin R A 1984 Formulation of personality disorders. In: Adams H E, Sutker P B (eds) Comprehensive handbook of psychopathology. Plenum, New York

Turner S M, Hersen M 1981 Disorders of social behaviour: a behavioural approach to personality disorders. In: Turner S M, Calhoun K S, Adams H E (eds) Handbook of behaviour therapy. Wiley, New York

Tyrer P, Alexander J 1979 Classification of personality disorder. British Journal of Psychiatry 135: 163–167

Widiger T A, Kelso K 1983 Psychodiagnosis of Axis II. Clinical Psychology Review 3: 491–510

Widom C S 1976 Interpersonal and personal construct systems in psychopaths. Journal of Consulting and Clinical Psychology 44: 614–623

Wiggins J S 1982 Circumplex models of interpersonal behaviour in clinical psychology. In: Kendall P C, Butcher J N (eds) Handbook of research methods in clinical psychology. Wiley, New York

Willner A H, Blackburn R 1986 Interpersonal reactions of violent offenders to threatening and affiliative situations. In preparation

Wolff S, Chick J 1980 Schizoid personality in childhood: a controlled follow-up study. Psychological Medicine 10: 85–100

World Health Organization 1978 Mental disorders: glossary and guide to their classification in accordance with the ninth revision of the International classification of diseases. World Health Organization, Geneva

11 *Edgar Miller*

Hysteria

INTRODUCTION

Hysteria is both one of the oldest and one of the least satisfactory of the nosological terms used in psychiatry. For those seeking an example to illustrate the conceptual confusions of traditional psychiatry hysteria is the ideal choice. This is presumably why Szasz (1961) in his book *The Myth of Mental Illness* based a lot of his argument on hysteria. It is not only those with radical views who have attacked hysteria. Even a psychiatrist as impeccably conventional as Slater (1976) has attacked the concept and the term has been dropped by the American Psychiatric Association's DSM III. On the other hand, as Lewis (1975) has noted, hysteria is a concept that has a nasty habit of outliving its obituarists.

That the term has survived so long, despite its well-recognized inadequacies, probably means that it reflects a useful role in referring to phenomena that are encountered in clinical practice. Even DSM III in dropping the term 'hysteria' has had to produce alternative labels for phenomena that might otherwise be described as hysterical. This chapter starts out by looking at the different types of hysteria that have been described. It sets out its own, more neutral definition of the term and goes on to argue that behaviour meeting this definition is encountered in practice. The various features associated with hysteria are then examined and, finally, theories of hysteria are critically examined.

Since hysterical behaviour as conceived in this chapter does not carry all the connotations that have sometimes been carried by the term, it could be argued that it might be better to employ an alternative term: either something like 'somatization disorder' as used in DSM III, or an entirely new term. The present writer is agnostic on this point. A new term might help avoid confusion produced by carrying old meanings. On the other hand, inventing new terms can create another set of confusions. For good or ill this chapter will stick with 'hysteria'.

THE CONCEPTS OF HYSTERIA

Given the considerable confusion surrounding 'hysteria' it is best to begin by looking at its referants. In fact it is a term that has a multitude of meanings and these have been set out by Kendell (1972, 1983a). Underlying the different types of hysteria are two basic meanings. These will be examined separately. In addition, hysteria overlaps with a number of other concepts and these also need to be considered.

Hysterical symptoms

A number of patients present with symptoms of a kind which, at first sight at least, would normally be associated with a disease process. Despite this it may prove impossible to establish any underlying pathology and careful consideration may reveal that the symptom does not match well-known anatomical or physiological principles. For example, the claimed loss of cutaneous sensation may not even remotely match the distribution of sensory innervation of the body. Such symptoms are commonly described as 'hysterical'.

Symptoms of this kind are also commonly referred to as 'conversion hysteria' or 'hysterical dissociation'. These terms pose difficulties because they derive from theoretical assumptions about the mechanisms alleged to produce the symptoms. In fact the confusion of descriptive term and supposed mechanism extends to 'hysteria' itself, based as it is on the Greek word for womb and the ancients' view that it was caused by a wandering womb. Given that this theory is now seen to be absurd and has not seriously been held for some time, it is now possible to regard 'hysteria' as a theoretically neutral term, and its use in this chapter is intended to be purely descriptive.

'Conversion hysteria' is a term derived from psychoanalysis and in classical Freudian theory hysteria arises from sexual conflicts at the oedipal stage of development. The incestuous quality of the libido at this stage is not resolved but is repressed and carried through into adult life. The psychic energy involved is then 'converted' into the hysterical symptom. As with most psychoanalytically derived hypotheses there are many variations on this basic theme, but these can be left until later.

At about the same time that Freud and Breuer were formulating their concept of conversion, Pierre Janet suggested that dissociation of consciousness could occur. What he meant by this was that elements of consciousness could fail to be integrated (or become 'dissociated'), resulting in a restriction of conscious awareness (Janet, 1907). This state is alleged to be temporary and can involve an amnesia for events occurring during the period of dissociation. The classical hysterical dissociative states consist of multiple personality, hysterical amnesias, fugues and trance states, whilst such things as sensory loss and paralyses are traditionally regarded as conversion reactions.

Apart from multiple personality, which is very rare, both conversion reactions and dissociative states involve the same key feature. They present with symptoms of a kind that, superficially at least, would normally be considered as the manifestations of organic disease yet these have no organic pathology. Multiple personality could be fitted into this as mimicking mental rather than physical illness. The differences lie in the exact nature of the symptoms and the putative causal mechanisms. It will be argued later that evidence for these causal mechanisms is, at best, very weak and so there is little to be gained from retaining terms implying the action of these mechanisms. There seems no a priori reason for regarding hysterical amnesia (allegedly a dissociative state) as needing to be labelled differently from hysterical paralysis (a conversion reaction) since these two have as much, or as little, in common with one another as hysterical amnesia and hysterical trance states (both dissociative reactions). In line with this analysis the rest of this chapter will be mainly concerned with hysterical symptoms, and the question of further subdivision is something to be established empirically.

Having thus combined hysterical conversion and hysterical dissociation, this is only a start in trying to cut through the conceptual confusion. Defining hysteria as the presence of symptoms in the absence of underlying pathology still leaves a number of other problems. Both hypochondriasis and malingering might also meet this definition. Conventional views of psychopathology distinguish between hysteria and malingering in that the malingerer deliberately and consciously sets out to fake symptoms of disease. In contrast, hysterical symptoms are alleged to be 'real' in the sense that the person with hysterical paralysis is actually unable to move the affected limbs. Distinguishing between hysteria and malingering on the basis of whether the motivation is conscious or unconscious is acceptable as part of a formal definition. It presents serious problems in practice. This is because judgements about the motivations of others and their conscious awareness are unreliable and provide an unsatisfactory basis on which to distinguish between individual patients. This is a point that will be considered in greater detail later.

The distinction between hypochondriasis and hysteria is also not easy, although the more extreme manifestations may be discriminable. In hypochondriasis (Kenyon 1976) the assumption is that the patient has an overconcern with bodily health and is thus likely to consult medical practitioners about relatively trivial symptoms which are assumed to indicate serious illness (as when a mild headache is alleged to be the first sign of a brain tumour). The hypochondriac's symptoms are often minor but there is considerable anxiety about their possible significance. Hysterical symptoms are typically grosser (e.g. blindness or complete paralysis below the waist) and, according to classical dogma, the patient exhibits 'la belle indifference'. In other words the patient fails to show an appropriate concern for the symptom. Again these distinctions can be blurred. There is a continuum from being overconcerned about a symptom, through having an appropriate concern, to having what, in the observer's opinion is 'la belle indifference'. Just where the lines are drawn is a very subjective matter. No matter what definition is used for hysteria it is difficult to find reliable and objective criteria with which to discriminate it from hypochondriasis on the one hand, or malingering on the other, if indeed such distinctions do have a sound basis.

The hysterical personality

This has been outlined by Kendell (1983b). The concept of the hysterical personality (possibly better described as the 'histrionic personality') arose earlier this century at a time when hysteria was assumed to be more or less exclusively a female disorder and the 'hysterical personality' allegedly described the characteristics of the woman prone to develop hysterical symptoms.

Chodoff & Lyons (1958) have summarized the most commonly described features of the hysterical personality as being overdramatic and histrionic. Other characteristics often given are egotistic, having a labile and shallow affect, bringing a superficial sexuality into non-sexual relationships whilst at the same time being frigid or anxious about the physical aspects of sexuality, as well as being suggestible and demanding. Describing a woman as having a 'hysterical personality' usually has pejorative overtones. In fact Kendell (1972) has suggested that female patients who irritate their doctors are labelled 'hysterical' whilst males who irritate are called 'psychopathic'.

The idea of the hysterical personality raises two fundamental questions. The first is whether the features associated with the alleged hysterical personality really do hang together to form a distinct trait or personality characteristic. This issue will not be pursued further since it is not germane to the main concern of this chapter, which is with hysterical symptoms. It can just be noted in passing that it is difficult to find strong evidence that a personality trait of this kind does exist. The second question is whether those subjects exhibiting hysterical symptoms also have features that would match the descriptions of the hysterical personality. This of course does seem unlikely if there is no good evidence for the personality trait in the first place. However, it would be wrong to dismiss this notion without considering any evidence. Chodoff & Lyons (1958) identified 17 cases of conversion hysteria from clinic records. These were cases where the recorded information was such as to demonstrate that the cases met certain predetermined criteria for conversion hysteria and where a detailed examination of mental state and personality were recorded. Of these 17 only three showed a reasonable approximation to the hysterical personality. Marsden (1986) has similarly reported that most patients with hysterical symptoms do not have a hysterical personality.

Other investigators have used personality questionnaires (especially the MMPI) and tried to establish whether patients with hysterical symptoms could be distinguished from controls in terms of their questionnaire responses. Lair & Trapp (1962) and Watson & Buranen (1979) are typical studies and both obtained no evidence suggesting that hysteria was associated with a particular personality profile.

It is always possible to criticize studies of personality in terms of the appropriateness or the validity of the means adopted to assess the personality features of interest. In consequence the hypothesis that patients with hysterical symptoms have a particular kind of personality is difficult to refute since the measures adopted will be less than wholly satisfactory. All that can be said is that attempts to examine this issue carefully have generally failed to provide supporting evidence. There is very little to support the hypothesis other than the general convictions of some clinicians. Until more compelling evidence is produced it seems safe to discount the concept of the hysterical personality and to regard it as having no proper place in the understanding of hysterical symptoms.

Other forms of hysteria

A number of other forms of hysteria have not yet been described (Kendell, 1983a) and these merit a few brief comments. One of these is *mass* or *epidemic hysteria*. This has been discussed in greater detail by Sirois (1982). Outbreaks of epidemic hysteria have occurred from time to time throughout history. These include the 'dancing manias' which broke out in the Rhine basin in the fourteenth century and the mass outbreaks of hysteria in nunneries in the sixteenth and seventeenth centuries. In a more modern episode, girls at a secondary school in Lancashire started to collapse with complaints of dizziness, weakness, headaches and other symptoms. This followed a much publicized outbreak of poliomyelitis in the neighbourhood with reports of people refusing to enter the town because they feared catching the disease. Such outbreaks of epidemic hysteria typically involve girls or young women. They take place in closed communities such as schools and convents and during times of stress or perceived threat.

Another type of hysterical manifestation is formed by those with *Briquet's syndrome* or *St Louis hysteria*, which is also referred to in DSM III as the somatization syndrome. This alleged syndrome was first described by the French physician Briquet in the last century but has been highlighted more recently by the St Louis school of psychiatry. It occurs almost exclusively in women and has an onset between puberty and the mid-twenties. The individual presents with a large number of symptoms related to different bodily systems, usually to different physicians at different times. The symptoms are dramatized (e.g. the headache is always described as 'excruciating', 'agonizing', or something similar). Physical causes for the problems are rarely found. The sufferer may also undergo several operations and they are alleged to have high rates of delinquent or antisocial behaviour.

Briquet's syndrome obviously overlaps to some degree with the Munchausen syndrome. There are also various other categories that have some similarity, or overlap with different manifestations of hysteria. Compensation neurosis (Miller H 1961), the Ganser syndrome and factitious disorders are but a few. Factitious disorders are where the individual presents with a symptom of organic disease but which is due to a deliberate deception. For example, the patient may have diarrhoea but this is self-induced with purgatives.

These various things all have in common the key feature of hysteria as described earlier. They involve the presentation of symptoms of a type usually associated with a disease process but for which no underlying pathology exists. The grounds on which they are distinguished from one another, or from more mainstream 'conversion' or 'dissociative' hysteria, are often arbitrary or trivial. It may well eventually be shown to be the case that not all manifestations of hysteria are the same and that some differentiation is therefore necessary. Apart from common usage there seems to be no strong reason at present to refrain from treating all hysterical symptoms as being essentially similar in kind and this general assumption will run through the rest of the chapter.

CRITICISMS OF THE CONCEPT OF HYSTERIA

As has been noted above, the concept of the hysterical personality is very weak and will be given no further consideration. This leaves the question of hysterical symptoms in their various manifestations. Hysteria, even in this sense, is open to considerable dispute. The attacks on the concept have been of two kinds: the conceptual and the empirical.

The earliest conceptualizations of hysteria obviously regarded it as a disease like measles or leprosy. This was the case with the wandering womb hypothesis of the ancients. Hollender (1972) has shown that as late as the nineteenth century gynaecologists still implicated the womb in hysteria, with impulses from the plexus of nerves supplying the womb thought to have adverse effects on the nervous system. Bringing in the mediation of the nervous system allowed that other organs could sometimes have a similar adverse effect, making it possible to account for the rare cases of hysteria in males. Although Freud looked for explanations in the psyche rather than the soma, the traditional Freudian view regards hysteria very much as a form of mental illness. As Slater (1976) has pointed out, there are problems with any disease-related view of hysteria. The key feature defining hysteria is the absence of pathological signs and it is illogical to have a disease concept with no pathology. This line of argument is explored by Szasz (1961) at greater length.

Without considering the arguments any further it can readily be conceded that a disease-based notion of hysteria is unsatisfactory and must be rejected. It is tempting to some to go on from that and draw the conclusion, wholly erroneous, that the term 'hysteria' has no meaning and should be dropped. An alternative and more defensible view of hysteria is that it is a dispositional concept (e.g. Ryle 1949). The term is useful not because it refers to any entity, such as a disease process, but because it identifies the coexistence of certain features (symptoms apparently physical for which no pathology can be found). The usefulness of the concept of hysteria in this sense depends on the occurrence of situations which meet these criteria. Whether such situations ever arise is an empirical rather than a conceptual issue.

The frequently cited study by Slater & Glithero (1965) involved the follow-up of 85 patients given the diagnosis of 'hysteria' at the National Hospital for Nervous Diseases in London in the early 1950s (see also Slater 1965). At the time of the follow-up 12 patients had died, which is an unusually large number for a sample with a mean age of around 40 years. In many of these it seemed likely that the disease causing death must have been present when the diagnosis of hysteria was made. Of the rest some had been considered to have a hysterical overlay on a real disease process right from the start, others later developed real illnesses with similar symptoms, and yet others developed serious psychiatric disorders like schizophrenia. This left only 21 subjects (25% of the original group) for whom no underlying pathology, physical or mental, had become apparent.

There are two major implications from this study. One is that a high proportion of those whose symptoms are described as hysterical do turn out later to have other problems which would throw the original description into doubt. Hysteria is a term that needs to be used with some caution. The other implication is even more serious. If Slater & Glithero (1965) could dispose of all but 25% of their sample in other ways, then might even more careful and extensive investigations have reduced this 25% much further, and possibly even to zero? In other words is 'hysteria' merely a label meaning that no satisfactory explanations for the symptoms have been found, but that a pathological explanation would exist if only the clinician were able to detect it?

There are reasons for being cautious about Slater & Glithero's findings and especially with regard to drawing the most extreme conclusions from them. One is that it was conducted on patients at the National Hospital for Nervous Diseases in London. This is a very prestigious postgraduate teaching hospital with a high proportion of secondary referrals. Their patients may not therefore be representative of those with hysterical problems in the general population and it is possible that clear-cut cases of hysteria may not be referred to that hospital very readily. In addition other follow-up studies have not led to such extreme results. Watson & Buranen (1979) followed up 40 cases considered to have hysterical symptoms over a 10-year period. These were compared with a matched group of 40 neurotic patients. During the follow-up there was no excess of physical illness or mortality in the hysterical group. Of the original hysterics only 25% were considered to have developed any indication that the original problem was not hysterical.

It is also sometimes possible to demonstrate quite clearly that the bodily system associated with a hysterical symptom does in fact function much better than if the symptom were truly part of a disease process. For example, the patient complaining of paralysis from the waist down will not raise the legs from the bed when lying on the back. When asked to fold the arms across the chest and sit up the patient may then carry this out using the very same stomach muscles that could not raise the legs. The clearest examples of this kind come from the forced choice testing of sensory symptoms. Those complaining of a complete sensory loss are put in the situation when they have to 'guess' which of two or three sensory stimuli has been applied. Those with hysterical sensory losses then often guess with levels of success that are very significantly below chance levels or show patterns of responding that are in other ways inconsistent with an inability to detect the stimuli (e.g. Grosz & Zimmerman 1965, Miller 1968, 1986).

To conclude this section, it does seem that despite Slater & Glithero (1965), or at least the most pessimistic interpretation that might be placed on their findings, there are people who do present with hysterical symptoms in the sense that these have been defined in this chapter. There are therefore phenomena that need to be understood and explained.

CHARACTERISTICS OF THOSE WHO PRESENT WITH HYSTERICAL SYMPTOMS

A number of features have been associated with hysterical symptoms or those who present with them. Some of these are also features of the hysterical personality. Although it is desirable, as has been argued above, to separate off the notion of the hysterical personality from a consideration of hysterical symptoms, some of those who have written about hysteria have not made this dissociation and so some overlap in discussion is unavoidable.

Gender

The derivation of the very word 'hysteria' from the Greek word for womb implies that hysteria is a problem of females. It is clearly not confined to women but it certainly is the case that published series contain a preponderance of women, even when subject selection is not confined to one sex (e.g. Lader & Sartorius 1968, Merskey & Buhrich 1975, Slater & Glithero 1965, Ziegler et al 1960). Given that there are few studies with large unselected series it is difficult to give any exact figure for the sex ratio. One study with a larger sample than most is that of Stefanis et al (1976), who reported that females outnumbered males in a ratio of about 3 : 1. Ratios both more and less extreme than this could be cited. It could also be that, as some have suggested (e.g. Merskey 1979), the alleged association between women and hysteria may lead examiners to identify hysterical problems more readily in females. Nevertheless, whatever the reason, there is a definite preponderance of women in those considered to have hysterical symptoms. It could also be that social and cultural factors might be related to the sex ratio but this is a point that will come up in the discussion of explanations of hysterical behaviour.

Despite the overall bias in favour of females there is also some indication that the sex ratio varies with the type of hysterical symptom. Whitlock (1967) points out that in his series with 20 males and 36 females just over a third of the males had fugues or amnesias whilst a very much lower proportion of the females had symptoms that could be described in that way. More or less the reverse situation held with dysphonia or mutism. This is in line with the present author's clinical experience, where hysterical amnesia is almost exclusively a male phenomenon. Hysterical fits appear to be another symptom with a particularly strong sex bias. As Whitlock's series shows, the latter are very much a female prerogative. Overall hysterical symptoms may be more common in females, but it has to be noted that when individual symptoms are examined there are examples where males predominate. This is a fact that makes it less likely that the overall preponderance of women is due to crude sex biases or prejudices amongst examiners, who are largely male.

Anxiety

A classic feature of hysteria is 'la belle indifference' or the patient's apparent lack of concern for what, on the face of it, might be quite a serious symptom. Of course, as Merskey (1979) indicates, this lack of concern or anxiety is just what might be expected if the individual is actually resolving some conflict by exhibiting the symptom. Psychodynamic models of hysteria have also regarded anxiety as being 'converted' into physical symptoms, thus reducing anxiety by the production of symptoms. However, in this latter case the anxiety that is relieved by the development of the symptom is not necessarily conscious anxiety.

There have been few investigations that have attempted to examine anxiety in hysterical patients in an experimental way. Of these the soundest is that of Lader & Sartorius (1968). They compared ten subjects with 'conversion symptoms' with two control groups: one composed of subjects with anxiety-based neurotic problems and the other of normal subjects. The measures used were both rating scales and psychophysiological indices of anxiety (based on palmar skin conductance). The results from both types of measure indicated that the hysterical group, rather than having low levels of anxiety, was at least as anxious as the other patient group containing people diagnosed as having anxiety states or phobias.

A similar report has come from Rice & Greenfield (1969), who found that their hysterical subjects showed excess physiological reactivity to anxiety-provoking stimuli, as indicated by the galvanic skin response and tension in the frontalis muscle. A problem with their report is that their small sample of only seven 'hysterical subjects' included some with symptoms only dubiously regarded as hysterical, e.g. spasmodic torticollis. Merskey (1979) cites a paper by Rosen (1951) allegedly showing a reduced response in physiological indices that might be assumed to reflect anxiety (e.g. a smaller response to the cold pressor test).

The evidence with regard to anxiety is not entirely satisfactory. On balance it goes against the idea that anxiety is lessened in those with hysterical symptoms, and this is certainly the conclusion that follows from the most methodologically adequate of the available investigations (that of Lader & Sartorius 1968). It must also be pointed out that these studies are measuring anxiety in general rather than anxiety about the hysterical symptom. This leaves the possibility that hysterical patients could show normal, or even raised levels of anxiety in general, and yet show 'la belle indifference' towards their specific hysterical symptom.

Sexual adjustment

Disturbances of sexual behaviour or sexual adjustment are a central feature in the notion of the hysterical personality (Chodoff & Lyons 1958) but have also been related to those with hysterical symptoms, especially if female. Winokur & Leonard (1961) attempted to obtain information about sexual behaviour in 14 women with Briquet's syndrome. They found that over a half had undergone gynaecological operations and almost a third had been sterilized before the age of 30 years. As a group their premarital sexual experience was not unusual but after marriage their frequency of sexual intercourse was low when compared to normative data from Kinsey et al (1953). Similarly Merskey & Trimble (1979) claimed a higher proportion of sexual maladjustment, mainly frigidity, in patients with 'conversion symptoms'.

Roy (1981, 1982) has also described data relating to sexual functioning in a sample of women with hysterical symptoms. As compared to a matched group of subjects with neurotic depression there was no difference in the proportion who were married or cohabiting, or who had been divorced or separated. About 15% in each group had sexual dysfunction (vaginismus or anorgasmia).

There are serious limitations in these investigations. The majority do not employ proper control groups and no one appears to have examined sexual functioning in males with hysteria. Even so, the rates of sexual disturbance are often quite high, indicating that sexual adjustment in hysterical patients may be poor. However, Roy's (1981) paper indicates that impairment may not be any higher than it is in those with neurotic depression. Thus it could be that sexual disorder is more common in patient samples in general but is not a particular characteristic of those with hysteria.

Depression

That a high proportion of patients with hysterical symptoms also seem to be depressed has been noted for some time. Almost 10% of the sample followed up by Slater & Glithero (1965) were regarded as having developed a depressive illness, as were 15% of Merskey & Buhrich's (1975) sample. An even higher rate was claimed by Ziegler et al (1960), with no less than 40 of their sample of 134 cases of 'conversion reaction' being regarded as having the clinical features of depression.

Roy (1980, 1982) describes a study of 50 patients with hysterical symptoms. All but six were considered depressed and these had a symptom duration of less than 6 months. The remaining six subjects without the features of depression were a 'chronic group' in that all had had their hysterical symptoms for longer than a year. Using the Wakefield Self-Assessment Depression Inventory (Snaith et al 1971) it was found that Roy's 44 'acute' hysterics had scores which were slightly, but not significantly, higher than a group of neurotic depressives.

Although the variation in the rate is quite wide it does appear that those with hysterical symptoms are more likely than would otherwise be expected to exhibit the features of depression. It may be that, as Roy's (1980) work suggests, depression is most marked when symptoms are first manifest but that as they persist the depression fades away.

Physical disorder

As has already been mentioned, Slater & Glithero (1965) found that about 60% of their sample had organic illnesses on follow-up. A number of other reports have looked at the relationship between hysterical problems and physical disease, and with very varied results. For example, Whitlock (1967) found that just over 60% of his sample had definite neurological disease that either preceded or accompanied the hysterical symptom. In Merskey & Burich's (1975) sample the proportion was just less than a half. On the other hand, Watson & Buranen (1979) discovered no excess of physical disease in their hysterical sample as compared with subjects with non-hysterical neurotic diagnoses. Roy (1979) studied a sample of 31 hysterics, of whom only one had organic brain disease.

One thing that might account for much of the discrepancy in the findings is the context in which the sample is obtained. In the case of Slater & Glithero (1965) and Merskey & Buhrich (1975) the samples came from a famous hospital specializing in neurological disease (the National Hospital in London). As argued above, this could lead to a very biased group of hysterics. Roy's (1979) subjects came from a psychiatric setting and he obtained a low rate of organic disease.

If there is a relation between hysterical symptoms and organic disease this could reflect a number of different underlying mechanisms. It could be that some allegedly hysterical symptoms really are the manifestation of an undetected physical disease. As argued above this is unlikely to account for all cases, especially where the symptom is clearly incompatible with known physiological principles. The link could be less direct. Organic disease of the brain might under some circumstances create or increase a disposition to develop hysterical symptoms under appropriate conditions. Another possibility is that the experience of real illness might provide a useful stimulus or model for the development of hysterical symptoms. In relation to this last point, it has been suggested that those who present with hysterical symptoms often mimic symptoms with which they are familiar, either through their own experience of illness or of illness in those who are close to them.

Evidence that hysterical patients may model symptoms with which they are familiar comes from studies of hysterical seizures. As Roy (1977) has shown, an appreciable proportion of these do have true epilepsy as well as exhibiting hysterical fits. That the hysterical seizures are not truly epileptic can be revealed by long-term continuous EEG recordings, which fail to show epileptiform EEG patterns during the 'fits'. Such findings are also consistent with the illness behaviour/sick role model of hysteria, which will be dealt with in a later section.

Other factors

Disturbances in upbringing have been related to the production of hysterical symptoms. Small & Nicholi (1982) studied children attending an elementary school where there had been an outbreak of mass hysteria. The 34 children admitted to hospital with symptoms were compared with the rest. Of those admitted almost half had experienced parental divorce and nearly 75% a death within the family. The corresponding rates in the controls were appreciably less. Zoccolillo & Cloninger (1985) looked at cases meeting both the Feighner criteria for Briquet's syndrome and the DSM III criteria for somatization disorder (which are very similar) and depressed controls. The hysterical group had suffered more childhood abuse and more removals from the parental home. The indications are therefore that a bad or disrupted upbringing may predispose to developing hysterical symptoms.

Another potentially significant factor is the patient's own experience of illness, either in themselves or those with whom they are in close contact. Such familiarity with real symptoms may provide a model for later hysterical problems. As indicated in the previous section there is an association between true epilepsy and the occurrence of hysterical fits (Roy 1982). If modelling of known symptoms does occur then those epileptics who later develop hysterical symptoms should be particularly prone to hysterical fits. When Roy (1982) examined this possibility nine out of ten true epileptics with later hysterical symptoms had hysterical seizures. There was even a tendency for the behaviour exhibited in the hysterical fits to approximate to that occurring in the true fits. Thus subjects with grand mal epilepsy had different hysterical manifestations from those with psychomotor seizures.

Finally, there is a suggestion that where hysterical symptoms are lateralized they are more likely to affect the left than the right side of the body (e.g. Galin et al 1977, Fleminger et al 1980). This finding was extended by Fleminger et al (1980), who showed that when it was suggested to female subjects (both neurotics and controls) that they would experience tingling in the hand this was more often reported for the left hand. As the various authors point out this can be related to a large body of work that has explored the possibility that different psychopathological conditions can be linked to one hemisphere of the brain rather than the other (Miller 1984).

EXPLANATIONS OF HYSTERICAL BEHAVIOUR

Why some individuals should present with hysterical symptoms has proved to be a considerable puzzle. A number of explanatory ideas have been put forward but many of these are too vague and ill-defined to lead to predictions that can be subjected to empirical test. This section sets out to examine the main lines along which explanations have been sought. These include the classical notions of conversion, dissociation, certain allegedly 'neurobiological' models, and the notion of abnormal illness behaviour. These ideas and the evidence relating to them will be outlined, but space does not permit all the variants of each model to be pursued. This limitation is not serious in its impact since it is not generally possible to differentiate between all the variants of each model on empirical grounds.

One common assumption runs through almost all the explanatory models. This is that the person with hysterical symptoms is not just deliberately faking or malingering. The hypothesis that the individual concerned is nothing more than a faker or dissimulator has attracted very little support, with Szasz (1974) being one possible exception. Nevertheless it merits much more detailed consideration than is given in most accounts of hysteria. This is because the assumption that they are not faking is of such fundamental importance in conceptualizations of hysteria.

Conversion

This is the classic psychoanalytic model, which has lent itself to the commonly used term 'conversion hysteria'. It arose out of Freud's earliest work on psychological disorders (Breuer & Freud 1895). As is the case with most psychoanalytic formulations, the idea of conversion has undergone modification and development (Merskey 1979). It is thus not possible to present a standard account. An early version had it that unresolved oedipal conflicts resulted in libido of an incestuous nature being carried through into adult life. This is then repressed and the psychic energy invested in it is rechannelled or 'converted' into hysterical symptoms. A more general version of the same basic principle is that any anxiety or conflict can lead to repression and conversion of the released energy into symptoms.

Most advocates of this model rely on uncontrolled clinical observations. For example, Ziegler et al (1960) found that about a third of their sample of subjects with 'conversion reactions' had depressive features. They also draw attention to the fact that many depressed patients report having pain with no physical cause. Putting these two things together they postulate that conversion may occur as a defence against more overt depression. Whichever version of the psychoanalytic model is adopted results in the problem that it is very difficult, if not impossible, to subject it to direct empirical test. All that can be done is to derive more specific hypotheses which bear a relation to the general model and then to test these.

A common assumption is that anxiety or anxiety-producing conflict is reduced by the psychic energy invested in it being converted to symptoms. It might then be expected that hysterics would show low levels of anxiety or 'la belle indifference', as has been claimed. As discussed earlier (pp. 253–254), experiments like that of Lader & Sartorius (1968) cast doubt on the notion that those with hysterical symptoms have low levels of anxiety and, if anything, even suggest the reverse. Another experimental approach has been used by Dalbo et al (1984). In their version of the psychodynamic model the conversion arises out of a conflict between a wish and the denial of that wish. Female subjects with hysterical symptoms, and controls, were presented with pictures and then given a delayed recognition test for those pictures. Not all the stimuli shown at the original presentation were included in the recognition test. These intercalated stimuli were either sexually related (to provide the conflict) or neutral. Hysterical subjects recognized the pictures with intercalated sexual stimuli best, whilst controls showed the reverse pattern. This result is only consistent with Dalbo et al's version of the conversion model if it is further assumed that stimuli arousing conflict in hysterics are not processed so efficiently thus allowing the other stimuli to be processed better and that the reverse happens in controls. Alternative explanations of the findings can also be readily proposed (e.g. in terms of different arousal levels). To be fair to Dalbo et al (1984), the major thrust of their paper was to rule out neurobiological models of hysteria, and it is certainly the case that their results do not readily fit such models, although they could be assimilated into neurobiological models, given other assumptions.

The psychoanalytic model of conversion is important historically and remains important in the thinking of many who write about hysteria. As with other psychodynamic formulations its appeal does not lie in its ability to generate supporting evidence of an empirical kind. Being based also on the notion of unconscious mental processes it is open to the same kinds of philosophical or conceptual objections that will be discussed in the next section in relation to the idea of dissociation.

Dissociation

As already indicated, the idea of dissociation is particularly associated with Janet (Janet 1907). The leading modern advocate of dissociation theory is Hilgard (1977). The basic assumption is that some aspects of what would otherwise be 'consciousness' are unintegrated or 'dissociated' from the rest and thus may not be accessible to normal awareness. Thus in the case of a subject with a dual personality, one personality may not know the nature or be aware of the second personality.

The concept of dissociation has some affinity with the usual psychodynamic idea of the unconscious and, indeed, the kind of logic used to argue for dissociation is very similar to that used to justify the presence of an unconscious mind. Nevertheless, there are differences. Hilgard (1977) regards the Freudian notion of the unconscious as a horizontal split in the mind. The unconscious mind lies under the conscious mind, with the forces of repression keeping them apart. The two operate according to different principles: the pleasure principle as opposed to the reality principle, in classical Freudian doctrine. What goes on in the unconscious is inaccessible to the conscious mind except in rather indirect and distorted ways. In contrast, dissociation implies a vertical split in the conscious mind. Some of the thoughts, memories, attitudes, etc. that might be part of the conscious mind become separated off or dissociated. At times, as in cases of multiple personality, the dissociated material may assume consciousness, with what is on the other side of the dissociation barrier being correspondingly lost from conscious awareness.

Advocates of dissociation, like Hilgard (1977), use it as a mechanism to explain many things and not just hysterical symptoms, although present concern is limited to hysteria. Many attempts have been made to provide an experimental demonstration of dissociation, and obviously the general plausibility of the process of dissociation has a bearing on its use to explain hysterical symptoms. Basically the relevant experiments are directed at showing that some form of cognitive activity of a kind usually associated with consciousness can take place without the subject being aware of this activity.

Hilgard (1977) has described a number of experiments of this kind, most of which have used the 'hidden observer' paradigm. For reasons which will become clear it is not necessary to consider this work in detail. One recent example of such work has been selected for description because it is one of the best of these experiments with regard to its methodological sophistication. Zamansky & Bartis (1985) hypnotized subjects and gave the suggestion that they would experience no odour, nor would they be able to see anything written on a piece of paper. Those subjects who both gave no indication of smelling ammonia when it was presented and who failed to read a number on a piece of paper were then given further instructions under hypnosis. These included the suggestion that 'you have a hidden part of you that knows reality' even though the part of the mind of which they were conscious might not be aware. They were told that after a suitable stimulus this 'hidden information' would become available to them. Most subjects could then identify the smell that they could not detect earlier, and report the number written on the piece of paper.

Experiments of this kind are open to a number of criticisms and many of these are acknowledged by Zamansky & Bartis themselves. Only the two most serious problems will be considered here. Zamansky & Bartis (1985) allow that it is always possible, as Spanos (1983) has suggested, that the results can be explained in terms of subjects responding to situational demands. Subjects just report that they cannot detect the smell or read the number when it is suggested that this cannot be done. As soon as they are informed that the information is now available they recall it from memory in the ordinary way. This is a problem faced by all experiments of this type and no one has thought of an effective way of controlling for the effects of social expectancy (i.e. subjects just cynically doing what the experimenter appears to want them to do). There seems to be no way round this methodological problem in experiments of this kind.

The second major difficulty is philosophical or conceptual. The basis of the argument for dissociation, and incidentally for the presence of an unconscious mind in the Freudian sense, is that subjects can apparently perform some mental operation without being aware of it (e.g. registering an odour without being able to report that it has been smelled). Even if such phenomena are allowed to occur, and not just appear to occur because of social expectancy or situational demands, the conclusion that there must be an unconscious mind or dissociated part of the mind does not necessarily follow. As philosophers following in the tradition set by Wittgenstein have indicated (e.g. Ryle 1949, White 1967), it does not mean because something can be done 'unconsciously' that there is an unconscious mind, or dissociated part of the mind, for the underlying psychological processes to go on in. Space does not permit a long philosophical discussion but the basic arguments are set out by White (1967).

In summary, there are grounds for being suspicious of the notion of dissociation itself. This in turn makes it unsatisfactory to explain hysterical symptoms by claiming that they are maintained by a dissociated part of the mind. Given that the considerable conceptual and methodological problems underlying research into dissociation do not lend themselves to ready solution it seems advisable to look for explanations of hysterical behaviour elsewhere.

Neurobiological theories

Yet another approach to understanding hysteria is provided by the so-called 'neurobiological' theories. The association between hysteria and cerebral pathology, considered in an earlier section (pp. 255–256), could be thought to reinforce the view that hysteria might be produced by some impairment or malfunctioning of the brain. As already noted, the existence of a link between hysteria and cerebral pathology does not necessarily mean a direct causal link between the two. For example, certain types of pathology which affect personality may result in the individual being less inhibited and so enhance an already existing tendency to respond to certain situations by developing hysterical symptoms. Furthermore, studies like that of Whitlock (1967) showing an association between hysteria and cerebral pathology always contain a number of hysterical subjects with no demonstrable brain pathology.

Ludwig (1972) and Whitlock (1967) provide examples of neurobiological theories. The details of these theories differ and they can be based on rather loose speculations from a variety of contexts. In Ludwig's (1972) case there is much speculation about certain reactions in animals described by ethologists such as the 'sham death' reflex. Nevertheless, a common feature of these theories is an appeal to physiological mechanisms involved in such things as vigilance, consciousness, selective attention and the inhibition of afferent stimulation. Thus the person with hysterical anaesthesia may not be aware of afferent input from the relevant part of the body or not be able to attend selectively to it:

A number of experiments based on this line of thinking have been described, based on studies of such things as evoked potentials. Much of the earlier work is reviewed by Whitlock (1967) and the results are, at best, conflicting, with more findings being negative than positive. More recent work has not really altered this picture, although one interesting finding has been reported by Guze (1967), who studied 17 'conversion hysterics' after their symptoms had resolved. He looked at changes in skin conductance following an auditory stimulus and found that those who habituated most readily were also those whose hysterical symptoms had resolved most rapidly and who had the more stable and well-adjusted personalities.

There is a basic conceptual problem with any neurobiological theory. By definition the hysterical symptoms must have no demonstrable organic cause. The patient may have organic pathology somewhere in the body (e.g. in the brain) but this must be such that it could not possibly explain the symptom(s) regarded as hysterical. This means that any link between disordered brain functioning and the hysterical symptom must necessarily be indirect. The postulated lesion or brain malfunction must then act by predisposing the individual to develop hysterical symptoms whose primary cause must be of some other type. Contrary to what some authorities have claimed, it is not possible to have neurobiological mechanisms as a primary cause, although such factors may be important in other ways, e.g. by enhancing vulnerability. In fairness it should also be noted that there are those such as Whitlock (1967) who have espoused neurobiological mechanisms but who also appear to recognize their limitations as fundamental explanations of hysteria.

Hysteria as faking

The theories of hysteria considered so far share a common fundamental assumption. This is that the hysterical patient is in some way different from the one who malingers and deliberately makes false claims about his health. The assumption is that in hysteria there is no conscious production of spurious symptoms. Because this is such a fundamental assumption it warrants close analysis. In other words it is important to consider a model of hysteria which states that hysterical symptoms are nothing more than deliberate faking or malingering.

If hysteria is different from faking the key difference lies in the fact that the hysterical patient is not deliberately and consciously misrepresenting himself (e.g. Stevens 1986). The hysteric is not conscious of the spurious nature of his symptoms in the same way as the malingerer. If the person with hysteria is involved in any deception he is deceiving himself as much as anyone else. This point is impossible to resolve empirically since the investigator does not have access to the contents of the individual's consciousness (see also Grosz & Zimmerman 1965). What is possible is to ask the related question as to whether the behaviour of those considered to have hysterical symptoms differs from that of subjects known to be deliberately faking the same symptoms.

Evidence relevant to this latter point does exist. Spanos et al (1985) found that subjects asked to play the role of a prime suspect in a murder case and being interviewed under hypnosis showed a strong tendency to assume the role of a person with multiple personalities under some circumstances (questions being posed in a certain way). Aplin & Kane (1985) also reported that subjects asked to simulate hearing loss gave results on audiometric testing very similar to those reported for subjects with hysterical hearing loss.

A more direct experimental test was carried out by Silberman et al (1985). Using subjects with multiple personalities they hypothesized that subjects asked to learn one set of material as one personality and another set under another personality would show less interference between the two sets of material than normal subjects learning the same things in the ordinary way. In general no between-group differences were found on the main dependent variables. The authors examined their data closely and claimed some minor qualitative differences. Even if the latter are considered to be of importance, and they are most unlikely to impress the sceptic, this does not mean, as Silberman et al claim, that the multiple personalities could not be faking. The subjects with multiple personality will have had considerable practice at trying to keep information in 'separate compartments' whilst the control group presumably did not. Any minor differences could then be potentially explained as the results of differing levels of practice. This point is potentially capable of resolution by giving extended practice of an appropriate nature to the control group.

Another methodological problem is less open to easy resolution. If hysterical patients are to be compared with subjects asked to fake symptoms deliberately, the two groups are inevitably going to differ in other ways. The control group will not have spontaneously adopted hysterical symptoms whilst the experimental group has. There must be some other factor present in the experimental group which has caused them to adopt the strategy of developing spurious symptoms. Any difference between the two groups, expecially if minor, could be put down to this other factor rather than to one group faking and the other not.

Whilst it is possible to determine whether hysterics behave exactly the same as known dissimulators, it is difficult to decide exactly what the results mean if differences appear. Differences need not necessarily mean that hysteria is different from faking, especially if they are small, since alternative explanations are available. As long as convincing differences fail to be found, and this is what appears to be the case so far, it is then reasonable to go on and question the practical value in maintaining that there is a difference between hysteria and deliberate dissimulation.

Illness behaviour and the sick role

A very different approach to the understanding of hysterical behaviour comes from the use of notions like 'illness behaviour' and the 'sick role'. Variations of this model have been put forward as early as Ziegler & Imboden (1962), with Kendell (1983a), Mayou (1976) and Pilowsky (1969) amongst others also espousing the same general theme. It utilizes the concepts of 'illness behaviour' and the 'sick role' as developed by sociologists like Mechanic (1962) and Parsons (1951).

Mechanic (1962) defined illness behaviour as the ways in which symptoms may be perceived, evaluated and acted upon by individuals. It has been shown that somatic symptoms (headache, backache, dizziness, etc.) are extremely common in the general population (e.g. Kellner & Sheffield 1973, Ingham and Miller 1976). Few people experiencing such symptoms consult their doctors. Whilst those who do consult do on average report their symptoms as being more severe there is still a very considerable overlap in severity between those who consult and those who do not. As Mechanic and others have pointed out, this implies that the ways in which symptoms are perceived and evaluated and the context in which they occur may be of considerable importance. Mechanic (1962, 1986) has discussed the factors that may affect the perception of symptoms.

Once illness has been recognized and made legitimate by the diagnosing physician the individual is justified in adopting the 'sick role' (Parsons 1951). Those who are regarded as sick can be relieved of certain responsibilities (having to go to work, perform household chores, etc.) and others may be under an obligation to be especially considerate towards them. The sick role carries its own obligations such as having to cooperate in treatment and possibly withdraw from activities that might normally be pleasurable.

These processes may be unduly distorted in hysteria. Pilowsky (1969) and Mayou (1976) have tended to stress illness behaviour in terms of the hysterical subject's alleged tendency to perceive and evaluate symptoms inappropriately. Thus a minor twinge or feeling of discomfort that most would ignore may then be elevated to the status of a major symptom, at least in the individual's view. Kendell (1983a) has stressed the rewards of adopting the sick role. As he argues, most people experience illness at some time, especially in childhood, and the benefits of the sick role may be particularly reinforcing, thus leading to further claims to illness in the future. Kendell's views come quite close to those of psychologists who have seen hysterical symptoms as behaviour learned according to the rules of operant conditioning (e.g. Munford 1978). Although illness behaviour and the sick role can be separated they can also be seen as stressing different aspects of the same overall process involving the social/psychological aspects of the individual's reaction to disease. For this reason they are being treated here as part of the same general model of hysteria.

Pilowsky's (1969) view of the hysterical patient misperceiving the nature of trivial symptoms does not seem an adequate explanation of the more bizarre manifestations, such as multiple personality or a total paralysis below the waist. These might be more convincing as an inappropriate adoption of the sick role. Misperception of symptoms would better fit hypochondriacal symptoms or even patients meeting the criteria for Briquet's syndrome with a history of multiple minor complaints affecting a number of different bodily systems.

There is very little empirical evidence that can be cited in relation to this approach to hysteria. Wilson-Barnett and Trimble (1985) gave a number of self-report scales, including an 'Illness Behaviour Questionnaire' to a sample with hysterical symptoms. The results were not very conclusive but did reveal that hysterical subjects had past histories of vague and undiagnosable medical problems which would be compatible with a tendency to misperceive the significance of trivial symptoms. The preponderance of women in samples of hysterics and the tendency to mimic symptoms with which the individual is familiar are things that could readily be accommodated within the illness behaviour/sick role model without too much difficulty, e.g. in terms of different socialization in women making certain reactions to symptoms more socially acceptable for them.

The overall model has both advantages and disadvantages. It is weak because it is relatively imprecise and with minor modifications can be stretched to fit a very wide range of things that might be true of hysteria. At its worst it is little more than an alternative description of hysterical behaviour. To describe the subject who spends most of his waking life in a wheelchair because of hysterical paralysis as inappropriately adopting the sick role could be regarded as almost tautologous. Although the notions of abnormal illness behaviour or inappropriately adopting the sick role are not very penetrating in themselves, they are concepts that are open to being unpacked into constituent parts and testable predictions can be derived from them. For example, do subjects with hysterical symptoms tend to make different attributions concerning minor aches and pains, and have they had more opportunity than most to learn the benefits of adopting the sick role? Although this general approach needs to be elaborated, and may eventually need to be considerably modified or even abandoned, it is of heuristic value in pointing to worthwhile lines of further investigation. Deriving satisfactory testable predictions from some of the other models of hysteria is much less easy. It is also possible to use the illness behaviour/sick role model without making any assumptions about the role of conscious awareness in symptom production, which is very useful given the difficulty in resolving the issue of conscious awareness.

CONCLUSIONS

After centuries of speculation, regrettably few conclusions can be drawn about hysteria. The very concept is itself still open to dispute. Whilst the idea of hysteria as any kind of illness or medical entity can certainly be rejected, people do undoubtedly present to medical services with symptoms such as amnesia, blindness and paralysis of limbs for which no organic cause can be found and, moreover, where such a cause seems highly improbable. This means that explanations have to be sought in psychological terms.

Some things are known about the characteristics of those who present with hysterical symptoms, such as their proneness to associated anxiety or depression. Understanding why and how hysterical symptoms are developed has not progressed very far and all the suggested models have serious limitations. Even though it may ultimately be shown to be misguided the illness behaviour/sick role model appears to be the most fruitful at present. This is because it side-steps the vexed question of the role of consciousness and prompts a set of questions for the further investigation of hysteria that at least have a good chance of being useful in advancing understanding. Even if this model eventually falls, and it probably cannot survive without at least major modification, its exploration offers the best hope of a springboard from which to develop a sounder understanding of hysterical behaviour.

REFERENCES

Aplin, D Y, Kane J M 1985 Variables affecting pure tone and speech audiometry in experimentally simulated hearing loss. British Journal of Audiology 19: 219–228

Breuer J, Freud S 1895 Studies in hysteria. In: Standard edition of the complete psychological works of Sigmund Freud, Vol 2. Hogarth Press, London

Chodoff P, Lyons H 1958 Hysteria, the hysterical personality and 'hysterical' conversion. American Journal of Psychiatry 114: 738–740

Dalbo A, Cedla A, Brighenti F, Semenza C, de Bertolini C 1984 Recognition memory in conversion hysteria: effect of sexual stimuli during learning. Acta Psychiatrica Scandinavica 70: 535–539

Fleminger J J, McClure G M, Dalton R 1980 Lateral response to suggestion in relation to handedness and the side of psychogenic symptoms. British Journal of Psychiatry 136: 562–566

Galin D, Diamond R, Braff D 1977 Lateralization of conversion symptoms: more frequent on the left. American Journal of Psychiatry 134: 578–580

Grosz H J, Zimmerman J 1965 Experimental analysis of hysterical blindness. Archives of General Psychiatry 13: 256–260

Guze S B 1967 The diagnosis of hysteria: what are we trying to do? American Journal of Psychiatry 124: 491–498

Hilgard E R 1977 Divided consciousness. Wiley, New York

Hollender M H 1972 Conversion hysteria: a post-Freudian reinterpretation of 19th century psychosocial data. Archives of General Psychiatry 26: 311–314

Ingham J G, Miller P M 1976 The determinants of illness declaration. Journal of Psychosomatic Research 20: 309–316

Janet P 1907 The major symptoms of hysteria. Macmillan, New York

Kellner R, Sheffield B F 1973 The one-week prevalence of symptoms in neurotic patients and normals. American Journal of Psychiatry 130: 102–105

Kendell R E 1972 A new look at hysteria. Medicine 30: 1780–1783

Kendell R E 1983a Hysteria. In: Russell G F M, Hersov L A (eds) Handbook of psychiatry, Vol 4: the neuroses and personality disorders. Cambridge University Press, Cambridge

Kendell R E 1983b The hysterical (histrionic) personality. In: Russell G F M, Hersov L A (eds) Handbook of psychiatry, Vol 4: the neuroses and personality disorders. Cambridge University Press, Cambridge

Kenyon F E 1976 Hypochondriacal states. British Journal of Psychiatry 129: 1–14

Kinsey A C, Pomeroy W B, Martin C E, Gebhard P H 1953 Sexual behavior in the human female. Saunders, Philadelphia

Lader M, Sartorius N 1968 Anxiety in patients with hysterical conversion symptoms. Journal of Neurology, Neurosurgery and Psychiatry 31: 490–495

Lair C V, Trapp P 1962 The differential diagnostic value of MMPI with somatically disturbed patients. Journal of Clinical Psychology 18: 146–147

Lewis A 1975 The survival of hysteria. Psychological Medicine 5: 9–12

Ludwig A M 1972 Hysteria: a neurobiological theory. Archives of General Psychiatry 27: 771–777

Marsden C D 1986 Hysteria — a neurologist's view. Psychological Medicine 16: 277–288

Mayou R 1976 The nature of bodily symptoms. British Journal of Psychiatry 129: 55–60

Mechanic D 1962 The concept of illness behavior. Journal of Chronic Diseases 15: 189–194

Mechanic D 1986 The concept of illness behaviour: culture, situation and personal predisposition. Psychological Medicine 16: 1–7

Merskey H 1979 The analysis of hysteria. Bailliere Tindall, London

Merskey H, Buhrich N A 1975 Hysteria and organic brain disease. British Journal of Medical Psychology 48: 359–366

Merskey H, Trimble M 1979 Personality, sexual adjustment and brain lesions in patients with conversion symptoms. American Journal of Psychiatry 136: 179–182

Miller E 1968 A note on the visual performance of a patient with unilateral functional blindness. Behaviour Research and Therapy 6: 115–116

Miller E 1984 Neuropsychology. In: McGuffin P, Shanks M F, Hodgson R F (eds) The scientific principles of psychopathology. Grune & Stratton, London

Miller E 1986 Detecting hysterical sensory symptoms: an elaboration of the forced choice method. British Journal of Clinical Psychology 25: 231–232

Miller H 1961 Accident neurosis. British Medical Journal 1: 919–925

Munford P R 1978 Conversion disorder. Psychiatric Clinics of North America 1: 377–390

Parsons T 1951 The social system. Free Press, Glencoe

Pilowsky I 1969 Abnormal illness behaviour. British Journal of Medical Psychology 42: 347–351

Rice D G, Greenfield N S 1969 Psychophysiological correlates of la belle indifference. Archives of General Psychiatry 37: 1383–1385

Rosen H 1951 The hypnotic and hypnotherapeutic control of severe pain. American Journal of Psychiatry 107: 917–924
Roy A 1977 Hysterical fits previously diagnosed as epilepsy. Psychological Medicine 7: 271–273
Roy A 1979 Hysterical seizures. Archives of Neurology 36: 447–449
Roy A 1980 Hysteria. Journal of Psychosomatic Research 24: 53–56
Roy A 1981 Sexual dysfunction and hysteria. British Journal of Medical Psychology 54: 131–132
Roy A 1982 Hysteria. Wiley, Chichester
Ryle G 1949 The concept of mind. Hutchinson, London
Silberman E K, Putnam F W, Weingartner H, Braun B G, Post R M 1985 Dissociative studies in multiple personality disorder: a quantitative study. Psychiatry Research: 15: 253–260
Sirois F 1982 Epidemic hysteria. In: Roy A (ed) Hysteria. Wiley, Chichester
Slater E T O 1965 Diagnosis of 'hysteria'. British Medical Journal 1: 1395–1399
Slater E T O 1976 What is hysteria? New Psychiatry 2: 14–15
Slater E T O, Glithero E 1965 A follow-up of patients diagnosed as suffering from 'hysteria'. Journal of Psychosomatic Research 9: 9–13
Small G W, Nicholi M 1982 Mass hysteria among schoolchildren: early loss as predisposing factor. Archives of General Psychiaty 32: 186–190
Snaith R P, Ahmed S N, Mehta S, Hamilton M 1971 Assessment of severity of primary depressive illness: the Wakefield self-assessment inventory. Psychological Medicine 1: 143–149
Spanos N P 1983 The hidden observer as an experimental creation. Journal of Personality and Social Psychology 44: 170–176
Spanos N P, Weekes J P, Bertrand L D 1985 Multiple personality: a social psychological perspective. Journal of Abnormal Psychology 94: 362–376
Stefanis C, Markidus M, Christodoulou G 1976 Observations on the evaluation of the hysterical symptomatology. British Journal of Psychiatry 128: 269–275
Stevens H 1986 Is it organic or functional: is it hysteria or malingering? Psychiatric Clinics of North America 9: 241–254
Szasz T S 1961 The myth of mental illness. Harper & Row, New York
Szasz T S 1974 The second sin. Routledge & Kegan Paul, London
Watson G C, Buranen C 1979 The frequency and identification of false positive conversion reactions. Journal of Nervous and Mental Diseases 167: 243–247
White A R 1967 The philosophy of mind. Random House, New York
Whitlock F A 1967 The aetiology of hysteria. Acta Psychiatrica Scandinavica 43: 144–162
Wilson-Barnett J, Trimble, M R 1985 An investigation of hysteria using the Illness Behaviour Questionnaire. British Journal of Psychiatry 146: 601–607
Winokur G, Leonard C 1961 Sexual life in patients with hysteria. Diseases of the Nervous System 24: 337–343
Zamansky H S, Bartis S P 1985 The dissociation of experience: the hidden observer observed. Journal of Abnormal psychology 94: 243–248
Ziegler F J, Imboden J B 1962 Contemporary conversion reactions. II. A conceptual model. Archives of General Psychiatry 6: 279–287
Ziegler F J, Imboden J B, Meyer B 1960 Contemporary conversion reactions: a clinical study. American Journal of Psychiatry 116: 901–909
Zoccolillo M, Cloninger C R 1985 Parental breakdown associated with somatization disorder. British Journal of Psychiatry 147: 443–446

12 Eating disorders

Peter J. Cooper and Zafra Cooper

INTRODUCTION

The eating disorders are generally taken to include the clinical categories of anorexia nervosa, bulimia nervosa and obesity. Strictly, these categories do not all have the same logical status, as the first two refer to psychiatric disorders involving disturbances in behaviour and mental state, whereas obesity refers to a purely physical condition of excess body fat. Obesity tends to be considered along with essentially psychiatric conditions because it is assumed that the disorder of body weight arises out of a disorder of eating which is, at least in part, psychologically determined. This assumption can be challenged on a number of grounds. In a recent study in which a large group of adoptees was divided into weight categories, a strong relationship was found between the adoptees' weight category and the body mass index (weight/height) of their biological parents. No relationship was found between adoptees' weight and the body mass index of their adoptive parents (Stunkard et al 1986). This suggests that genetic factors are of considerable aetiological significance in obesity. It could, nevertheless, be argued that, in addition to inherited constitutional factors, psychological factors are also of causal significance in obesity in so far as they are responsible for leading some people to overeat. Over the past 20 years or so there has been considerable research interest in elucidating the role of psychological variables in obesity (Striegel-Moore & Rodin 1986). This work has been largely predicated on the assumption that obese people do overeat, in the sense that they eat significantly more than their normal-weight counterparts. The investigations of this hypothesis have been hampered by methodological difficulties. In particular, the limited food choice and general constraints of laboratory studies make it difficult to generalize from the findings of such research; and there are problems in accurately and non-intrusively measuring food intake in naturalistic studies. The findings of these investigations are conflicting. Of 29 laboratory studies reviewed by Spitzer & Rodin (1981), nine found obese people to have a higher food intake than non-obese people, whereas 20 found no difference between these two groups. The balance of evidence from the field studies is in the opposite direction: in three studies no difference was found, whereas in five the obese subjects were found to eat more than the normal-weight subjects.

Despite the meagre evidence that obese people eat more than non-obese people, there has been a great deal of research directed at identifying those aspects of the eating style of the obese which lead to their being overweight. This work has not produced consistent results (Stunkard & Kaplan 1977, Striegel-Moore & Rodin 1986). Some investigators have found obese subjects to eat more quickly than non-obese subjects (Hill & McCutcheon 1975, Dodd et al 1976). However, rate of eating changes over the course of a meal, presumably as a function of satiety, and studies which have included measures of the rate of eating continuously throughout a meal have found no difference between overweight and normal-weight individuals (Dodd et al 1976, Mahoney 1975, Warner & Balagura, 1975). Also, no differences have been found between these two groups in terms of number of mouthfuls eaten per time period (Mahoney 1975, Warner & Balagura 1975). Thus the evidence that obese people have particular disturbances in eating style is far from persuasive. The idea is further undermined by the finding that behavioural programmes designed to modify eating style have not led to substantial and enduring weight loss in a great many obese people (Dubbert & Wilson 1983, Brownell & Wadden 1986).

A related area of enquiry has been the attempt to demonstrate that obese people are peculiarly susceptible to certain cues to eat. In particular, Schachter (1971) proposed that the initiation of eating in normal-weight people was influenced largely by internal cues, such as gastric motility signalling hunger and satiety; whereas, the eating of obese people was influenced largely by external cues, such as time of day and food palatability. This hypothesis has generated considerable research which has clarified the factors leading to eating in both obese and lean people. It appears that external responsiveness with respect to eating is a dimension on which individuals vary, but that overweight people as a group are not necessarily more 'external' than normal-weight people. Palatability and variety of food choice do indeed stimulate eating, but no more so for those who are obese than others (Striegel-Moore & Rodin 1986). Another cue, emotional arousal, has been shown in laboratory work to lead obese people to eat more than normal-weight controls (Slochower 1985); but the significance of this finding to the development or maintenance of obesity is far from clear.

The evidence that obesity is a disorder with a significant psychological component is weak. The condition presents as an essentially physical disorder of body weight and the role of disturbed eating in its aetiology and maintenance is, at best, unproven. It is therefore not reasonable to regard obesity as an eating disorder in the sense that anorexia nervosa and bulimia nervosa are clearly such disorders. The remainder of this chapter will therefore be concerned with the latter two conditions.

HISTORICAL DEVELOPMENT

Accounts of self-induced weight loss can be traced back to the Middle Ages (Hammond 1879). However, the first clinical description of anorexia nervosa was provided in 1694 by an English physician, Richard Morton (see Strober 1986). He suggested the name 'phthisis nervosa' for a disorder he had encountered in two of his patients involving food avoidance, extreme emaciation, amenorrhoea and overactivity. Morton regarded the disorder as neurological in origin, but recognized the influence of psychological factors. He reported that one of these patients, 'a skeleton only clad with skin', died from 'a multitude of cares and passions of the mind'. The term 'anorexia nervosa' was introduced into the medical literature in 1874 by Sir William Gull, Physician Extraordinary to Queen Victoria. Gull described a 'peculiar form of disease' occurring mostly in young women, and characterized by extreme emaciation. He clearly regarded anorexia nervosa as essentially a psychological disorder. In 1914, the German pathologist Morris Simmonds reported a case of emaciation and amenorrhoea in a girl whose pituitary gland had atrophied. For the next 25 years most cases of anorexia nervosa were thought to be suffering from Simmond's disease and were treated with pituitary extracts. Eventually it became clear that the pituitary disorder produces symptoms not found in anorexia nervosa (such as lassitude and lack of pubic hair) and the two disorders were recognized as distinct. In the 1940s and 1950s theories of psychological causality flourished, the most influential early writer being Hilda Bruch (1973). Since then, there has been a remarkable consistency in the conceptualization of the disorder, with authorities in the field of varying theoretical orientations presenting accounts of the central psychopathological features in very similar terms (Russell 1970, Crisp 1980, Garfinkel & Garner, 1982). This consistency is immediately apparent when one considers the relative ease with which it is possible to specify generally acceptable diagnostic criteria for the condition (see below).

Bulimia nervosa is a far newer clinical concept. Towards the end of the 1970s reports began to emerge of people with a disorder characterized principally by episodes of uncontrolled eating. These people closely resembled patients with anorexia nervosa but were generally of normal weight. The disorder attracted a variety of names, including 'the dietary chaos syndrome' (Palmer 1979), 'the abnormal normal weight syndrome' (Crisp 1979) and 'bulimarexia' (Boskind-Lodahl 1976). The two terms which have subsequently gained widest acceptance have been 'bulimia nervosa' (Russell 1979), the term usually used in Britain, and 'bulimia', the term included in DSM III, the third edition of the *Diagnostic and Statistical Manual* of the American Psychiatric Association (1980). The use of the term 'bulimia' to refer to the disorder is unfortunate because it confuses a behaviour (gross overeating) with a constellation of psychological characteristics in which bulimic episodes invariably occur. The final version of the revisions to DSM

III currently being made will remove this ambiguity by adopting the term 'bulimia nervosa'. Unfortunately, the British and American concepts of this disorder have differed more than just in name, since they have been associated with quite different sets of diagnostic criteria.

DIAGNOSTIC CRITERIA

There is wide agreement about the necessary clinical features for a diagnosis of anorexia nervosa. Table 12.1 provides one specification of formal diagnostic criteria. It is based on a report by Garrow et al (1975) which in turn owes much to the criteria originally provided by Russell (1970). Other criteria, such as those of Feighner et al (1972) and DSM III (1980), differ from these criteria in detail and emphasis, but clearly are attempting to define the same clinical population. The most striking feature of this disorder is the self-induced weight loss. As can be seen from the table, no precise criterion of extent of weight loss is provided. Garfinkel & Garner (1982), in their definitive account of anorexia nervosa, regard this as desirable because it prevents the definition from being arbitrarily restrictive.

Table 12.1 Diagnostic criteria for eating disorders

Anorexia nervosa (Garrow et al 1975):
1. Self-inflicted severe loss of weight, using one or more of the following devices: (a) avoidance of foods considered to be 'fattening' (especially carbohydrate-containing foods); (b) self-induced vomiting; (c) abuse of purgatives; and (d) excessive exercise
2. A secondary endocrine disorder of the hypothalamic anterior pituitary gonadal axis manifest in the female as amenorrhoea and in the male by a diminution of sexual interest and activity
3. A psychological disorder that has as its central theme a morbid fear of being unable to control eating and hence becoming too fat

Bulimia (DSM III 1980):
1. Recurrent episodes of binge eating (rapid consumption of a large amount of food in a discrete period of time, usually less than two hours)
2. At least three of the following:
    (i) consumption of high-caloric, easily ingested food during a binge
    (ii) inconspicuous eating during a binge
    (iii) termination of such eating episodes by abdominal pain, sleep, social interruption, or self-induced vomiting
    (iv) repeated attempts to lose weight by severely restrictive diets, self-induced vomiting, or use of cathartics or diuretics
    (v) frequent weight fluctuations greater than ten pounds due to alternating binges and fasts
3. Awareness that the eating pattern is abnormal and fear of not being able to stop eating voluntarily
4. Depressed mood and self-depreciating thoughts following eating binges
5 The bulimic episodes are not due to anorexia nervosa or any known physical disorder

Bulimia nervosa (Russell 1979):
1. The patients suffer from powerful and intractable urges to overeat
2. They seek to avoid the 'fattening' effects of food by inducing vomiting or abusing purgatives or both
3. They have a morbid fear of becoming fat

Some criteria do, however, specify a weight loss of 25%; but this ignores the problems of an obese person losing 25% of body weight and presenting at normal weight. It also creates problems when applied to young girls. The requirement of a 'secondary endocrine disorder' is desirable, according to Garfinkel & Garner (1982), because it eliminates those who may be engaging in fairly stringent but normal dieting. This is a somewhat dubious point because the degree of dietary restriction, and indeed, the extent of weight loss necessary to produce the endocrine disorder is not the same for every individual. Also, a variety of factors, such as athletic activity and psychological and physical stress, can contribute to the development of amenorrhoea (Wakeling 1985). In any event, it is doubtful whether, amongst those who fulfil the other two criteria, those who are still menstruating differ from those who are not, in terms of prognosis and outcome. The third criterion specified refers to what can be termed the specific psychopathology of the eating disorders; that is, the extreme concerns about shape and weight which are so widely accepted as a central and necessary feature of anorexia nervosa. These concerns have been variously characterized as 'a morbid fear of fatness' (Russell 1970), 'a pursuit of thinness' (Bruch 1973), and 'a weight phobia' (Crisp 1967).

The appropriate diagnostic criteria for bulimia nervosa are less clear. The central feature common to all existing criteria is episodes of loss of control over eating. Which other clinical features should be regarded as necessary is a matter about which there is considerable current debate (Fairburn & Garner 1986). The table provides the diagnostic criteria of the DSM III (1980) category of bulimia; and the criteria for bulimia nervosa originally delineated by Russell (1979). These two sets of criteria are clearly intended to define a similar patient population; but in fact they identify partially overlapping groups of people. This is, in part, because the DSM III criteria are over-inclusive. Thus, a symptom, the presence of bulimic episodes, is sufficient for the diagnosis of the full syndrome of bulimia; while one of the central features, behaviour intended to compensate for having overeaten, is only recognized as possibly contributing to the diagnosis. In addition, a key feature, concern about shape and weight, is omitted altogether. One unfortunate result of this over-inclusiveness and lack of specificity is that the significant minority of depressed patients who overeat (Paykel 1977) could satisfy these criteria for a diagnosis of bulimia. There are further problems with the DSM III criteria, which are elaborated elsewhere (Fairburn & Garner 1986, Cooper & Cooper 1987). Problems with Russell's criteria for bulimia nervosa have resulted in a subsequent revision (Russell 1985a). First, he modified the second criterion to include a wider range of measures designed to control weight or to compensate for overeating. The new criterion reads ' . . . devices aimed at counteracting the "fattening" effect of food'. This is a reasonable revision as it has become clear that patients who experience episodes of uncontrolled excessive eating and have the characteristic concerns about shape and weight present with a wider range of weight control measures than specified in the original criteria. Second, Russell attempted to clarify the relationship between bulimia nervosa and anorexia nervosa by adding the requirement that there should have been a previous overt or 'cryptic' episode of anorexia nervosa. There are two problems with this requirement. First, it is not clear what is meant by the term 'cryptic'. Russell (1986) has recently clarified this somewhat by defining a 'cryptic episode' as one in which a period of some weight loss follows an episode of dietary restriction. This definition is unsatisfactory because it is so broad as to include the very large number of women who diet without experiencing significant weight loss. The second problem is that epidemiological research (Fairburn & Cooper 1982, 1984a), and descriptions of patient series (Pyle et al 1981, Fairburn & Cooper 1984b) indicate that at least half of those who meet Russell's original criteria for bulimia nervosa have no history of anorexia nervosa, however broadly defined.

There is no current agreement about which of these diagnostic criteria should be used in clinical practice and research. This lack of consensus concerning diagnostic criteria for bulimia nervosa creates considerable difficulties in interpreting the research literature. Indeed, comparison between the findings of British and American studies is sometimes impossible. This unsatisfactory state of affairs has been remedied by the new criteria specified in DSM III-R (1987). These criteria include a definition of bulimic episodes in which loss of control is a necessary feature, as well as the recognition of a wide range of methods of compensating for overeating. Finally, extreme concerns about shape and weight are included as a necessary criterion. These new criteria will eliminate the major differences in diagnostic practice which have proved so problematic.

EPIDEMIOLOGY

Studies of the incidence and prevalence of anorexia nervosa are beset with methodological difficulties. Uncertainties concerning the definition of a 'case', and the fact that many people with frank anorexia nervosa do not regard themselves as having a problem, make it difficult to derive accurate prevalence figures for anorexia nervosa from the community studies. Case-register studies are difficult to interpret because they do not include mild cases which have escaped detection; and because they are contaminated by the vicissitudes of diagnostic and referral practices. The latter point is well illustrated by a case-register study covering three distinct geographical areas: north-east Scotland, Monroe County in New York, and Camberwell in London (Kendell et al 1973). The estimates of the incidence of anorexia nervosa varied from 0.37 per 100 000 per year in Monroe County to 1.6 per 100 000 per year in north-east Scotland. A consistent finding of the case-register studies is that there has been a sharp rise in the number of cases coming to specialist attention over the past two or three decades

(Szmukler 1985). For example, Szmukler et al (1986) recently reported that the rate of anorexia nervosa in north-east Scotland, based on records of contacts with the in-patient and out-patient psychiatric services, had risen from 1.60 per 100 000 per year for the period 1966 to 1969, to 4.06 per 100 000 per year for the period 1978 to 1982. A similar increase has been observed in America (Jones et al 1980). It is very probable that these well-documented changes in the number of cases being referred for treatment reflect a genuine increase in the incidence of the disorder. However, it is also quite possible that these changes have occurred because of a greater awareness of the condition and a concomitant increase in likelihood of specialist referral.

There have been several community studies of the prevalence of anorexia nervosa (Szmukler 1985). In Britain, Crisp et al (1976) conducted a five to six year retrospective survey of nine schools, seven private and two state run. Their estimate of prevalence was one case of anorexia nervosa per 100 girls aged over 16 in the private schools; and roughly one-fifth this rate amongst the girls in the state schools. A more recent survey has largely confirmed these findings (Szmukler 1983, Mann et al 1983). In this study the estimated prevalence rate of anorexia nervosa in six private schools was one case per 90 girls aged 16–18. A similar difference between state and private schools was found, as had been reported by Crisp and colleagues. An additional finding of this study was that, amongst the girls in the private schools, in addition to the cases of anorexia nervosa, a further 5% were identified with a so-called 'partial syndrome'.

Anorexia nervosa is a disorder which predominantly affects young women, only 5–10% of cases being male. The modal age of onset is 16, although pre-pubertal cases do occur and cases with an onset well into adult life also arise. The disorder is over-represented in girls from upper socio-economic families. Garfinkel et al (1980) are one group amongst many who have reported this social class bias; but they later noted (Garfinkel & Garner 1982) that in recent years the social class distribution of their cases was coming to reflect more closely the background population. This finding has not been confirmed by the case-register studies of incidence referred to earlier (Jones et al 1980, Szmukler et al 1986). There is a striking elevation of the prevalence of anorexia nervosa amongst those for whom a slim body shape has a special significance, such as ballet students and modelling students (Garner & Garfinkel 1980). The disorder arises predominantly in Western countries and developed non-Western societies such as Japan; and it is extremely rare in other cultures. Until recently the disorder was also rare amongst American blacks, but it appears to be increasing in this group (Hsu 1987).

Nothing is known of the incidence of bulimia nervosa. The diagnostic concept is too new for case-register studies to be of use; and there have been no community studies which could cast any light on the inception rate. Nevertheless, it is generally accepted that the incidence of the disorder has increased dramatically in recent years. Although individual case histories can be found in the annals of psychiatry, and patients with 20- and 30-year histories are sometimes seen, it was only towards the end of the 1970s that reports began to emerge of large numbers of these patients presenting for treatment.

Russell's (1979) original account of the disorder constituted a report of 30 cases which he had collected over six and a half years. This suggested that the condition might be extremely rare. However, two studies in the early 1980s, both of which used the media to identify probable cases of bulimia nervosa, indicated that the condition was a significant source of undetected morbidity (Fairburn & Cooper 1982, 1984a). There have been a number of attempts to estimate the prevalence of bulimia nervosa and DSM III bulimia and their constituent components (Szmukler 1985). This work has produced conflicting findings, largely because of weaknesses in the methodology (Fairburn 1984). In particular, the great majority of the surveys have used simple self-report questionnaires with key concepts, such as 'a binge', inadequately defined. Those studies which have used two-stage designs, following a phase of screening by questionnaire with a clinical interview, have been compromised by the high attrition rate of subjects (e.g. Clarke & Palmer 1983). A tentative estimate of prevalence was provided by one study in which a questionnaire was administered to a large group of women attending a family-planning clinic (Cooper & Fairburn 1983). It was found that, during the previous two months, 20.0% reported having experienced an episode of uncontrollable and excessive eating; and 2.9% had used self-induced vomiting as a means of weight control. The point prevalence of probable bulimia nervosa was estimated to be 1.9%. A similar survey conducted on American college students using DSM III criteria produced very comparable findings (Pyle et al 1983). Using a criterion of weekly bulimic episodes and weekly self-induced vomiting or laxative abuse, the prevalence of the bulimic syndrome amongst the women students was estimated to be 1.4%. The American authors have recently published a replication of this study, in which they found a three-fold increase in this prevalence rate (Pyle et al 1986). However, the inference made that the incidence of bulimia is rising is not legitimate given the differences in methods used in the two studies. A replication of the British study reported above found the same prevalence rate as had been reported originally, thus failing to confirm an increased prevalence (Cooper et al 1987a).

Bulimia nervosa is largely confined to women. Although there have been reports of male patients, the samples reported have been small (Gwirtsman et al 1984, Hertzog et al 1984, Robinson & Holden 1986, Turnbull et al 1987). From the published case series it appears that around 1% of cases presenting for treatment are men (Cooper 1985). This is precisely the sex ratio estimated in one media-based survey (Fairburn & Cooper 1984a). The age of patients at presentation is somewhat older than those with anorexia nervosa, most being in their twenties, although a wide age range is affected. The social class distribution of patients has not been systematically studied, but it appears to be broader than that of patients with anorexia nervosa.

CLINICAL FEATURES

The clinical features of anorexia nervosa have been clearly described by numerous authorities in the field, such as Russell (1970), Bruch (1973), Crisp (1980) and Garfinkel & Garner (1982). As noted earlier, there is wide agreement about what constitutes the central clinical features. More uncertainty surrounds the core disturbances in bulimia nervosa. The first detailed account of clinical features was provided by Russell (1979). This account was followed by three American reports of patients with bulimia, which largely confirmed Russell's findings (Pyle et al 1981, Hertzog 1982, Mitchell et al 1985). Although these reports provided a considerable amount of valuable clinical information, there has been only one account of a series of patients which was systematically assessed using standardized measures (Fairburn & Cooper 1984b).

The clinical features of the eating disorders comprise features specific to these disorders and features more generally associated with psychological disturbance.

Specific psychopathology

Eating habits

Patients with anorexia nervosa markedly restrict their food intake. This involves a selective avoidance of food regarded as 'fattening' leading, generally, to a high-protein, low-carbohydrate diet. Frequently they monitor their calorie intake closely and set a rigid calorie limit, usually in the region of 600–800 calories per day. The term 'anorexia' is a misnomer because, except in long-standing cases, appetite for food persists. There is often an obsessional component to the eating habits of patients with anorexia nervosa: they may eat exactly the same food every day, cut up their food into very small pieces, or engage in other ritualistic practices associated with eating. Associated with the efforts to restrict food intake there is a preoccupation with food and eating. Patients frequently spend hours pouring over recipe books, cook elaborate meals for others, and choose jobs which involve working with food.

About half of those with anorexia nervosa alternate between episodes of dietary restriction and bulimic episodes (Garfinkel et al 1980, Casper et al 1980, Strober 1981). During such bulimic episodes food that is normally avoided tends to be consumed, sometimes in large quantities. These episodes lead to considerable distress and are a source of profound guilt and shame. Usually bulimic episodes are followed by self-induced vomiting. A number of consistent differences have been found between the bulimic subgroup and the restricting subgroup of patients with anorexia nervosa as regards presenting symptoms and history. Indeed, some regard these differences as of sufficient importance to merit the inclusion of this dichotomy in the specification of formal diagnostic criteria (Garfinkel & Kaplan 1986).

Patients with anorexia nervosa engage in a variety of weight control measures in addition to dietary restriction. As noted, many induce vomiting, some abuse laxatives, diuretics and appetite suppressants, and many exercise vigorously.

The principal complaint of patients with bulimia nervosa is that they have lost control of their eating. Thus they all report episodes of gross overeating which are experienced as outside of voluntary control. The actual quantity consumed in a bulimic episode varies greatly between patients, and absolute amount consumed is not therefore useful as a defining feature of these episodes. Despite this variability in amount eaten, patients have no difficulty in distinguishing such episodes from mere overeating (Abraham & Beumont 1982). What is of primary importance is not how much is eaten but whether it is experienced as excessive and uncontrolled. The frequency of bulimic episodes also varies greatly between patients. In one patient series, at presentation half the patients reported that such episodes were occurring at least daily (Fairburn & Cooper 1984b). It is not unusual to see patients who are experiencing bulimic episodes many times a day.

Bulimic episodes are fairly uniform in nature. They are invariably secret and food is often eaten quickly with little attention being paid to its taste. Usually they consist of those items patients are at other times attempting to exclude from their diet. Typically, bulimic episodes alternate with attempts to maintain a rigid diet. Strict dieting may be disrupted by dysphoric mood states and boredom (Johnson & Larson 1982, Davis et al 1985, Cooper & Bowskill 1986); and by the belief that some dietary rule has been transgressed. The precise psychological and physiological precursors of bulimic episodes have not been systematically studied.

The body weight of patients with bulimia nervosa is usually within the normal range, reflecting a balance between the episodes of overeating and various compensatory behaviours designed to counteract the effects of bulimic episodes. The most common method of weight control is self-induced vomiting, which frequently terminates bulimic episodes. In the patient series mentioned above, three-quarters were vomiting at least once a day and nearly half reported vomiting at least twice a day. Some patients vomit as much as 30 times a day. Many practice a flushing-out procedure when vomiting, which involves drinking water and then vomiting, with this process repeated until the contents of the stomach emerge as clean water. Vomiting is generally accomplished by inducing the gag reflex with the fingers; but around a quarter of these patients learn to vomit spontaneously. Vomiting is a source of considerable guilt and self-disgust and is almost always practised secretly. It may go undetected for many years.

Self-induced vomiting is habit-forming. While it relieves the abdominal discomfort which results from overeating and lessens the risk of weight gain, it also appears to encourage overeating and therefore further vomiting. Purgatives are also used by some patients to control their weight. Like vomiting, purgative use can become habit-forming; and since tolerance develops, some patients increase their consumption progressively. As in anorexia nervosa a variety of other methods of weight control are also practised by some patients.

Beliefs and attitudes

A central feature of the eating disorders is certain overvalued ideas concerning the importance of shape and weight. Thus, patients with anorexia nervosa place an abnormal degree of significance on the pursuit of a thin body shape; and they have an exaggerated fear of weight gain. Accompanying these extreme concerns, there is often a complete denial that they have any problems. Since Bruch declared that a disturbance of body image was pathognomic in anorexia nervosa (Bruch 1962), there has been a considerable amount of empirical work concerned with establishing whether patients with eating disorders overestimate their body size (Garner & Garfinkel 1981, Slade 1985). Two main methods of assessment have been used: the movable calliper technique, which provides data on particular body regions; and the image-distorting technique, which provides data on patients' perception of their whole body. Using both techniques, as a group patients have usually been found to overestimate their body size; and in most studies this overestimation has been greater than that found in controls. However, many patients have been found to be accurate in their estimation of their body size and some have been found to underestimate their size. Moreover, many people with no eating disorder have been found to overestimate their size. Marked overestimation in patients has been found to be rare. Factors associated with overestimation have not been well studied. It has been tentatively suggested that body size overestimation might occur amongst women who are depressed and who place a high value on slimness, as a specific manifestation of self-depreciation (Taylor & Cooper 1986).

Patients with bulimia nervosa display similar concerns to those with anorexia nervosa about their shape and weight. In patients with bulimia nervosa the discrepancy between their actual body weight and desired weight is generally no greater than amongst normal young women; however, the discrepancy between their estimation of their body size and their desired size is significantly greater than amongst a control population (Cooper & Taylor 1987). Thus they tend both to overestimate their body size significantly more than do controls, and to have a desired size significantly smaller than that of controls. Patients with bulimia nervosa recognize that they have problems, but tend to present them in terms of their disturbed eating habits rather than their beliefs and values about shape and weight. It has been argued that these overvalued ideas concerning shape and weight constitute the core psychopathological disturbance in the eating disorders (Fairburn et al 1986a). A discussion of the role of these ideas in the maintenance of these conditions is provided below.

General psychopathology

General neurotic symptoms are common in anorexia nervosa. There have been no systematic investigations of the frequency of general neurotic symptoms in newly presenting patients. Depressive symptoms have, however, been particularly thoroughly examined in one study (Eckert et al 1982). Using self-report scales of depressive symptomatology, patients with anorexia nervosa were found as a group to have a level of symptoms mid-way between the scores of patients with a primary diagnosis of anxiety and those with a diagnosis of depression. These authors concluded that, as a group, the patients with anorexia nervosa were mildly to moderately depressed, manifesting a 'clinically significant level of depression'. The level of depression was found to be positively associated with disturbances in eating habits and attitudes. Other symptoms reported as present in anorexia nervosa, but not systematically investigated, are lability of mood, and anxiety symptoms related to situations which involve eating (Fairburn & Hope 1988). Obsessional symptoms are also common. Indeed, these patients have been found to have high scores on questionnaires assessing obsessive-compulsive symptomatology (Smart et al 1976, Solyom et al 1982). However, this finding is not of diagnostic significance as some have argued, because patients with a primary diagnosis of depression show similar high scores on these questionnaires (Kendell & DiScipio 1970). In more chronic cases, hopelessness and suicidal ideation are sometimes present. Suicide is the most likely cause of death amongst those who die prematurely because of the disorder (Hsu 1980).

The nature, frequency and severity of the neurotic symptoms occurring in a consecutive series of patients with bulimia nervosa has been systematically studied (Fairburn & Cooper 1984b, Cooper & Fairburn 1986). A wide range of symptoms occur; and, in terms of global indices of severity, such as the total score on the Present State Examination (Wing et al 1974) and the Montgomery and Asberg Depression Rating Scale (Montgomery & Asberg 1979), patients with bulimia nervosa as a group are very similar to patients with a primary diagnosis of depression. Depressive symptoms are particularly common: in particular, depressed mood, guilt, self-depreciation and hopelessness. Significant concentration impairment is also common. Similarly, anxiety symptoms occur in the majority of patients, these arising predominantly in situations involving exposure to high-calorie foods.

Physical factors

One of the most obvious and striking features of anorexia nervosa is the state of semi-starvation of these patients. This emaciation has wide-ranging effects on patients' physiology and also on their physical health (Mitchell 1986a). Some of these consequences of the emaciation interact with the central psychological disturbances. For example, slow gastric motility, arising from the low weight and reduced caloric consumption, leads patients to complain of fullness, bloating and abdominal pain; and these symptoms are taken as evidence for the need for further dietary restriction. Recently it has been argued that many aspects of the psychopathology of anorexia nervosa could be a direct result of starvation (Garner et al 1985). This argument is largely based on an experimental study of the effects of starvation conducted over 30 years ago (Keys et al 1950). The study involved restricting the caloric intake of 36 healthy male volunteers. Following base-line assessment, for six months or more these men ate roughly half their normal daily food intake and, on average, they lost 25% of their original body weight. There was a plethora of psychological repercussions. Of particular note was the fact that the men became markedly preoccupied with thoughts about food and eating, spending considerable periods of time planning how they would eat their allocation of food. As a consequence of these preoccupations, they experienced significant concentration impairment. They also became peculiarly concerned about how their food was served, demanding unusual concoctions and markedly increasing their consumption of salt and spices. A few of the men lost control of their eating and appeared to experience frank bulimic episodes. Stealing and hoarding of food, seen in some patients with anorexia nervosa, also developed in some of the men. In addition to these effects on eating, there were profound emotional changes in most of the subjects. Depressed mood was common; and lability of mood also occurred in some of the men. Social withdrawal and apathy were common, as was irritability. All of these symptoms are seen in anorexia nervosa and, to varying degrees, could be a direct consequence of the emaciation. A question of considerable interest is the extent to which these symptoms are reversed by simply restoring body weight to within the normal range. Although it is well known that hospitalization and refeeding result in significant improvements in aspects of the psychopathology (Russell 1985a), there has been no report of a systematic demonstration of this effect.

There are a number of physiological abnormalites and medical complications in bulimia nervosa (Mitchell 1986b). Unlike anorexia nervosa, where most of these disturbances are the result of emaciation, most of those seen in bulimia nervosa result from specific behaviours, such as vomiting, purgative abuse and the bulimic episodes themselves. The most significant medical complications arise from electrolyte disturbance caused by purgation. The psychological correlates of the physical disturbances have not been investigated and are not understood. It appears that some features of the non-specific psychopathology of bulimia nervosa may be related to the disturbed eating habits. The drowsiness, sleep disturbance, weakness, anergia and lability of mood reported by these patients may all be secondary to repeated overeating and purgation.

AETIOLOGY AND MAINTENANCE

While the aetiology of the eating disorders is not known, it is widely accepted that a combination of biological, psychological and social factors are of importance (Garfinkel & Garner 1982, Agras & Kirkley 1986). There has been a considerable amount of theoretical speculation about the significant aetiological factors, but there are little firm data.

Although a number of factors broadly related to personality have been suggested as predisposing individuals to anorexia nervosa, there has been little such speculation in the case of bulimia nervosa. One of these factors, especially emphasized by Bruch (1973), is difficulties in autonomous functioning and an associated sense of ineffectiveness. Crisp (1980), on the other hand, has emphasized how those predisposed to develop anorexia nervosa are unprepared for maturity and how the symptoms of the disorder represent a flight from adolescent concerns and responsibilities. However, problems with autonomy and with coming to terms with adult sexuality are by no means unique to patients with anorexia nervosa; and they may, indeed, reflect no more than a general predisposition to psychological disorder. Both Bruch and Crisp also emphasize the compliant, perfectionist and dependent nature of these patients' personalities, aspects also highlighted by Slade (1982) as setting conditions for the development of anorexia nervosa. However, there are enormous problems in establishing firmly a relationship between such characteristics and the development of anorexia nervosa. First, the measures of personality used in the research have frequently been of questionable validity; and second, as Garfinkel & Garner note, it is difficult to draw meaningful conclusions about premorbid personality characteristics because it is so difficult to separate out possible predisposing factors from those which might arise as a consequence of a disorder with such significant and wide-ranging physical and psychological repercussions. It should also be noted that even factors which are thought to be associated with the disorder may not be specific to anorexia nervosa in the sense of being peculiar to this disorder. Thus, despite the fact that many of the dimensions mentioned above, such as ineffectiveness and maturity fears, have been found on the Eating Disorder Inventory (Garner et al 1983) to differentiate patients with anorexia nervosa from normal controls, psychiatric outpatients with no eating disorder have also been found to have high scores on this measure; and those with high levels of general psychological disturbance have been found to be no different on many of the subscales from patients with anorexia nervosa (Cooper et al 1985).

Eating disorders run in families. Thus the prevalence of these disorders in the relatives of probands has been found to be significantly higher than the expected rate in the general population (Strober & Humphrey 1987). Much of the research on which this conclusion is based is methodologically weak; but two recent studies of family aggregation have been conducted particularly well. Gershon et al (1984) found a 6% life-time morbid risk for eating disorders in the first-degree relatives of 24 anorexia nervosa probands, compared with a 1% risk in the families of normal controls. Similarly, Strober et al (1985) found a significant excess of eating disorders in the first- and second-degree relatives of patients with anorexia nervosa compared with non-anorexic psychiatric controls: indeed, a case of anorexia nervosa or bulimia was found in 27% of the families of the anorexia nervosa probands, compared with 6% of the control families. There are also a number of reports, reviewed by Garfinkel & Garner (1982), of anorexia occurring in twins. In one recent rigorously conducted study of 34 pairs of twins and one set of triplets with an anorexia nervosa proband (Holland et al 1984), a 55% concordance rate was found for monozygotic twins compared with a 7% concordance for dizygotic twins. The authors consider alternative explanations for these findings, favouring an account in terms of a genetic predisposition which could become manifest under adverse conditions such as stringent dieting or emotional stress.

The family aggregation findings are explicable in both genetic and environmental terms. The data on the pathogenesis of family influences in the eating disorders has recently been reviewed by Strober & Humphrey (1987). A major problem with this work is that the findings are derived exclusively from families of patients; and, as such, it is not possible to conclude anything about the causal role of any family disturbances identified. The mothers of patients with eating disorders have been described as particularly intrusive and overprotective, anxious and perfectionist; and the fathers as passive, obsessional and ineffectual. These impressions have little empirical basis, because it has not been demonstrated that these characteristics are specific to the parents of those with eating disorders; nor, indeed, that they are present in these parents to any significant degree. Although some recent systematic examinations of the families of patients with bulimia have found that they perceive their families as more disturbed in various ways than controls (Humphrey 1986), it has not been shown that these perceptions are a function of their eating disorder rather than of nonspecific psychological disturbance as might be found in a group of young patients with other psychological disorders. Indeed, unless some practicable means of conducting prospective research can be evolved, it is unlikely that studies of the families of patients with eating disorders will reveal anything about the aetiology of the disorder. They may well, of course, produce important findings relevant to the maintenance of these conditions and to their treatment.

A family history of affective disorder is common amongst patients with eating disorders. Thus, the rate of affective disorder amongst the relatives of anorexia nervosa probands is as high as amongst relatives of patients with depression (Strober et al 1985, Strober and Katz 1987). Preliminary evidence indicates that this association also obtains for patients with bulimia nervosa (Hudson et al 1983a, Strober and Katz 1987). Patients with eating disorders also commonly have a personal history of affective disorder. In a recent review of a number of studies estimating life-time prevalence, Strober & Katz (1987) conclude that these studies are consistent in finding a high rate of affective disorder, ranging from 25% to 80%. As these reviewers note, a major problem with the interpretation of these studies is that the chronology of symptoms in patients with eating disorders is not always clear; and in many cases depressive symptoms may arise as a secondary response to disturbances in eating. However, some studies have made particularly careful analysis of the order in which symptoms have arisen. For example, Piran et al (1985) reported that amongst 18 patients with anorexia nervosa with a life-time history of major depression, affective symptoms post-dated the onset of the eating disorder in 34%, occurred within the same year in 22%, and preceded the emergence of the eating disorder by at least one year in 44%. Comparable analyses have been made with similar results in patients with bulimia (Hudson et al 1983a, Lee et al 1985, Walsh et al 1985). Thus, it appears that a vulnerability to depression may increase predisposition to eating disorders; and an episode of depression may contribute to the initiation of its symptoms.

As mentioned above, eating disorders are particularly prevalent in social subgroups where a particular value is placed on a slim body shape (Garner & Garfinkel 1980). This observation, together with other related evidence, has led to considerable speculation about the role of societal pressures in the aetiology of the eating disorders (Striegel-Moore et al 1986). Indeed, the shift in societal preference in recent decades towards a thinner female body shape has been offered as a possible explanation for the increasing prevalence of anorexia nervosa (Garfinkel & Garner 1982). It is suggested that this increase is a result of greater numbers of young women dieting. Whilst this explanation is highly persuasive, it is obviously not complete. Not all ballet dancers, modelling students or young women who diet to be slim develop eating disorders; and as yet the factors which render dieters vulnerable to develop anorexia nervosa or bulimia nervosa have not been systematically investigated.

To date, the evidence about factors of possible aetiological significance have furthered understanding of the eating disorders in a limited and piecemeal way. However, as with many psychological disorders, attempts to account for maintenance have proved more profitable. Three views on maintenance can be distingished. The least well developed of these is an account in terms of anxiety reduction (Rosen & Leitenberg 1982, 1985). This view regards bulimia nervosa as analogous to obsessive-compulsive disorders, with purging fulfilling an anxiety-reduction function similar to that of compulsive hand-washing or checking rituals. The central tenet of this account is, therefore, that 'the driving force of this disorder may be vomiting rather than bingeing' (Rosen & Leitenberg 1982). This account of maintenance clearly applies only to a subset of those with eating disorders: that is, those who engage in purging behaviour and who do so in immediate response to overeating. The exposure and response-prevention treatment which has been developed from these ideas thus has a correspondingly limited application. As yet, this account of the maintenance of bulimia has been submitted to little empirical examination. Three small series of patients treated with exposure and response-prevention techniques have been reported (Rosen & Leitenberg 1982, Leitenberg et al 1984, Wilson et al 1986); and they provide tentative support for the efficacy of this form of therapy. However, the small number of reported cases, the high rate of patient attrition, the tendency to combine this treatment with other forms of management, and the absence of a controlled comparison, do not allow firm conclusions to be drawn about the efficacy of the treatment or the validity of the anxiety-reduction account of maintenance.

Two other views of the maintenance of eating disorders have been extensively elaborated: they have been regarded as an affective disorder; and their maintenance has been accounted for in cognitive behavioural terms. Both these views have been applied equally to anorexia nervosa and bulimia nervosa; and both have significant implications for treatment.

The affective disorder conceptualization

Five lines of evidence have been advanced to support the contention that the eating disorders are 'closely related to' or 'a form of' affective disorder (Hudson et al 1983a). These arguments relate to the course of these disorders, their response to certain biological tests, their phenomenology, the tendency of these patients to have a family history of affective disorder, and the response of patients with eating disorders to anti-depressant medication. Each of these lines of evidence will be considered in turn.

There have been a number of studies of the outcome of anorexia nervosa (Hsu 1980, Szmukler & Russell 1986). One such study has attracted a considerable amount of attention (Cantwell et al 1977). The investigators followed up 16 patients for an average of five years after treatment. At follow-up, only one patient was regarded as still 'possibly manifesting a full anorexic syndrome'. However, 12 of the patients met criteria for a diagnosis of affective disorder. The authors concluded from their study that at least some cases of anorexia nervosa 'may be a variant of affective disorder'. Although there have been numerous other follow-up studies, none provide clear support for this conclusion. Whilst it is indeed the case that depressive symptoms are common at follow-up, these symptoms are closely associated with the presence and severity of persisting symptoms reflecting the specific psychopathology of anorexia nervosa. In fact, apart from the study by

Cantwell and colleagues, there is no evidence to suggest that anorexia nervosa evolves into another psychiatric condition; and all the evidence points to a variable outcome with a tendency for the psychopathology of anorexia nervosa to 'breed true'. There are no follow-up data of any note on patients with bulimia nervosa and it is not therefore possible to evaluate whether the course of this condition supports the argument that the eating disorders are a form of affective disorder.

The second line of argument concerns the status of certain putative biological markers of depression. In particular, much has been made of the fact that the rate of cortisol non-suppression (established by the so-called dexamethasone suppression test, DST) for patients with eating disorders is similar to that found in patients with a primary diagnosis of depression. Thus high rates of non-suppression have been found in patients with anorexia nervosa (e.g. Gerner & Wilkins 1983, Hudson & Hudson 1984, Gold et al 1986) and in patients with bulimia (e.g. Gwirtsman et al 1983, Hudson et al 1983b, Mitchell et al 1984, Lindy et al 1985, Kiriike et al 1986, Hughes et al 1986a). However, as Swift et al (1986) have recently noted, the validity of such measures as markers of depression remains controversial, and interpretation of their application to eating disorders is therefore highly problematic. Aside from this general objection, this line of argument has been undermined by some recent findings concerning the effects of the experimental manipulation of diet. Mullen at al (1986) restricted the calorie intake of 14 female volunteers selected for an absence of current or past eating or mood disturbance. Although the subjects were kept on the diet for only two weeks and they lost an average of only 4.3 kg in body weight, there was a marked change in their responses to dexamethasone, with 'a significant switch from suppression to non-suppression'. This change was independent of any mood change. The authors concluded that these results suggest that the dexamethasone findings in patients with depression may be secondary to loss of appetite and loss of weight. This conclusion has not been supported by a recent study of the relationship between weight change and cortisol non-suppression in depressed patients, in which no relationship was found (Schweitzer et al 1986). However, the findings of the experimental study are sufficiently dramatic to make it unreasonable to conclude anything at present about the relationship between eating disorders and affective disorders from the DST findings in patients with anorexia nervosa. This still leaves to be explained the DST findings in patients with bulimia nervosa. However, they cannot be regarded as indicating a relationship with affective disorder until it is demonstrated that they are not secondary to the frequent weight fluctuations these patients experience; and that they are not a function of these patients' grossly disturbed eating habits; and, indeed, that the DST is a valid marker of depression.

The third line of evidence adduced in support of the affective disorder account derives from the fact that patients with eating disorders present with a number of depressive symptoms. The general finding using a wide range of assessment instruments is that patients with both anorexia nervosa and bulimia nervosa present with mild to moderate levels of depressive symptoms (Strober & Katz 1987). In the case of anorexia nervosa there are considerable difficulties is assessing depression, because many of the dimensions of interest such as dysphoria, sleep disturbance, anergia, concentration impairment, loss of appetite and sexual interest, and so on, are affected by the malnutrition per se. In the light of this it is especially noteworthy that one detailed study of the depressive symptoms of anorexia nervosa discussed earlier (Eckert et al 1982) found the level of depressive symptomatology to be closely associated with a variety of coexisting complications, such as the degree of disturbance in eating habits, the presence of bulimic episodes, the degree of body size overestimation, and the extent of weight loss. Furthermore, the depressive symptoms were found to decrease markedly with restoration to a normal body weight. These findings suggest that the depressive symptoms are generally likely to be secondary to the core eating and weight disturbances.

In the case of bulimia nervosa, only one study has made a detailed comparison of the depressive symptoms of these patients with those with a diagnosis of primary depressive disorder (Cooper & Fairburn 1986). In terms of a global index of severity provided by the total score on the Montgomery and Asberg Depression Rating Scale, there was no difference between the two groups of patients. However, there were differences on more than half the individual symptoms; and significant differences in terms of the frequency of a number of symptoms on the Present State Examination. Indeed, discriminant function techniques revealed that there was a different inter-relationship between the symptoms for the two groups. Furthermore, when the content of the depressive symptoms amongst the patients with bulimia nervosa was examined, they were found to be clearly related to the specific psychopathology of the disorder. Thus the pathological guilt present in virtually all the patients was related to minor dietary indiscretions or deceitful eating practices; the concentration impairment present in two-thirds was invariably a function of ruminations about food, eating, weight and shape; and the mood disturbance present in the majority was directly related to the loss of control over eating.

The depressive symptoms of bulimia nervosa therefore appear to take a specific form and to be secondary to the core disturbance. This conclusion is supported by a study of outcome (Fairburn et al 1985). Twenty-two patients with bulimia nervosa were assessed before and after psychological treatment directed solely at their disturbed eating habits. When the patients were categorized into 'good', 'moderate', or 'bad' outcome groups, based entirely on their eating habits, outcome was found to be closely associated with the post-treatment severity of depressive symptomatology: those whose eating had improved were significantly less depressed than before treatment; and those whose eating had not improved remained depressed. Since treatment outcome was unrelated to pre-treatment mental state, these data run counter to the argument that the depressive symptoms are of primary significance in bulimia nervosa. This body of data strongly suggests that the depressive symptoms in bulimia nervosa are generally a secondary response to these patients' disturbed eating habits.

The fourth line of evidence advanced in support of the affective disorder conceptualization of eating disorders is the fact that there is a high rate of affective disorder amongst the first-degree relatives of patients with eating disorders. As noted above, this finding has been replicated on a number of occasions in the case of anorexia nervosa; and similar findings are emerging for bulimia nervosa. However, a raised rate of disorder B amongst the relatives of patients with disorder A is not evidence for an equivalence or even for a common constitutional basis. Indeed, in one family history study in which the relatives of patients with anorexia nervosa were found to have a high rate of affective disorder, the rate of eating disorders amongst the relatives of patients with affective disorder was also examined (Strober et al 1985, Strober & Katz 1987). The cross-prevalence data did not support the conclusion that these disorders were part of a genetic spectrum, in that the rate of eating disorders amongst the relatives of patients with affective disorder was low. Thus the view that eating disorders and affective disorders are accounted for by the same mechanisms of genetic transmission is not supported by the family history data.

The final line of evidence cited in support of the affective disorder account derives from the results of treatment with antidepressant medication. As noted by Russell (1985b), antidepressant drugs are commonly prescribed in clinical practice to patients with anorexia nervosa who present with severe or persistent depressive symptoms. However, the evidence to support such practice is weak. Some data have been provided demonstrating that some patients given antidepressants do improve (Mills et al 1973, Needleman & Waber, 1976). However, these studies were uncontrolled and failed to demonstrate that the benefits were not a result of non-specific factors such as hospital admission. There has been only one double-blind controlled trial of an antidepressant (Halmi et al 1986). Three treatment regimes were compared: amitriptyline, cyproheptadine, and placebo. The principal outcome measures were speed and extent of weight gain. There was no difference on these measures between the two active drugs; and the placebo group showed a perfectly satisfactory rate of weight gain. There was also no difference between the three groups in terms of the alleviation of depressive symptoms: depression improved significantly for all groups and this improvement was closely associated with the extent of weight gain. Neither this study nor any other has examined the longer-term effects of antidepressant medication on these patients' weight, or indeed on any other aspect of their psychopathology. Two authoritative reviews of the role of drug treatment in the management of anorexia nervosa concluded that there is no drug which approximates to the impressive short-term results obtained from hospitalization and skilled nursing care; and that there is no case for the general use of any particular medication (Szmukler 1982, Russell 1985b).

Although the case for the use of antidepressant medication in anorexia nervosa is weak, there is far more support for this form of treatment for patients with bulimia. A series of double-blind controlled trials has demonstrated the superiority of tricyclic antidepressants and monoamine oxidase inhibitors over a placebo in the management of these patients (Pope et al 1983, Mitchell & Groat 1984, Walsh et al 1984, Hughes et al 1986b, Agras et al 1987). However, there are two problems in interpreting the findings of these studies. First, all of these studies were of very brief duration. Since transient fluctuations in symptom severity are to be expected, it is the long-term effects of treatment which are of importance, and the short-term results of brief trials are of little clinical or theoretical significance. The one study which did include a longer follow up (Pope et al 1985) involved continuing and active treatment, with all patients receiving a multitude of different drugs. Although the outcome of the patients was in general good, it is unclear to what this effect should be ascribed. The second problem concerns the nature of the patient populations included in these trials. All used the DSM III criteria for bulimia and not the narrower criteria for bulimia nervosa. As such, they may have included cases of atypical depression with appetite increase (Paykel 1977); that is, patients who would not fulfil criteria for a diagnosis of bulimia nervosa because the characteristic concerns about shape and weight are absent, and should more properly be designated as cases of depression. Indeed, the single double-blind controlled trial which did include patients who fulfilled Russell's 1979 criteria for bulimia nervosa found the tetracyclic mianserin to have no specific effect on these patients' eating habits, attitudes to shape and weight, or their mental state (Sabine et al 1983). It must be added that even if antidepressant medication were found to be effective for a significant proportion of patients with bulimia nervosa, this would not be of diagnostic significance. Tricyclic antidepressants are known to have a wide range of effects in a number of psychological disorders, and drug response clearly constitutes an inadequate basis for deriving a diagnosis.

There is little basis for the affective disorder view of eating disorders, in that the evidence for eating disorders being a form of affective disorder is weak. However, there is clearly a strong association between eating disorders and depression: a high rate of depressive disorder has been found amongst the close family relatives of patients with eating disorders; and a personal history of depressive disorder appears to be common amongst these patients. However, as argued earlier, these data suggest that a vulnerability to affective disorder may predispose individuals to develop an eating disorder, or it may contribute to its maintenance; but they do not support the idea that the eating disorders are in some sense a manifestation of an affective disorder. It is also worth noting that the affective disorder view of eating disorders in fact does little to illuminate the factors and processes involved in the maintenance of these disorders, in that it simply changes the problem of accounting for their specific maintenance into one of accounting for the maintenance of affective disorder.

The cognitive behavioural conceptualization

The argument for a cognitive behavioural conceptualization of anorexia nervosa and bulimia nervosa has been extensively elaborated in recent reviews (Garner & Bemis 1982, Fairburn et al 1986a). The essential tenet of this view is that the central psychopathological disturbance in these patients is their overvalued ideas about shape and weight. Indeed, it is argued, most of the other clinical features of these disorders can be understood in terms of this core psychopathology. According to this view, the belief that shape and weight are of fundamental importance and must be kept under strict control is not merely symptomatic of these disorders, but is of primary importance in their maintenance. The specific features of eating disorders, such as frequent weighing, sensitivity to changes in shape and weight, extreme dieting, self-induced vomiting and purgative abuse, and abnormal attitudes towards food and eating, are also presented as comprehensible given these core beliefs concerning shape and weight.

The cognitive behavioural account of eating disorders regards the relatively uniform beliefs and values of these patients as implicit unarticulated rules by which they assign meaning and value to their experience. The way they evaluate themselves and their behaviour, their perceptions and aspirations, are regarded as being determined by these values. Thus their self-worth is seen as being evaluated in terms of their shape and weight: they view fatness as odious and reprehensible, they see slimness as attractive and desirable, and the maintenance of self-control is of prime importance. In addition, some attach extreme importance to weight loss. It is clear that such beliefs are not radically different from views which are widely held and reinforced by prevailing social values. They differ from these more generally held attitudes by being exaggerated, rigidly held and imbued with great personal significance; and it is these qualities, it is argued, which make them dysfunctional. It is further argued that the absolute and exaggerated nature of these concerns about shape and weight reflect the operation of certain dysfunctional styles of reasoning (Garner & Bemis 1985, Fairburn et al 1986a). These are similar to those described by Beck and colleagues (1979) as operating in depression, and they include dichotomous thinking, overgeneralization and errors of attribution. Examples include the belief that food can be categorized as 'fattening' and 'non-fattening'; the belief that minor dietary indiscretions are indicative of a total lack of self-control; and the belief that success and failure are totally determined by bodily appearance.

The cognitive behavioural view of the maintenance of eating disorders regards much of the behaviour of these patients as arising from unexamined thoughts which arise from these patients' implicit values about shape and weight. The most obvious of these is frequent weighing. These thoughts could also account for the habitual use of exercise and purgatives to control weight; and also, of course, the attempts to adhere to a rigid diet.

Although the cognitive behavioural conceptualization of eating disorders has considerable prima face validity, there is very little direct evidence to support it. A major reason for this has been the absence of an appropriate measure of the core psychopathology of these disorders. This situation has been remedied recently by the development of the Eating Disorders Examination (Cooper & Fairburn 1987). This measure, a comprehensive interview assessment of the full range of the specific psychopathology of eating disorders, will enable an empirical examination of the predictions of the cognitive account. One fundamental prediction is that a change in the core dysfunctional attitudes is a prerequisite for full and lasting recovery (Fairburn 1985, Garner & Bemis 1985). Although this prediction is still to be tested, there has been considerable interest in the generation of cognitive behavioural treatments for anorexia nervosa (Garner & Bemis 1985, Garner 1986) and for bulimia nervosa (Fairburn 1985). Surprisingly, there has not been a single report of the systematic application of this form of treatment to patients with anorexia nervosa. There have been numerous systematic case reports attesting to the efficacy of this treatment for patients with bulimia nervosa (Wilson 1986, Garner et al 1987); but few controlled trials (Kirkley et al 1985, Fairburn et al 1986b). Although there is now a considerable body of evidence demonstrating that this treatment, particularly when administered in an individual rather than a group format, leads to substantial improvement in the great majority of these patients, it has not been clearly demonstrated that this form of treatment is superior to other forms of psychological management or, indeed, to other forms of physical treatment. Neither has it been shown that cognitive treatments produce more cognitive change than non-cognitive ones; and, as already noted, nor has it been established that a change in the characteristic beliefs and values is a necessary requirement for an enduring change in patients' eating habits.

Dietary restraint

Bulimic episodes present two problems for a cognitive behavioural conceptualization of eating disorders. First, given these patients' implicit values concerning shape and weight, it would be predicted that their fear of weight gain would simply lead to constant dieting, with success reinforcing further dietary restriction. Second, it would be predicted that if for some reason a patient did break their diet, they would simply recommence dieting. The clinical features of bulimia nervosa and of the bulimic subgroup of patients with anorexia nervosa are not consistent with either of these predictions. These patients do not successfully adhere to their dietary regimes; and when their diets are broken, rather than minimizing the indiscretion, they go to the other extreme and overeat. It has recently been argued that it is dietary restriction itself which is responsible for the episodes of loss of control over eating; and that the link between dieting and bulimic episodes is a cognitive one (Polivy et al 1984, Polivy & Herman 1985). It has been found in laboratory research that, under certain predictable circumstances, subjects who are restricting their food intake will overeat or 'counter-regulate'. One such circumstance is the belief that certain dietary rules have been transgressed: that is, in contrast to unrestrained eaters, restrained eaters tend to eat more following the prior consumption of a large number of calories than following a small number of calories (Herman & Mack 1975, Hibscher & Herman 1977, Herman et al 1979, Ruderman & Wilson 1979). This effect has also been produced by simply manipulating the subjects' beliefs about the calorie content of the previously consumed food (Polivy 1976, Spencer & Fremouw 1979, Woody et al 1981). Other factors found to produce counter-regulation in dieters are dysphoric mood states and the consumption of alcohol (Wardle & Beinhart 1981, Polivy et al 1984). These factors are thought to operate by disrupting dieters' motivation to deprive themselves of food. According to this view, dieters place themselves in a state of physiological deprivation by using cognitive rather than physiological regulators of food intake (Herman & Polivy 1984). Once the cognitive constraints on eating are removed by some disinhibiting factor, hunger and other physiological forces aimed at correcting the deprivation take over and lead to overeating. This essentially laboratory phenomenon has been presented as an analogy for bulimic episodes (e.g. Polivy et al 1984). The evidence in support of this is indirect and weak: it is rare to find bulimic episodes in the absence of attempts at dietary restriction (Polivy & Herman 1985); amongst community samples, the greater the degree of dietary restraint the more probable the occurrence of bulimic episodes (Wardle 1980), and the more severe the bulimic episode the greater the degree of restraint (Hawkins & Clement 1980); and amongst patients with bulimia nervosa, the majority report that the onset of their bulimic episodes coincided with a period of dietary restriction (Fairburn & Cooper 1984b, Mitchell et al 1985); and bulimic episodes are commonly precipitated by patients eating 'forbidden' foods (Abraham & Beumont 1982) or by emotional distress (Davis et al 1985, Cooper & Bowskill, 1986). These findings all provide indirect support for the hypothesis that dietary restraint is implicated in the development of bulimic episodes as they arise in patients with bulimia nervosa and anorexia nervosa. However, more direct evidence is required before it can be accepted. In particular, it has not been demonstrated in a systematic longitudinal study that at least some people who restrict their food intake subsequently lose control of their eating. If this were to be demonstrated, then the further question would arise of what factors operate to increase the likelihood of dieting leading to disturbed eating habits. Furthermore, the basic laboratory research on counter-regulation has to be questioned because all the studies cited above used as their criterion of dietary restriction the Restraint Scale of Herman & Mack (1975), which has been shown to confound dietary restriction per se with fluctuations in body weight (Drewnowski et al 1982, Blanchard & Frost 1983, Ruderman 1983). A number of psychometrically pure measures of dietary restraint have recently been developed (Stunkard & Messick 1985, Wardle 1986) which will allow the conclusions from the laboratory research reviewed above to be re-evaluated.

CONCLUSION

There has been a considerable increase in interest in eating disorders in recent years. This owes much to the recent emergence of bulimia nervosa as a common and disabling disorder; and there has been a great deal of research concerned with elucidating its clinical features, establishing its epidemiology, and developing and evaluating treatments. All aspects of this work are at an early stage. Although the general psychopathology of bulimia nervosa has been studied in some detail, the disturbed beliefs and values which constitute a central feature of this disorder and of anorexia nervosa have not been adequately examined in either condition; and the relation between the particular disturbed behaviours in these disorders and particular dysfunctional attitudes remains unexplored. This area of enquiry constitutes a major challenge for psychopathologists in the coming years. A related area of interest concerns the role of depression in the development and maintenance of these disorders. A number of important associations have already been identified. However, in order to gain understanding of the psychological processes underlying these relationships it will be necessary to develop research strategies to complement the cross-sectional and retrospective clinical studies conducted to date. Longitudinal research on high-risk groups holds particular promise. To achieve an understanding of the eating disorders these lines of enquiry need to be pursued in parallel with social and biological research.

REFERENCES

Abraham S F, Beumont P J V 1982 How patients describe bulimia or binge eating. Psychological Medicine 12: 625–635

Agras W S, Kirkley B G 1986 Bulimia: theories of etiology. In: Brownell K D, Foreyt J P (eds) Handbook of eating disorders: physiology, psychology and treatment of obesity, anorexia and bulimia. Basic Books, New York

Agras W S, Dorian B, Kirkley B, Arnow B, Bachman J 1987 Imipramine in the treatment of bulimia: a double-blind controlled study. International Journal of Eating Disorders 6: 29–38

American Psychiatric Association 1980 DSM-III: Diagnostic and statistical manual of mental disorders, 3rd edn. American Psychiatric Association, Washington, DC

American Psychiatric Association 1987 DSM-III R: Diagnostic and statistical manual of mental disorders: revised 3rd edn. American Psychiatric Association, Washington, DC

Beck A T, Rush A J, Shaw B F, Emery G 1979 Cognitive therapy of depression: a treatment manual. Guilford Press, New York

Blanchard F A, Frost R O 1983 Two factors of restraint: concern for dieting and weight fluctuation. Behaviour Research and Therapy 21: 259–267

Boskind-Lodahl M 1976 Cinderella's stepsisters: a feminist perspective on anorexia nervosa and bulimia. Signs: Journal of Women, Culture and Society 2: 342–356

Brownell K D, Wadden F A 1986 Behaviour therapy for obesity: modern approaches and better results. In: Brownell K D, Foreyt J P (eds) Handbook of eating disorders: physiology, psychology and treatment of obesity, anorexia and bulimia. Basic Books, New York

Bruch H 1962 Perceptual and conceptual disturbances in anorexia nervosa. Psychosomatic Medicine 24: 187–194

Bruch H 1973 Eating disorders: obesity, anorexia nervosa, and the person within. Basic Books, New York

Cantwell D P, Sturzenberger S, Burroughs J, Salkin B, Green J K 1977 Anorexia nervosa: an affective disorder. Archives of General Psychiatry 34: 1087–1093

Casper R C, Eckert E D, Halmi K A, Goldberg S C, Davis J M 1980 Bulimia: its incidence and clinical importance in patients with anorexia nervosa. Archives of General Psychiatry 37: 1030–1034

Clarke M G, Palmer R L 1983 Eating attitudes and symptoms in university students. British Journal of Psychiatry 142: 299–304

Cooper P J 1985 Eating disorders. In: Watts F (ed) New developments in clinical psychology. Wiley, Chichester

Cooper P J, Bowskill R 1986 Dysphoric mood and overeating. British Journal of Clinical Psychology 25: 155–156

Cooper P J, Cooper Z 1987 The nature of bulimia nervosa. Pediatric Reviews and Communications 1: 217–237

Cooper P J, Fairburn C G 1983 Binge-eating and self-induced vomiting in the community: a preliminary study. British Journal of Psychiatry 142: 139–144

Cooper P J, Fairburn C G 1986 The depressive symptoms of bulimia nervosa. British Journal of Psychiatry 148: 268–274

Cooper Z, Fairburn C G 1987 The Eating Disorders Examination: a semi-structured interview for the assessment of the specific psychopathology of eating disorders. International Journal of Eating Disorders 6: 1–8

Cooper P J, Taylor M J 1987 Body image disturbance in bulimia nervosa. British Journal of Psychiatry (in press)

Cooper Z, Cooper P J, Fairburn C G 1985 The specificity of the Eating Disorder Inventory. British Journal of Clinical Psychology 24: 124–130

Cooper P J, Charnock D, Taylor M J 1987a The prevalence of bulimia nervosa. British Journal of Psychiatry 15: 684–686

Cooper P J, Taylor M J, Cooper Z, Fairburn C G 1987b The development and validation of the Body Shape Questionnaire. International Journal of Eating Disorders 6: 485–494

Crisp A H 1967 The possible significance of some behavioural correlates of weight and carbohydrate intake. Journal of Psychosomatic Research 11: 117–131

Crisp A H 1979 Fatness, metabolism and sexual behaviour. In: Carenza L, Zichella L (eds) Emotion and reproduction. Academic Press, London

Crisp A H 1980 Anorexia nervosa: let me be. Academic Press, London

Crisp A H, Palmer R L, Kalucy R S 1976 How common is anorexia nervosa? A prevalence study. British Journal of Psychiatry 128: 549–558

Davis R, Freeman R, Solyom C 1985 Mood and food: an analysis of bulimic episodes. Journal of Psychiatric Research 19: 331–335

Dodd D K, Birky H J, Stalling R B 1976 Eating behaviour of obese and non-obese females in a normal setting. Addictive Behaviours 1: 321–325

Drewnowski A, Riskey D, Desor J A 1982 Feeling fat yet unconcerned: self-reported overweight and the Restraint Scale. Appetite 3: 273–279

Dubbert P M, Wilson G T 1983 Failures in behavioural therapy for obesity: causes, correlates and consequences. In: Foa E B, Emmelkamp P M S (eds) Failures in behavioural therapy. Wiley, New York

Eckert E D, Goldberg S C, Halmi K A, Casper R C, Davis J M 1982 Depression in anorexia nervosa. Psychological Medicine 12: 115–122

Fairburn C G 1984 Bulimia: its epidemiology and management. In: Stunkard A J, Stellar E (eds) Eating and its disorders. Raven Press, New York
Fairburn C G 1985 Cognitive-behavioural treatment for bulimia. In: Garner D M, Garfinkel P E (eds) Handbook of psychotherapy for anorexia nervosa and bulimia. Guilford Press, New York
Fairburn C G, Cooper P J 1982 Self-induced vomiting in the community: an undetected problem. British Medical Journal 284: 1153–1155
Fairburn C G, Cooper P J 1984a Binge-eating, self-induced vomiting and laxative abuse: a community study. Psychological Medicine 14: 401–420
Fairburn C G, Cooper P J 1984b The clinical features of bulimia nervosa. British Journal of Psychiatry 144: 238–246
Fairburn C G, Garner D M 1986 The diagnosis of bulimia nervosa. International Journal of Eating Disorders 5: 403–419
Fairburn C G, Hope R A 1987 Disorders of eating and weight. In: Kendell R E, Zealley A K (eds) Companion to Psychiatric Studies. Churchill Livingstone, Edinburgh (in press)
Fairburn C G, Cooper P J, Kirk J, O'Connor M 1985 The significance of the neurotic symptoms of bulimia nervosa. Journal of Psychiatric Research 19: 135–142
Fairburn C G, Cooper Z, Cooper P J 1986a The clinical features and maintenance of bulimia nervosa. In: Brownell K D, Foreyt J P (eds) Handbook of Eating Disorders: Physiology, psychology and treatment of obesity, anorexia and bulimia. Basic Books, New York
Fairburn C G, Kirk J, O'Connor M, Cooper P J 1986b A comparison of two psychological treatments for bulimia nervosa. Behaviour Research and Therapy 24: 629–643
Feighner J P, Robins E, Guze S B, Woodruff R A, Winokur G, Munoz R 1972 Diagnostic criteria for use in psychiatric research. Archives of General Psychiatry 26: 57–63
Garfinkel P E, Garner D M 1982 Anorexia nervosa: a multidimensional perspective. Brunner/Mazel, New York
Garfinkel P E, Kaplan A S 1986 Anorexia nervosa: diagnostic conceptualisation. In: Brownell K D, Foreyt J P (eds) Handbook of eating disorders: physiology, psychology and treatment of obesity, anorexia and bulimia. Basic Books, New York
Garfinkel P E, Moldofsky H, Garner D M 1980 The heterogeneity of anorexia nervosa. Archives of General Psychiatry 37: 1036–1040
Garner D M 1986 Cognitive therapy for anorexia nervosa. In: Brownell K D, Foreyt J P (eds) Handbook of eating disorders: physiology, psychology and treatment of obesity, anorexia and bulimia. Basic Books, New York
Garner D M, Bemis K 1982 A cognitive-behavioural approach to anorexia nervosa. Cognitive Research and Therapy 6: 123–150
Garner D M, Bemis K 1985 Cognitive therapy for anorexia nervosa. In: Garner D M, Garfinkel P E (eds) Handbook of psychotherapy for anorexia nervosa and bulimia. Guilford Press, New York
Garner D M, Garfinkel P E 1980 Socio-cultural factors in the development of anorexia nervosa. Psychological Medicine 10: 647–656
Garner D M, Garfinkel P E 1981 Body image in anorexia nervosa: measurement, theory and clinical implications. International Journal of Psychiatry in Medicine 11: 263–284
Garner D M, Garfinkel P E, Schwartz D, Thompson M 1980 Cultural expectation of thinness in women. Psychological Reports 47: 483–491
Garner D M, Olmsted M P, Polivy J 1983 Developmental and Validation of a multidimensional eating disorder inventory for anorexia nervosa and bulimia. International Journal of Eating Disorders 2: 15–34
Garner D M, Rockert W, Olmsted M P, Johnson C, Coscina D 1985 Psychoeducational principles in the treatment of bulimia and anorexia nervosa. In: Garner D M, Garfinkel P E (eds) Handbook of psychotherapy for anorexia nervosa and bulimia. Guilford Press, New York
Garner D M, Fairburn C, Davis R 1987 Cognitive-behavioural treatment of bulimia nervosa: a critical appraisal. Behaviour Modification (in press)
Garrow J S, Crisp A H, Jordan H A et al 1975 Pathology of eating, group report. In: Silverstone T (ed) Dahlem Konferenzen, Life Sciences Research Report 2. Berlin
Gerner R H, Wilkins J N 1983 CSF cortisol in patients with depression, mania or anorexia nervosa and in normal subjects. American Journal of Psychiatry 140:92–94

Gershon E S, Schreiber J L, Hamovit J R et al 1984 Clinical findings in patients with anorexia nervosa and affective illness and their relatives. American Journal of Psychiatry 141: 1419–1422

Gold P W, Gwirtsman H, Augerinos P C et al 1986 Abnormal hypothalamic–pituitary–adrenal function in anorexia nervosa. New England Journal of Medicine 314: 1335–1342

Gwirtsman H E, Roy-Byrne P, Yager J, Gerner R H 1983 Neuroendocrine abnormalities in bulimia. American Journal of Psychiatry 140: 559–563

Gwirtsman H E, Roy-Byrne P, Lerner L, Yager J 1984 Bulimia in men: report of three cases with neuroendocrine findings. Journal of Clinical Psychiatry 45: 78–81

Halmi K A, Eckert E, LaDu T J, Cohen J 1986 Anorexia nervosa: treatment efficiency of cyproheptadine and amitriptyline. Archives of General Psychiatry 43: 177–181

Hammond W A 1879 Fasting girls: their physiology and pathology. Putnam, New York

Hawkins R C, Clement P F 1980 Development and construct validation of a self report measure of binge-eating tendencies. Addictive Behaviours 5: 219–226

Herman C P, Mack D 1975 Restrained and unrestrained eating. Journal of Personality 43: 647–660

Herman C P, Polivy J 1984 A boundary model for the regulation of eating. In: Stunkard A J, Stellar E (eds) Eating and its disorders. Raven Press, New York

Herman C P, Polivy J, Silver R 1979 Effects of an observer on eating behaviour: the evolution of sensible eating. Journal of Personality 47: 85–99

Hertzog D B 1982 Bulimia: the secretive syndrome. Psychosomatics 23: 481–484

Hertzog D B, Norman D K, Gordon C, Pepose M 1984 Sexual conflict in 27 males with bulimia. American Journal of Psychiatry 141: 989–990

Hibscher J A, Herman C P 1977 Obesity, dieting, and the suppression of obese characteristics. Journal of Comparative and Physiological Psychology 91: 374–380

Hill S W, McCutcheon N 1975 Eating responses of obese and non-obese humans during dinner meals. Psychological Medicine 37: 395–401

Holland A J, Hall A, Murray R, Russell G F M, Crisp A H 1984 Anorexia nervosa: a study of 34 twin pairs and one set of triplets. British Journal of Psychiatry 145: 414–419

Hsu L K 1980 Outcome of anorexia nervosa: a review of the literature. Archives of General Psychiatry 37: 1041–1046

Hsu L K G 1987 Are the eating disorders becoming more common in blacks? International Journal of Eating Disorders 6: 113–124

Hudson J I, Hudson M S 1984 Endocrine dysfunction in anorexia nervosa and bulimia: comparison with abnormalities in other psychiatric disorders and disturbances due to metabolic factors. Psychiatric Developments 4: 237–272

Hudson J I, Pope H G, Jonas J M, Yurgelun-Todd D 1983a Family history study of anorexia nervosa and bulimia. British Journal of Psychiatry 142: 133–138

Hudson J I, Pope H G, Jonas J M, Laffer P S, Hudson M S, Melby J M 1983b Hypothalamic pituitary adrenal axis hyperactivity in bulimia. Psychiatric Research 8: 111–118

Hughes P L, Wells L A, Cunningham M S 1986a The dexamethasone suppression test in bulimia before and after successful treatment with desipramine. Journal of Clinical Psychiatry 47: 515–517

Hughes P L, Wells L A, Cunningham C I, Istrup D M 1986b Treating bulimia with desipramine, Archives of General Psychiatry 43: 182–186

Humphrey L L 1986 Family relations in bulimic-anorexic and nondistressed families. International Journal of Eating Disorders 5: 223–232

Johnson C, Larson R 1982 Bulimia: an analysis of moods and behaviour. Psychosomatic Medicine 44: 341–351

Jones D J, Fon M M, Babigian H M, Hutton H E 1980 Epidemiology of anorexia nervosa in Monroe County, New York: 1960–1976. Psychosomatic Medicine 42: 551–558

Kendell R G, DiScipio W 1970 Obsessional symptoms and obsessional personality traits in patients with depressive illness. Psychological Medicine 1: 65–72

Kendell R E, Hall D J, Hailey A, Babigian H M 1973 The epidemiology of anorexia nervosa. Psychological Medicine 3: 200–203

Keys A, Brozek J, Hanschel A, Michelson O, Taylor H L 1950 The biology of human starvation. University of Minnesota Press, Minneapolis

Kiriike N, Nishiwaki S, Izumiya Y, Kawakita Y 1986 Dexamethasone suppression test in bulimia. Biological Psychiatry 21: 328–332

Kirkley B G, Schneider J A, Agras W S, Bachman J A 1985 Comparison of two group treatments for bulimia. Journal of Consulting and Clinical Psychology 53: 43–48

Lee W F, Rush A J, Mitchell J E 1985 Depression and bulimia. Journal of Affective Disorders 9: 231–238

Leitenberg A, Gross J, Peterson J, Rosen J C 1984 Analysis of an anxiety model and the process of change during exposure plus response prevention treatment of bulimia nervosa. Behaviour Therapy 15: 3–20

Lindy D C, Walsh T B, Reese S P, Gladis M, Glassman A H 1985 The dexamethasone test in bulimia. American Journal of Psychiatry 142:1375–1376

Mahoney M J 1975 The obese eating style: bites, beliefs and behaviour modifications. Addictive Behaviors 3: 129–134

Mann A H, Wakeling A, Wood U, Monck E, Dobbs R, Szmukler G I 1983 Screening for abnormal eating attitudes and psychiatric morbidity in an unselected population of 15-year-old school girls. Psychological Medicine 13: 573–580

Mills I H, Wilson R J, Eden M A M, Lines J G 1973 Endocrine and social factors in self-starvation amenorrhoea. In: Robertson R F (ed) Symposium: Anorexia nervosa and obesity. Royal College of Physicians, Edinburgh

Mitchell J E 1986a Anorexia nervosa: medical and physiological aspects. In: Brownell K D, Foreyt J P (eds) Handbook of eating disorders: physiology, psychology and treatment of obesity, anorexia and bulimia. Basic Books, New York

Mitchell J E 1986b Bulimia: medical and physiological aspects. In: Brownell K D, Foreyt J P (eds) Handbook of eating disorders: physiology, psychology and treatment of obesity, anorexia and bulimia. Basic Books, New York

Mitchell J E, Groat R 1984 A placebo-controlled double-blind trial of amitriptyline in bulimia. Journal of Clinical Psychopharmacology 4:186–193

Mitchell J E, Pyle R L, Hatsukami D, Boutacoff C I 1984 The dexamethasone suppression test in patients with bulimia. Journal of Clinical Psychiatry 45: 508–511

Mitchell J E, Hatsukami D, Eckert E D, Pyle R L 1985 Characteristics of 275 patients with bulimia. American Journal of Psychiatry 142: 482–485

Montgomery S A, Asberg M 1979 A new depression scale designed to be sensitive to change. British Journal of Psychiatry 134: 382–389

Mullen P E, Linsell C F, Parker D 1986 Influence of sleep disruption and caloric restriction on biological markers of depression. Lancet ii: 1051–1055

Needleman H L, Waber D 1976 Amitriptyline therapy in patients with anorexia nervosa. Lancet 2: 580

Palmer R L 1979 The dietary chaos syndrome: a useful new term? British Journal of Medical Psychology 52: 187–190

Paykel E S 1977 Depression and appetite. Journal of Psychosomatic Research 21: 401–407

Piran N, Kennedy S, Garfinkel P E, Owens M 1985 Affective disturbance in eating disorders. Journal of Nervous and Mental Diseases 173: 395–400

Polivy J 1976 Perception of calories and regulation of intake in restrained and unrestrained subjects. Addictive Behaviors 1: 237–243

Polivy J, Herman C P 1985 Dieting and bingeing: a causal analysis. American Psychologist 40: 193–201

Polivy J, Herman C P, Jazwinski C, Olmsted M P 1984 Restraint and binge-eating. In: Hawkins R C, Fremouw W, Clement P (eds) Binge-eating; theory, research and treatment. Springer, New York

Pope H G, Hudson J I, Jonas J M, Yurgelun-Todd D 1983 Bulimia treated with imipramine: a placebo-controlled double-blind study. American Journal of Psychiatry 140: 554–558

Pope H G, Hudson J I, Jonas J M, Yurgelun-Todd D 1985 Antidepressant treatment of bulimia: a two-year follow-up study. Journal of Clinical Psychopharmacology 6: 320–327

Pyle R L, Mitchell J E, Eckert E D 1981 Bulimia: a report of 34 cases. Journal of Clinical Psychiatry 42: 60–64

Pyle R L, Mitchell J E, Eckert E D, Halvorson P A, Neuman P A, Goff G M 1983 The incidence of bulimia in freshman college students. International Journal of Eating Disorders 2: 75–85

Pyle R L, Halvorson P A, Neuman P A, Mitchell J E 1986 The increasing prevalence of bulimia in freshman college students. International Journal of Eating Disorders 5: 631–647

Robinson P H, Holden N L 1986 Bulimia nervosa in the male: a report of nine cases. Psychological Medicine 16: 795–803
Rosen J C, Leitenberg H 1982 Bulimia nervosa: treatment with exposure and response prevention. Behavior Therapy 13: 117–124
Rosen J C, Leitenberg H 1985 Exposure plus response prevention treatment of bulimia. In: Garner D M, Garfinkel P E (eds) Handbook of psychotherapy for anorexia nervosa and bulimia. Guilford Press, New York
Ruderman A 1983 Obesity anxiety and food consumption. Addictive Behaviors 8: 235–242
Ruderman A J, Wilson G T 1979 Weight, restraint, cognitions and counter-regulation. Behaviour Research and Therapy 17: 581–590
Russell G F M 1970 Anorexia nervosa: its identity as an illness and its treatment. In: Price J H (ed) Modern trends in psychological medicine. Butterworths, London
Russell G F M 1979 Bulimia nervosa: an ominous variant of anorexia nervosa. Psychological Medicine 9: 429–448
Russell G F M 1985a Anorexia nervosa and bulimia nervosa. In: Russell G F M, Hudson L (eds) Handbook of psychiatry: the neuroses and personality disorders. Cambridge University Press, Cambridge
Russell G F M 1985b Do drugs have a place in the management of anorexia nervosa and bulimia nervosa? In: Sandler M, Silverstone T (eds) Psychopharmacology and food. Monograph No 7. British Association for Psychopharmacology, Oxford
Russell G F J 1986 The diagnostic formulation in bulimia nervosa. Paper read at the Second International Conference on Eating Disorders. New York
Sabine E J, Yonace A, Farrington A J, Barratt K H, Wakeling A 1983 Bulimia nervosa: a placebo-controlled double-blind therapeutic trial of mianserin. British Journal of Clinical Pharmacology 15: 195S–202S
Schachter S 1971 Emotion, obesity and crime. Academic Press, New York
Schweitzer I, Maguire R P, Tiller J W G, Gee A H, Harrison L E, Davis B M 1986 The effects of weight change on the dexamethasone suppression test in depressed and anorexic patients. British Journal of Psychiatry 149: 751–755
Slade P D 1982 Towards a functional analysis of anorexia nervosa. British Journal of Clinical Psychology 21: 167–179
Slade P D 1985 A review of body image studies in anorexia nervosa and bulimia nervosa. Journal of Psychiatric Research 19: 255–265
Slochower J 1985 Excessive eating: the role of emotions and environment. Human Sciences Press, New York
Smart D E, Beumont P J V, George G C W 1976 Some personality characteristics of patients with anorexia nervosa. British Journal of Psychology 128: 57–60
Solyom L, Freeman R J, Miles J E 1982 A comparative psychometric study of anorexia nervosa and obsessive neurosis. Canadian Journal of Psychiatry 27: 282–286
Spencer J A, Fremouw W J 1979 Binge-eating as a function of restraint and weight classification. Journal of Abnormal Psychology 88: 262–267
Spitzer L, Rodin J 1981 Human eating behavior: a critical review of studies in normal weight and overweight individuals. Appetite 2: 293–329
Striegel-Moore R H, Rodin J 1986 The influence of psychological variables on obesity. In: Brownell K D, Foreyt J P (eds) Handbook of eating disorders: physiology, psychology and treatment of obesity, anorexia and bulimia. Basic Books, New York
Striegel-Moore R H, Silberstein L R, Rodin J 1986 Towards an understanding of risk factors for bulimia. American Psychologist 41: 246–265
Strober M 1981 The significance of bulimia in juvenile anorexia nervosa: exploration of possible etiologic factors. International Journal of Eating Disorders 1: 28–43
Strober M 1986 Anorexia nervosa: history and psychological concepts. In: Brownell K D, Foreyt J P (eds) Handbook of eating disorders: physiology, psychology and treatment of obesity, anorexia and bulimia. Basic Books, New York
Strober M, Humphrey L 1987 Familial contributions to the etiology and course of anorexia nervosa and bulimia. Journal of Consulting and Clinical Psychology (in press)
Strober M, Katz J 1987 Depression in the eating disorders: a review and analysis of descriptive, family and biological findings. In: Garner D M, Garfinkel P E (eds) Diagnostic issues in anorexia nervosa and bulimia nervosa. Brunner/Mazel, New York (in press)

Strober M, Morrell W, Burroughs J, Salkin B, Jacobs C 1985 A controlled family study of anorexia nervosa. Journal of Psychiatric Research 19: 239–246

Stunkard A J, Kaplan D 1977 Eating in public places: a review of reports on the direct observation of eating behaviour. International Journal of Obesity 1: 89–101

Stunkard A J, Messick S 1985 The Three Factor Eating Questionnaire to measure dietary restraint, disinhibition and hunger. Journal of Psychosomatic Research 29: 71–84

Stunkard A J, Sorensen T I A, Hanic C et al 1986 An adoption study of human obesity. New England Journal of Medicine 314: 193–198

Swift W J, Andrews D, Barklage N E 1986 The relationship between affective disorders and eating disorder: a review of the literature. American Journal of Psychiatry 143: 290–299

Szmukler G I 1982 Drug treatment of anorexic states. In: Silverstone T (ed) Drugs and appetite. Academic Press, London

Szmukler G I 1983 Weight and food preoccupation in a population of English school girls. In: Bargamon G J (ed) Understanding anorexia nervosa and bulimia. Fourth Ross Conference. Ross Laboratories, Ohio

Szmukler G I 1985 The epidemiology of anorexia nervosa and bulimia. Journal of Psychiatric Research 19: 143–153

Szmukler G I, Russell G F M 1986 Outcome and prognosis of anorexia nervosa. In: Brownell K D, Foreyt J P (eds) Handbook of eating disorders: physiology, psychology and treatment of obesity, anorexia and bulimia. Basic Books, New York

Szmukler G I, McCance C, McCrane L, Carlson I H 1986 Anorexia nervosa: a case register study from Aberdeen. Psychological Medicine 16: 49–58

Taylor M J, Cooper P J 1986 Body size overestimation and depressed mood. British Journal of Clinical Psychology 25: 153–154

Turnbull J D, Freeman C P L, Barry F, Annandale A 1987 Physical and psychological characteristics of five male bulimics. British Journal of Psychiatry 150: 25–29

Wakeling A 1985 Neurobiological aspects of feeding disorders. Journal of Psychiatric Research 19: 191–201

Walsh B T, Stewart J W, Roose S P, Gladis M, Glassman A H 1984 Treatment of bulimia with phenelzine: a double-blind placebo-controlled trial. Archives of General Psychiatry 41: 1105–1109

Walsh B T, Roose S P, Glassman A H, Gladis M A, Sadik C 1985 Depression and bulimia. Psychosomatic Medicine 47: 123–131

Wardle J 1980 Restraint and binge eating. Behaviour Analysis and Modification 4: 201–209

Wardle J 1986 The assessment of restrained eating. Behaviour Research and Therapy 24: 213–215

Wardle J, Beinhart H 1981 Binge eating: a theoretical review. British Journal of Clinical Psychology 20: 97–109

Warner K E, Balagura S 1975 Intermeal eating patterns of obese and non-obese humans. Journal of Comparative and Physiological Psychology 89: 778–783

Wilson G T 1986 Cognitive-behavioural and pharmacological therapies for bulimia. In: Brownell K D, Foreyt J P (eds) Handbook of eating disorders: physiology, psychology and treatment of obesity, anorexia and bulimia. Basic Books, New York

Wilson G T, Rossiter E, Kleinfield E I, Lindholm L 1986 Cognitive-behavioural treatment of bulimia nervosa: a controlled evaluation. Behaviour Research and Therapy 24: 277–288

Wing J K, Cooper J E, Sartorius N 1974 The measurement and classification of psychiatric symptoms. Cambridge University Press, Cambridge

Woody E Z, Costanzo P R, Leifer H J, Conger J 1981 The effects of taste and calorie perceptions on the eating behaviour of restrained and unrestrained subjects. Cognitive Research and Therapy 5: 381–390

13   *Ray J. Hodgson*

Alcohol and drug dependence

INTRODUCTION

In 1965 a World Health Organization Committee provided us with a much-quoted definition of drug dependence. It is 'a state, psychic and sometimes also physical, resulting from the interaction between a living organism and a drug, characterised by behavioural and other responses that always include a compulsion to take the drug on a continuous or periodic basis in order to experience its psychic effects, and sometimes to avoid the discomfort of its absence' (Eddy et al 1965). This is a reasonable starting point even though we need further information about the 'behavioural and other responses' which characterize dependence and also what is meant by compulsion. The World Health Organization further attempted to categorize all the drugs that can lead to dependence on the basis of similarities in effects and similarities in the behavioural patterns that develop with excessive use. The following nine categories, or classes of dependence-producing substances, were proposed:

1. The alcohol–barbiturate group: drugs that lower the level of arousal of the central nervous system, leading to sedation and sleep.
2. Amphetamines and amphetamine-like substances: drugs that stimulate the central nervous system, reducing fatigue and the need for sleep.
3. Cannabis (marijuana, hashish): drugs that produce a 'high' in regular users that is generally pleasurable and associated with unusually vivid sensations.
4. Cocaine: a natural extract from the leaves of the South American coca shrub, which is both a stimulant and a euphoria-producing drug.
5. Hallucinogens (LSD and related substances): drugs that produce perceptual distortions, a sense of ecstatic detachment and euphoria.
6. Khat: a stimulant used primarily in Yemen and Ethiopia.
7. Opiates or opioids: a wide variety of natural and totally synthetic substances that have morphine-like effects, relieving pain and inducing a state of indifference to threatening situations.
8. Volatile solvents: glue, gasoline and cleaning fluids which, when inhaled or sniffed, produce a state of intoxication similar to alcoholic drunkenness but which sometimes result in hallucinogenic 'trips'.

9. Tobacco: a plant used for smoking, sniffing or chewing, associated with both stimulating and relaxing effects.

In this chapter the focus will be upon psychological processes and theories in general rather than any one drug in particular. The emphasis will be on similarities; nevertheless, it should be remembered that drugs do differ in their reinforcement potential, method of administration, cost and availability, as well as their social acceptability. A comprehensive model should address these differences as well as the many similarities. It should be added that our favourite drug, alcohol, will be mentioned more frequently than other drugs, but the assumption is being made that theories about alcohol consumption will turn out to be relevant to other forms of drug use and misuse.

A PSYCHOLOGICAL MODEL OF DRUG DEPENDENCE

Several hypotheses or working assumptions can be derived from a psychological or social learning view of dependence (Hodgson & Stockwell 1985). These hypotheses will be briefly considered before delving in more depth into the processes involved in the development of, and recovery from, drug and alcohol dependence.

Drinking alcohol is mainly functional. The use of drugs often appears to be irrational, mindless and beyond all reason. According to a psychological model, however, drug use is nearly always a function of the expected consequences, whether these are increased sociability, a pleasant glow or avoidance of future withdrawal symptoms. Such a view seems to conflict with the frequently cited evidence that alcohol and drug use can result in increased anxiety, hostility and guilt as well as adverse social consequences (Stockwell et al 1982). This 'addiction paradox' is similar to the 'neurotic paradox' noted by Mowrer more than twenty years ago (Mowrer 1960) and can be explained in a number of ways. First, short-term consequences tend to influence behaviour more powerfully than long-term consequences. Second, pleasant effects which occur only intermittently can have a powerful influence on behaviour. The one-armed bandit is a good example of an intermittent reinforcer which, nevertheless, encourages hopeful expectations. Third, expected consequences are always relative. An increase in anxiety as a result of drinking will be tolerated if the alternative is even worse. Fourth, behaviour is influenced by expected consequences which might be very different from the actual consequences. Finally, some consequences might be ignored or repressed if thinking about them is too distressing (Bandura 1977).

Drug use is learned and will be influenced by social, cognitive and psychophysiological processes. Through observational learning and communications, we learn about drug use from parents, peers, books, films and the media. Some of the expected consequences of drug use will be learned in this way. Others are learned through direct experience. The likelihood that a person will have direct experience of heavy drug use will depend upon a wide range of psychosocial factors, including occupation, personality, subculture, price and availability. Since drugs alter the state of the central nervous system, it has been suggested that an adaptive or homeostatic process gradually develops in order to counteract the effects of alcohol (Kalant et al 1971, Solomon 1977, Gross 1977). It has also been proposed that this homeostatic process, or neuroadaptation (Edwards et al 1981) results in both tolerance and withdrawal symptoms (Kalant 1973). In the face of a massive body of research there can now be no doubt that some such adaptive processes are involved in excessive alcohol and drug use.

A learned habit or life style can become a learned compulsion. If a heavy drug user begins to experience problems to do with health, finance, personal relationships, self-esteem, mood swings, or any of the wide variety of unpleasant consequences associated with drugs, then a set of negative expectations will develop. These will become part of the balance sheet or pay-off matrix (Orford 1985), so that the drug user has strong reasons to want drugs and also strong reasons to resist. They have developed an approach–avoidance conflict which will then be experienced as a compulsion. To say that some heavy drug using appears to be a learned compulsion is simply to put a label upon this process.

Cognitive control. Within a psychological model great emphasis is placed upon the development of cognitive control skills and the ways in which such an ability can be impaired (e.g. Bandura 1977, Hodgson 1984). The gardener, writer and problem drinker will make plans, set both short-term and long-term goals, and make pledges or commitments. They will deliberately attempt to achieve desirable objectives. Sometimes, however, a state of 'learned helplessness' afflicts the gardener, the writer and the problem drinker, as a result of repeated failures (Seligman 1976). In this state, motivation is sapped, emotionality heightened and pessimism prevails. Problem drinkers and drug users often describe such a state when no attempt is made to stop because they have learned from past experience that it is futile to try.

The relapse process will change as dependence increases. Although relapse is a continuous process, it can be arbitrarily divided into three phases. Phase 1 involves mainly psychosocial cues such as arguments, anxiety, criticism, social pressure and frustration (Litman et al 1979, Marlatt & Gordon 1980). Phase 2 involves the person's reactions to taking just a small dose. We can make the prediction from a learning-theory model that a small dose will prime a desire for more (Hodgson et al 1979) and also that learned helplessness will tend to be experienced. Finally, Phase 3 will involve the expectation of withdrawal symptoms and drug use which is motivated by desire to escape from or avoid them. From a purely theoretical point of view, we can make the prediction that Phase 1 is involved for all problem drinkers, but that Phases 2 and 3 become increasingly involved as drinking becomes more and more excessive.

Having briefly outlined the major assumptions of the psychological model of drug dependence the various psychological processes will now be considered in more detail.

COGNITIVE FACTORS

The use of drugs is very closely related to expectations about the consequences of consumption. For example, a factor analytical study by Brown et al (1980) revealed six independent factors when drinkers were asked about the expected effects of alcohol. According to this study drinkers expect alcohol to transform experiences in a positive way, to enhance social and physical pleasure, to enhance sexual performance and experience, to increase power and aggression, to increase social assertiveness and to reduce tension. Which of these expectancies predominates will of course depend upon the occasion, the person and the social context. The strength of such expectancies often outweighs the actual effects of intoxication, a phenomenon which has been clearly demonstrated by experimental work making use of a balanced placebo design (Marlatt & Rosenow 1980). This design involves four conditions which allow for the effects of the drug to be compared with the effects of expectancies. In research on alcohol consumption, for example, the conditions would be:
1. Given alcohol and told that the drink contains alcohol.
2. Given alcohol but told that the drink is a soft drink.
3. Given a soft drink and told that the drink is a soft drink.
4. Given a soft drink but told that the drink contains alcohol.

Using this design it has been shown that, in males, the belief that they had consumed alcohol tended to reduce social anxiety whether or not the drink actually contained alcohol (Wilson & Abrams 1977), whereas women who believe that they are intoxicated show increased social anxiety (Abrams & Wilson 1979). Other studies have similarly demonstrated for moderate doses that learned expectancies can be as important as intoxication in the influence that they have on aggression (Lang et al 1975), on sexual disinhibition (Wilson & Lawson 1976) and also on the amount consumed by problem drinkers (Marlatt et al 1973).

In both social drug users and also those who are more severely dependent it has been shown that expectations about the effects of taking a drug and the effects of not taking a drug are important predictors of both intention and drug-taking behaviour. For example, Brown (1985) has shown that alcoholics' expectations of positive effects from drinking predicted drop out from treatment. The expectation that alcohol reduces tension predicted relapse better than factors such as marital status, employment status, living environment, participation in aftercare programmes, social support and level of reported stress. One method of studying the influence of these outcome expectancies in the field of addiction was pioneered by Mausner & Platt (1971) in studying changes in smoking behaviour. In order to assess the influence of the consequences of drug taking they argued that expectations about a particular consequence as well as the value of that consequence must both be considered. One person may believe that drug misuse will ruin his marriage but does not care (high expectancy–low value). Another who values his marriage may be unaffected by such an expectancy because he believes that his marriage will survive his drug taking (low expectancy–high value). Mausner & Platt devised a questionnaire which listed forty possible consequences of continuing to smoke and stopping smoking. The smoker was asked to rate both his expectation that a particular outcome would occur and also the value or utility of each outcome. An overall subjective expected utility (SEU) score was then computed. The smokers were contacted five days later and there was a significant relationship between the SEU scores and the extent to which subjects had reduced their smoking. In other words, those who reduced were the ones who expected more favourable outcomes from stopping smoking.

A number of studies carried out by Bauman (1980, Bauman et al 1985) confirmed the usefulness of the SEU methodology. They asked 12- and 13-year-olds to select from a list of 54 consequences those that they expected to occur if, in the future, they were to use marijuana. They were then asked to rate the importance or utility of each as well as subjective probability. An overall SEU score derived from these ratings predicted self-reported marijuana use, this time not five days later but one year later. Sutton (1987) has reviewed the usefulness of the subjective expected utility model of addictive behaviour as well as two clearly related models, namely: Fishbein & Ajzen's Behavioural Intention Model (1975), and the Health Belief Model (Becker 1974). He concludes that 'these approaches are a rich source of ideas that may be used to further our understanding of addictive behaviour. To date, these theories have not been widely used in this area and their potential has been largely untapped'.

When considering the way in which addictive behaviour changes over time it is useful to focus upon both outcome expectancies and efficacy expectancies. Whether drug users reduce their consumption is related to both outcome expectancies and also to their confidence that they can cope. These efficacy expectations are important predictors of future actions (Bandura 1985) and several studies have demonstrated that efficacy expectations have an important influence on addictive behaviour. Rist & Watzl (1983) carried out an investigation of efficacy expectations in hospitalized alcoholics and demonstrated that those who expected to be able to cope with a variety of high-risk situations were less likely to relapse during the three months after discharge. A study of smokers came to very similar conclusions (Condiotti & Lichtenstein, 1981). Whether addicts relapse after treatment is a function of severity of dependence (Edwards et al 1983, Babor et al 1987), but in a study of alcoholics (Heather et al 1983) and also in a study of smokers (Killen et al 1984) a self-efficacy measure turned out to be a better predictor of outcome than measures of degree of dependence.

Clearly, there is now sufficient evidence to indicate that cognitive processes are important factors that must be included in a comprehensive model of dependence and that there are ways of assessing both outcome and efficacy expectations which are both reliable and valid. Since cognitive factors are so crucial, it is reasonable to suppose that methods of treatment and prevention should place a great deal of emphasis upon cognitions.

In the next section the importance of associative learning or classical conditioning will be considered, since there is now a body of evidence which has important implications for models of addiction and also for methods of treating addictions.

ASSOCIATIVE LEARNING

When considering the early stages of drug and alcohol misuse psychological factors have always been emphasized, whereas most explanations of the later stages, involving tolerance and physical dependence, have tended to invoke pharmacological or physiological concepts. The more-or-less implicit assumption of such models is that the core of dependence and the cure for dependence will be chemical or medical, and not psychological. More recently a growing body of evidence has demonstrated that a comprehensive model of tolerance and physical dependence must include the principles of associative learning or classical conditioning which have been elucidated by psychologists during the last fifty years. In the most well-known example of classical or Pavlovian conditioning an animal responds to a signal or cue (e.g. a bell) with an anticipatory response (e.g. salivation) in order to prepare for a particular activity or event (e.g. eating). This simple process of associative learning enhances our ability to prepare for action and to cope with a variety of threatening and disturbing events. Before considering the relevance of such conditioning to the field of drug dependence the concepts of tolerance and compensatory adaptive responses will be introduced.

Tolerance occurs, following drug use, when the same dose begins to have a reduced psychophysiological effect and therefore a larger dose is needed to achieve the same effect. The development of such tolerance, which can lead to more excessive drug use, is usually explained by invoking the concept of a compensatory-adaptive response which counteracts the effect of the drug. This adaptive response is a homeostatic process which opposes the toxic effect of the drug. For example, insulin produces hypoglycaemia or a low blood sugar level and the compensatory-adaptive response produces hyperglycaemia or a high blood sugar level. A key question, which has only recently been answered, is whether the compensatory or opponent process can be conditioned to associated cues. If such conditioning is an important element in the development of addiction then perhaps the compensatory adaptive process can be deconditioned or unlearned. This would have very important implications for the treatment of drug, alcohol and cigarette dependence. An early demonstration of a conditioned response to a drug which appeared to provide evidence for conditioned compensatory adaptive responses was produced by Subkov & Zilov (1937), who noted that cues associated with the administration of adrenaline caused a decrease in heart rate (bradycardia), whereas adrenaline itself caused tachycardia. There are now numerous demonstrations of this phenomenon (Table 13.1).

Table 13.1 The effects of a variety of drugs and the compensatory conditioned responses (CR). Reproduced with permission from MacRae et al (1987)

Drug	Drug effect	CR
Amphetamine	↑ O_2 consumption	↓ O_2 consumption
Atropine	↓ Salivation	↑ Salivation
Caffeine	↑ Salivation	↓ Salivation
Chlordiazepoxide	Hypothermia	Hyperthermia
Chlorpromazine	↓ Activity	↑ Activity
Dinitrophenol	↑ O_2 consumption	↓ O_2 consumption
Dinitrophenol	Hyperthermia	Hypothermia
Adrenaline	Tachycardia	Bradycardia
Adrenaline	↓ Gastric secretion	↑ Gastric secretion
Adrenaline	Hyperglycaemia	Hypoglycaemia
Ethanol	Hypothermia	Hyperthermia
Glucose	Hyperglycaemia	Hypoglycaemia
Histamine	Hypothermia	Hyperthermia
Insulin	Hypoglycaemia	Hyperglycaemia
Lithium chloride	↓ Drinking	↑ Drinking
Lithium chloride	↓ Salivation	↑ Salivation
Methyl dopa	↓ Blood pressure	↑ Blood pressure
Midazolam	↓ Activity	↑ Activity
Morphine	Bradycardia	Tachycardia
Morphine	Analgesia	Hyperalgesia
Morphine	Hyperthermia	Hypothermia
Morphine	↓ Activity	↑ Activity
Morphine	↑ Intestinal transit time	↓ Intestinal transit time
Nalorphine	Tachycardia	Bradycardia
Naloxone	Antagonism of opiate analgesia	Analgesia

If tolerance results from compensatory-adaptive responses which can be conditioned, then it follows that tolerance should be more pronounced when a drug is administered in the presence of cues which have previously been associated with the drug administration. An early example of such an effect was provided by Adams et al (1969), who demonstrated that rats exhibited tolerance to the analgesic effects of morphine only if the injection of the drug occurred in the same environment as previous injections. Siegel and his colleagues have replicated and extended these studies and it is now very clear that tolerance is strongly affected by associative learning (Siegel 1983, MacRae et al 1987).

These findings lead directly to the hypothesis that tolerance should be reduced or extinguished when a conditional stimulus is presented without the drug administration. For example, if a placebo substance is injected then the cues associated with the drug administration would occur without the psychophysiological effects of the drug. This is an extinction paradigm, since the conditional stimulus is experienced without the unconditional response. Under these circumstances the compensatory-adaptive response should be extinguished, and consequently so should tolerance. A number of recent experiments have shown that this does in fact occur (MacRae et al 1987). Tolerance to a variety of effects of morphine, amphetamine, ethanol and midazolam (a short-acting benzodiazepam) can be extinguished. The very important implications of these findings will be considered in the later section on treatment.

In the next section the relapse process will be considered in some detail, beginning with the influence of compensatory-adaptive responses.

THE RELAPSE PROCESS

Mark Twain noted that 'Giving up smoking is easy. I've done it hundreds of times'. The implication of this statement also applies to alcohol and drug dependence. It is relatively easy to stop but very difficult to maintain this resolve over a long period.

There are many factors which influence the relapse process, and one of them is closely related to the development of compensatory-adaptive processes described above. It is usually argued that tolerance and withdrawal symptoms are closely related phenomena. Compensatory-adaptive responses result in tolerance when a drug is administered, and withdrawal symptoms when the drug is stopped. If compensatory-adaptive responses occur in the presence of drug cues then the resulting psychophysiological state will be very similar to withdrawal symptoms. There is reasonably good evidence that this does occur. For example, addicts can experience withdrawal symptoms if they are offered heroin by a friend. Similar observations have been made in experimentally addicted animals. One experimenter who listened to tape-recorded music when injecting monkeys with morphine discovered that the music could elicit withdrawal symptoms. When the animal had been drug-free for several months the experimenter played the tape-recorded music and noted that the animal 'became restless, had piloerection, yawned, became diuretic, showed rhinorrhea, and again sought out the drug injection' (Ternes, pp. 167–168, quoted by MacRae et al 1987). On the assumption that the music was not of the type that always produces this dramatic effect, it would appear that such a conditioning phenomenon can contribute to the relapse process. There are now a number of investigations which have confirmed this common clinical observation, that drug-associated cues can elicit withdrawal symptoms (Siegel 1983). These studies have shown that when addicts are confronted with drug-associated stimuli in the laboratory (e.g. injection paraphernalia for the intravenous drug user) they display definite symptoms of drug withdrawal. It is very likely that these conditioned responses contribute to the relapse process even though other psychosocial processes are probably more important.

The most cost-effective and sensible way to initiate an investigation of the relapse process is to simply ask people about the personal and environmental events leading up to a recent relapse. Marlatt and his colleagues used this strategy across a range of people with addictive and compulsive complaints (Marlatt & Gordon 1980). They concluded that there are three primary high-risk situations: *negative emotional states* were predominant in 35% of all relapses in the sample. A description of the series of events leading up to a relapse would be placed in this category if a negative mood state was reported which was not linked to an interpersonal situation. Anger caused by an unexpected bill or an impersonal event would fall into this category, whereas anger resulting from a marital conflict would be placed in the next category. *Interpersonal conflict* (16% of relapses) refers to situations involving current or relatively recent conflict, usually within a family, between friends or at work. *Social pressure* (20%) covers both direct and indirect pressure in situations where there is verbal persuasion or simply an expectation that everybody will drink. There are two other intrapersonal categories which should be included within a broad model, at least for alcoholics and compulsive gamblers. The first is labelled simply 'urges and temptations'. The second is labelled 'testing personal control' and is linked to the thought that 'Surely, I can now take one or two drinks and then stop' (Litman et al 1979). This body of evidence is very valuable when attempting to understand or treat addictive problems even though the data are based upon subjective attributions and memory of disturbing events.

One way of asking questions about the context in which relapse or recovery occurs is to assess the personal and environmental variables that are prevalent during the follow-up period after treatment. For example, Moos and his colleagues identified two groups of patients on the basis of their drinking history during the two years following treatment. Patients were assigned to a recovered group ($n = 55$) if they showed no signs of problem drinking when assessed at six months and two years. They were compared to a relapsed group ($n = 58$) which included those who were hospitalized for treatment of alcoholism or whose drinking was associated with problems, or was so severe that they could not be classified as recovered moderate drinkers (Bromet et al 1977, Cronkite & Moos 1980). One set of variables that had some predictive significance was concerning the patient's intake symptoms, the type of treatment programme and level of co-operation. However, all of these factors taken together with sociodemographic characteristics accounted for less than 20% of the variance at the two-year follow-up (Cronkite & Moos 1980). Another set of variables covered the nature of the alcoholics' social environment, family relationships, work environment and life stresses that were experienced during the follow-up period, as well as their preferred coping styles. These post-treatment factors independently accounted for 10–30% of the variance in outcome functioning. Of course, the direction of effects is debatable. Does poor outcome result in poor relationships and an increase in the number of life stresses, or is the major influence the other way around. Undoubtedly, there is a reciprocal relationship; nevertheless, in a series of longitudinal analyses it was found that social factors, life events and coping style were significant predictors of outcome, even after controlling the prior levels of functioning, supporting the view that these factors appear to have an important influence on relapse and recovery (Billings & Moos 1982).

Other studies have also demonstrated the importance of family cohesion and occupational status in relapse and recovery (e.g. Orford & Edwards 1977, Polich et al 1980). Furthermore, two treatment investigations, to be described later, suggest that relapse can be prevented by either a direct attack on social, family and occupational relationships (e.g. Azrin 1976) or by focusing upon the development of effective coping strategies (Chaney et al 1978).

The perspective that is emerging from this work is represented in Figure 13.1. According to this simple model, relapse is a function of high-risk events occurring against a background of sensitizing and protective personal

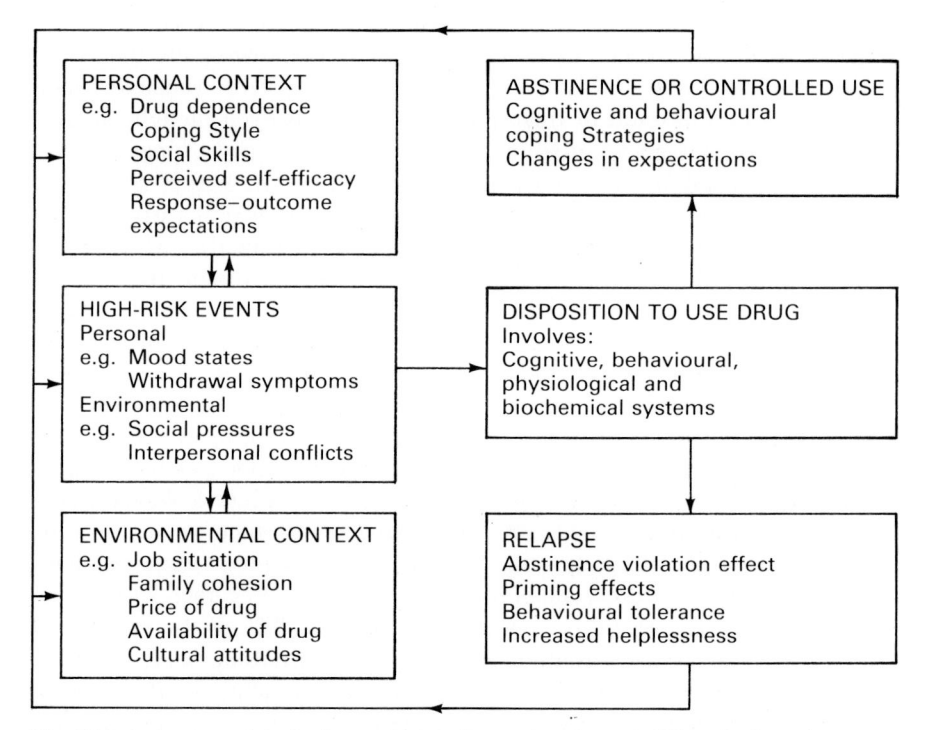

Fig. 13.1 A simple model of relapse which indicates that the probability of relapse is a function of high-risk, personal or environmental events occurring within a personal and environmental context.

and environmental conditions. Relapse can arbitrarily be divided into three stages. Stage 1 involves taking the first dose of a drug after a period of abstinence. The second stage occurs after the first dose has been consumed, and it has been suggested that a psychophysiological response, associated with craving, is primed or kindled (Ludwig et al 1974). Stage 3 involves prolonged heavy drinking and is associated with an altered psychophysiological state and feelings of helplessness, as well as changes in relationships and environments.

A question that has led to a great deal of controversy is whether or not priming effects do occur and, if so, whether this a psychophysiological or a purely cognitive phenomenon. A number of investigations have focused upon these questions during the last twenty years (e.g. Merry 1966, Marlatt et al 1973). Hodgson et al (1979) compared eleven problem drinkers designated as 'severely dependent', since they reported several months of almost daily withdrawal, relief-type drinking and a 'narrowed drinking repertoire', with nine 'moderately dependent' who had experienced less extensive withdrawal experiences. All were in-patients of the Bethlem Royal Hospital Treatment Unit while participating in the study. Three hours after a relatively high priming dose (150 ml vodka), the severely dependent group consumed available alcoholic drinks faster than after a small priming dose (15 ml vodka) or no priming dose. The reverse was the case for moderately dependent drinkers, and the contrast between the two groups was highly significant. A more recent study of priming effects has confirmed this finding, and demonstrated that the actual alcoholic content of the priming dose overrides the subject's belief as to its content for severely, but not the moderately, dependent drinkers (Stockwell et al 1982).

A number of conclusions can tentatively be drawn from these two priming experiments. Firstly, and perhaps most importantly, assessments of severity of dependence turned out to be crucial. In both experiments nothing of interest would have emerged if the degree of dependence had been ignored. Secondly, priming effects do occur, but more strongly, in the severely dependent drinker. Thirdly, the priming effects that we have observed do appear to be influenced by psychophysiological cues.

Even though priming effects do occur it is still probable that, during all the stages of relapse, cognitive variables play a very important part. Marlatt (1982) emphasizes the importance of such a cognitive process, which he labels the 'Abstinence Violation Effect' (AVE). If a drug user is committed to total abstinence then one small dose (e.g. one cigarette) breaks this rule and leads to the abandonment of the rule. The abstinence violation effect is postulated to occur during the following conditions: 'Prior to the first lapse, the individual is personally committed to an extended or indefinite period of abstinence. The intensity of the AVE will vary as a function of several factors, including the degree of prior commitment or effort expended to maintain abstinence, the duration of the abstinence period (the longer the period, the greater the effect) and the subjective value or importance of the prohibited behaviour to the individual' (ibid., p. 342).

The relative emphasis that should be given to the cognitive and psychophysiological processes involved at various stages of relapse is still in doubt, and the answers have important treatment implications.

TREATMENT STRATEGIES

Recent pharmacological discoveries have ensured that the typical alcoholic or drug addict who is admitted to a hospital or detoxification unit will probably not experience very severe withdrawal symptoms. Within a couple of weeks his nervous system will be almost back to normal. The main problem with all addictions is not in stopping but in remaining abstinent or developing permanent control. Treatment must, therefore, be directed towards preventing relapse. There are four broad approaches to the treatment of drug dependence, with some evidence to suggest that all four can be effective.

Drug substitution

The use of methadone taken orally as a substitute for injected heroin is one example of drug substitution. Dole & Nyswander, who pioneered the use of methadone as a treatment, believed that it counteracted the craving that occurred during withdrawal and also that a sufficient dose of methadone produced a 'heroin blockade' (Dole & Nyswander 1976). In sufficient doses, they argued, it would prevent the euphoric and sedative effects of heroin by blocking the sites in the brain that respond to opioid substances. Because methadone is taken by mouth rather than by injection, the effects wear off very slowly; consequently, it can be taken just once a day. Moreover, since methadone produces fewer sharp fluctuations in mood, the experience and behaviour of an addict maintained on the substitute drug are relatively normal. There is still a great deal of debate about the usefulness of methadone, but the criticism voiced by some — that methadone maintenance is like 'treating an addiction to Scotch with bourbon' — is an oversimplification.

Nicotine chewing-gum is the other drug substitute for which there is some good evidence of effectiveness (Russell et al 1983, NIDA Monograph 1985). Nicotine in chewing-gum is slowly absorbed through the membranes of the mouth and throat, unlike the rapid absorption from a cigarette. Nevertheless, craving for a cigarette appears to be counteracted by the gum, especially during the early stages of withdrawal. Furthermore, it is then much easier to give up the gum than it is to give up cigarettes.

Many people, especially the less severely dependent, are able to give up their addictions without the use of a substitute drug; this, of course, is always preferable if it can be done. Oral methadone, nicotine chewing-gum, and other drugs should be viewed as useful components of treatment. They are not as addictive or pleasurable as injected or inhaled drugs and so they are ideal for the addict who worries about withdrawal symptoms and needs to give up in stages.

Coping with craving

People who are dependent upon drugs, alcohol and cigarettes are often resigned to the fact that they cannot cope with craving. When it starts to build up, for whatever reason, they feel helpless and powerless to resist. In recent years research has, therefore, been directed towards methods of helping people to cope with craving and temptation.

Alan Marlatt and his colleagues have been able to help alcoholics by having them identify high-risk situations and then repeatedly practise ways of dealing with these situations (Chaney et al 1978). High-risk events could involve social pressures, negative moods, stressful interactions with other people, or a small dose of alcohol. Coping strategies might be to avoid being 'overwhelmed' by thinking about just one hour at a time; concentrating on the long-term benefits of abstinence; going for a walk or digging in the garden in order to ride out the craving; being assertive with other people, perhaps telling them not to put temptation in your way; or practising relaxation or meditation.

Examples of the high-risk situations that were covered by Chaney and his colleagues include the following:

'You are eating at a good restaurant with some friends on a special occasion. The waitress comes over and says "Drink before dinner?" Everyone else orders one. All eyes seem to be on you.'

'You get up on Saturday morning and realize that you don't have anything planned to do during the day. You sit around for a while but you begin to feel bored and restless.'

The problem-solving approach outlined by Chaney et al involves eight $1\frac{1}{2}$-hour sessions in which the goal is to focus upon specific relapse situations such as the ones above and generate ways of coping. These coping strategies are then rehearsed. This psychological intervention was compared with a similar treatment which concentrated upon the problems but not the solutions. The problem-solving treatment was also compared with traditional psychiatric treatment. The outcome of this trial turned out to be very encouraging. A verbal role-playing measure (the situational competency test) showed significant improvement in the training group compared to the two control groups and, furthermore, the one-year post-treatment follow-up indicated that the problem-solving approach decreased the duration and severity of relapse episodes. One finding that should be the subject of further research was the very high correlation between the situational competency test and treatment outcome at the one-year follow-up. This supports the body of work on efficacy expectations mentioned earlier. It would appear that problem-solving and rehearsal should be one component of a comprehensive treatment strategy, although a recent review of relapse prevention programmes concludes that overall the results are mixed (Brownell et al 1986).

Cue exposure

A similar but slightly different method of treatment involves repeated exposure to real-life temptations. This cue exposure approach is analogous to the methods that have been shown to very effective in the treatment of phobias and obsessional-compulsive disorders, where the basic goal of therapy is to provoke the urge to escape or indulge in a compulsive ritual but then resist the urge until it goes away (Rachman & Hodgson 1980). The first application of cue exposure in the field of alcohol and drug dependence resulted in a very interesting finding (Hodgson & Rankin 1976). This individual case study focused upon the priming effect of a few drinks (e.g. Hodgson et al 1979, Stockwell et al 1982). A number of cues were related to the desire to drink but one of the most potent of these was the consumption of a moderate amount of alcohol. Once the patient had consumed four vodkas he experienced a very strong craving for more drink. Over a three-week period he was, therefore, exposed repeatedly to this situation by giving him four vodkas and then providing support as he resisted continuing drinking. Although craving was initially moderately high it diminished over time and lessened at an increasing rate across sessions, so that at the end of the twelfth session virtually no craving was present immediately after cue exposure. Furthermore, these exposure sessions, carried out within the hospital environment, appeared to strengthen the ability to cope in other situations outside the hospital. Fourteen months after treatment this patient was re-admitted for a series of booster sessions and this time a higher dose of alcohol was used, with the focus being upon the craving or desire to drink which was experienced on the morning after the night before (Hodgson & Rankin 1982). The results of this extended study with a five-year follow-up were consistent with the following hypotheses:

> Cue exposure can prime the urge to drink, even within a hospital environment. When the urge is primed by a heavy-drinking session, then the associated cues tend to be 'psychophysiological' in nature, since they involve a cognitive component (e.g. 'What will happen if I don't drink?') and a physiological component (e.g. tremor). Repeated cue exposure leads to extinction of craving and subsequent reality testing until expectations match up with reality. (Hodgson & Rankin 1982, p. 219)

Finally, a controlled trial was carried out on ten other severely dependent problem drinkers in order to test further the hypothesis that cue exposure leads to a decline in craving (Rankin et al 1983). Ten severely dependent alcoholics had six sessions of this 'in vivo' cue exposure experience. To control for non-specific factors five of the subjects also had six sessions of imaginal cue exposure in which they were asked to picture themselves resisting drink in tempting situations. The rise and fall of craving over the sessions of 'in vivo' cue exposure indicated that craving did eventually habituate, the effect being particularly evident in those subjects who were given imaginal exposure before the 'in vivo' sessions. A speed of drinking craving test confirmed these overall results and we concluded that 'in vivo' exposure resulted in a dramatic modification of craving whereas imaginal cue exposure did not.

This work suggests that cue exposure, perhaps in combination with problem solving or coping skills training, is one approach to dependence that must be given serious consideration. In our studies we were attempting to prevent relapse after drinking begins, but there is also some evidence that exposure to drinking situations whilst remaining totally abstinent also has a beneficial effect (Blakey & Baker 1980).

If we ask why cue exposure is effective then we must look to basic psychological theories. Recent extinction theories have placed a great deal of emphasis upon cognitive processes, especially the development of expectations. It may be that cue exposure leads to a change in both outcome and efficacy expectations (Hodgson & Rankin 1982). On the other hand, the work of Siegel and his colleagues suggests the hypothesis that repeated exposure to the interoceptive and external cues associated with drinking would lead to the extinction of compensatory adaptive processes (Siegel 1983). This is an important area of debate.

Social interventions

A simple model of relapse such as that presented in Figure 13.1 leads to the prediction that social and interpersonal factors should be given a great deal of attention if treatment is to be very comprehensive. One approach, which Azrin and his colleagues have called 'community reinforcement' (Hunt & Azrin 1973), focuses upon employment, marriage and social activities in an attempt to make sobriety more rewarding. They argue that, if a problem drinker is interacting well with his community, then sobriety will be reinforced and excessive drinking will be curtailed. Azrin and his colleagues have now completed three studies which, taken together, do demonstrate that modifying vocational, marital, social and recreational activities can have a strong beneficial effect on drinking (Hunt & Azrin 1973, Azrin 1976, Azrin et al 1982). The social counselling procedures involved arranging social interactions with non-drinkers or moderate drinkers and reducing interactions with friends who were known to have a drinking problem. A former tavern was converted into a self-supporting social club for clients and friends. This club provided a juke box, card games, dances, picnics, films and other types of social activities. Furthermore, alcoholic beverages were strictly forbidden. Patients without jobs were helped to obtain one. Married patients were counselled with the aim of improving their interactions and making the drinking of alcohol incompatible with the improved relationship. Positive results were obtained in all three studies and, even though Antabuse was also used in two of them, these exceptionally good results do suggest that one focus of treatment should be the links between the person and his social environment.

CONCLUSIONS AND IMPLICATIONS

A psychological model of dependence emphasizes the influence of cognitive, psychophysiological and social learning processes in the development of drug dependence, as well as in continued use, excessive use, relapse and recovery. Outcome and efficacy expectancies are at the heart of this model and a wide range of variables such as price and availability of drugs, social pressure to use drugs and placebo effects can best be understood in terms of their effects on expectancies. Even the effects of psychophysiological phenomena are moderated by expectancies. Withdrawal symptoms, for example, do not always result in craving. Through instrumental and associative learning a drug user develops acquired motivational states, compensatory adaptive responses and subjective expected utilities and probabilities linked to particular situations or events. The aims of both prevention and treatment strategies are to halt or reverse these processes.

Developing coping skills and improving social relationships will influence both outcome and efficacy expectancies, so that temptations are more likely to be avoided or confronted. Not all temptations or cues can be avoided and this is why cue exposure should logically be an integral part of treatment. Exposure to tempting social situations and to small doses of a drug should facilitate a change in expectancies and possibly extinguish compensatory adaptive processes. The radical proposal which is suggested by this psychological model is that good treatment should involve exposure to drugs and to tempting situations.

Many psychological concepts and processes have not been covered in this chapter, even though they should be considered within a comprehensive model. Personality, family processes, operant principles and cultural attitudes would need to be included; nevertheless, the concepts described above provide one way of incorporating these and other psychological processes into a cognitive and social learning model.

REFERENCES

Abrams D B, Wilson G T 1979 Effects of alcohol on social anxiety in women: cognitive versus physiological processes. Journal of Abnormal Psychology 88: 161–173

Adams W J, Yeh S Y, Woods L A, Mitchell C L 1969 Drug-test interaction as a factor in the development of tolerance to the analgesic effect of morphine. Journal of Pharmacology and Experimental Therapeutics 168: 251–257

Azrin N H 1976 Improvements in the community reinforcement approach to alcoholism. Behaviour Research and Therapy 14: 339–348

Azrin N H, Sisson R W, Meyers R, Godfrey M 1982 Alcoholism treatment by Disulfiram

and community reinforcement therapy. Journal of Behavioural Therapy and Experimental Psychiatry 13: 105–112
Babor T F, Cooney N L, Laverman R J 1987 The drug dependence syndrome concept as a psychological theory of relapse behaviour: an empirical evaluation. British Journal of Addiction 82: 393–405
Bandura A 1977 Social learning theory. Prentice-hall, Englewood Cliffs, NJ
Bandura A 1985 Social foundations of thought and action. Prentice-Hall, Englewood Cliffs, NJ
Bauman K E 1980 Predicting adolescent drug use: the utility structure and marijuana. Praeger, New York
Bauman K E, Fisher L A, Bryan E S, Chenoweth R L 1985 Relationship between subjective expected utility and behavior: a longitudinal study of adolescent drinking behavior. Journal of Studies on Alcohol 46: 32–38
Becker M H (ed) 1974 The health belief model and personal health behavior. Slack, NJ
Billings A G, Moos R H 1982 Work stress and the stress-buffering roles of work and family resources. Journal of Occupational Behaviour 3: 215–232
Blakey R, Baker R 1980 An exposure approach to alcohol abuse. Behavior Research and Therapy 18: 319–325
Bromet E, Moos R H, Bliss F, Wuthman C 1977 Post-treatment functioning of alcoholic patients: its relation to program participation. Journal of Consulting and Clinical Psychology 45: 829–842
Brown S A 1985 Reinforcement expectancies and alcohol treatment outcome after one year. Journal of Studies on Alcohol 46: 304–308
Brown S A, Goldman M S, Inn A, Anderson L R 1980 Expectations of reinforcement from alcohol: their domain and relation to drinking patterns. Journal of Consulting and Clinical Psychology 48: 418–425
Brownell K D, Marlatt G A, Lichtenstein E, Wilson G T 1986 Understanding and preventing relapse. American Psychologist 41: 765–782
Chaney E F, O'Leary M R, Marlatt G A 1978 Skill training with alcoholics. Journal of Consulting and Clinical Psychology 46: 1092–1104
Condiotti M M, Lichtenstein E 1981 Self-efficacy and relapse in smoking cessation programs. Journal of Consulting and Clinical Psychology 49: 648–658
Cronkite R C, Moos R H 1980 The determinants of post-treatment functioning of alcoholic patients: a conceptual framework. Journal of Consulting and Clinical Psychology 48: 305–316
Dole V P, Nyswander M E 1976 Methadone maintenance treatment: a ten-year perspective. Journal of the American Medical Association 235: 2117–2119
Eddy N B, Halbach H, Isbell H, Seevers M A 1965 Drug dependence: its significance and characteristics. Bulletin of the World Health Organization 32: 721–733
Edwards G, Arif A, Hodgson R 1981 Diagnosis and classification of drug- and alcohol-related problems: a WHO memorandum. WHO Bulletin 3865. WHO, Geneva
Edwards G, Duckitt A, Oppenheimer E, Sheehan M, Taylor C 1983 What happens to alcoholics? Lancet 2: 269–271
Fishbein M, Ajzen I 1975 Belief, attitude, intention and behavior: an introduction to theory and research. Addison-Wesley, Reading, Mass
Grabonski J, Hall S M 1985 Pharmacological adjuncts in smoking cessation. NIDA Research Monograph 53
Gross M M 1977 Psycholobiological contributions to the alcohol dependence syndrome: a selective review of recent research. In: Edwards G (ed) Alcohol related disabilities. WHO, Geneva
Heather N, Rollnick S, Winton M 1983 A comparison of objective and subjective measures of alcohol dependence as predictors or relapse following treatment. British Journal of Clinical Psychology 22: 11–17
Hodgson R J 1984 Social learning theory. In: McGuffin P, Shanks M, Hodgson R (eds) The scientific principles of psychopathology. Academic Press, London
Hodgson R, Rankin H 1976 Cue exposure and the treatment of alcoholism. Behaviour Research and Therapy 14: 305–307
Hodgson R J, Rankin H J 1982 Cue exposure and relapse prevention. In: Hay W M, Nathan P E (eds) Clinical Case Studies in the Behavioural Treatment of Alcoholism. Plenum Press, New York

Hodgson R J, Stockwell T R 1985 The theoretical and empirical basis of the alcohol dependence model: a social learning perspective. In: Heather N, Robertson I, Davies P (eds) The misuse of alcohol. Croom Helm, London

Hodgson R J, Rankin H J, Stockwell T R 1979 Alcohol dependence and the priming effect. Behaviour Research and Therapy 17: 379–387

Hunt G M, Azrin N H 1973 A community-reinforcement approach to alcoholism. Behavior Research and Therapy 11: 91–104

Kalant H 1973 Biological models of alcohol tolerance and physical dependence. In: Gross M M (ed) Alcohol intoxication and withdrawal: experimental studies. Plenum, New York

Kalant H, LeBlanc A E, Gibbins R J 1971 Tolerance to and dependence on some non-opiate psychotropic drugs. Pharmacological Review 23: 135–191

Killen J D, Maccoby N, Taylor C B 1984 Nicotine gum and self-regulation training in smoking relapse prevention. Behaviour Therapy 15: 234–248

Lang A R, Goeckner D J, Adesso V J, Marlatt G A 1975 Effect of alcohol on aggression in male social drinkers. Journal of Abnormal Psychology 84: 508–518

Litman G, Eiser J R, Taylor C 1979 Dependence, relapse and extinction: a theoretical critique and behavioural examination. Journal of Clinical Psychology 35: 192–199

Ludwig A M, Wickler A, Stark L H 1974 The first drink: psychobiological aspects of craving. Archives of General Psychiatry 30: 539–547

MacRae J R, Scoles M T, Siegel S 1987 The contribution of Pavlovian conditioning to drug tolerance and dependence. British Journal of Addiction 82: 371–380

Marlatt G A 1982 Relapse prevention: a self-control program for the treatment of addictive behaviors. In: Stuart R B (ed) Adherence, compliance and generalisation in behavioural medicine. Bruner/Mazel, New York

Marlatt G A, Gordon J R 1980 Determinants of relapse: implications for the maintenance of behaviour change. In: Davidson P O, Davidson S M (eds) Behavioural medicine: changing health lifestyles. Brunner/Mazel, New York

Marlatt G A, Rosenow D 1980 Cognitive processes in alcohol use: expectancy and the balanced placebo design. In: Mello N (ed) Advances in substance abuse: behavioural and biological research. JAI Press, Greenwich, Conn

Marlatt G A, Demming B, Reid J B 1973 Loss of control drinking in alcoholics. An experimental analogue. Journal of Abnormal Psychology 81: 233–241

Mausner B, Platt E S 1971 Smoking: a behavioural analysis. Pergamon, New York

Merry J 1966 The 'loss of control myth'. Lancet 1: 1257–1258

Mowrer O H 1960 Learning Theory and Behaviour. Wiley, New York

Orford J 1985 Excessive appetites. Wiley, Chichester

Orford J, Edwards G 1977 Alcoholism: a comparison of treatment and advice. Maudsley Monograph No 26. Oxford University Press, London

Polich J M, Armor D J, Braiker H B 1980 The course of alcoholism. Four years after treatment. Wiley, New York

Rachman S J, Hodgson R J 1980 Obsessions and Compulsions. Prentice-Hall, Englewood Cliff, New Jersey

Rankin H J, Hodgson R J, Stockwell T R 1983 Cue exposure and the treatment of alcohol dependence. Behaviour Research and Therapy 21: 435–446

Rist F, Watzl H 1983 Self-assessment of relapse risk and assertiveness in relation to treatment outcome of female alcoholics. Addictive Behaviours 8: 121–127

Russell M A H, Merriman R, Stapelton J, Taylor W 1983 Effect of nicotine chewing gum as an adjunct to general practitioners' advice against smoking. British Medical Journal 287: 1782–1785

Seligman M E P 1976 Learned helplessness and depression in animals and men. In: Spence J T et al (eds) Behavioural approaches to therapy. General Learning Press, Morristown, New Jersey

Siegel S 1983 Classical conditioning, drug tolerance and drug dependence. In: Israel Y, Glaser, F B, Kalant H, Popham R E, Schmidt W, Smart R G (eds) Research Advances in Alcohol and Drug Problems, Vol 7, pp 207–246. Plenum, New York

Solomon R L 1977 An opponent process theory of acquired motivation. The effective dynamics of addiction. In: Maser J D, Seligman M E P (eds) Psychopathology: experimental models. Freeman, San Francisco

Stockwell T R, Hodgson R, Rankin H, Taylor C 1982 Alcohol dependence, beliefs and the priming effect. Behaviour Research and Therapy 20: 513–522

Subkov A A, Zilov G N 1937 The role of conditioned reflex adaptation in the origin of hyperergic reactions. Bulletin de Biologie et de Medecine Experimentale 4: 294–296

Sutton S 1987 Social-psychological approaches to understanding addictive behaviours: attitude-behaviour and decision-making models. British Journal of Addiction Special Issue on Psychology and Addiction. Hodgson R (ed)

Ternes J W 1977 An opponent process theory of habitual behavior with special reference to smoking. NIDA Research Monograph 17: 157–182

Wilson G T, Abrams D B 1977 Effects of alcohol on social anxiety and physiological arousal: cognitive versus pharmacological processes. Cognitive Therapy and Research 1: 195–210

Wilson G T, Lawson D M 1976 Expectancies, alchohol and sexual arousal in male social drinkers. Journal of Abnormal Psychology 85: 587–594

14

Keith Hawton

Sexual dysfunctions

INTRODUCTION

Interest in sexual dysfunctions has increased greatly during the past two decades among both researchers and clinicians. There are at least three reasons for this. First, attitudes to sexuality have altered such that there is now more general concern with satisfactory sexual function and the resolution of sexual difficulties. Second, relatively effective means of treating sexual dysfunctions have been developed. The most notable contribution has been by Masters & Johnson, who in 1970 published their new approach to treating couples with sexual dysfunctions. This has had a highly significant impact on clinical practice. Further developments since 1970 have resulted in the refinement of their approach, and in new methods for other client groups, for example individuals without partners and people whose sexual problems are the result of physical disorders. Third, increasingly sophisticated methods including new laboratory techniques for investigating dysfunctional subjects have allowed substantial gains in terms of understanding both the physiological and psychological basis of sexual dysfunctions.

This chapter is divided into two sections. In the first the nature of sexual dysfunction is considered, including a description of the major dysfunctions and their prevalence. The second section is devoted to the causal explanations for sexual dysfunctions, with attention to evidence from empirical studies and the effects of treatment.

THE NATURE OF SEXUAL DYSFUNCTIONS

The definition of sexual dysfunction

It is difficult to provide an adequate general definition of sexual dysfunction. 'Persistent impairment of the normal patterns of sexual interest or response' is one used by the author (Hawton 1985), while recognizing that it is not entirely adequate for two reasons. First, it is virtually impossible to indicate precise limits of 'normality' in sexual functioning because the range of sexual behaviour among men and women in the general population is vast (Kinsey et al 1948, Kinsey et al 1953). Second, an individual's expectations and needs, which may be profoundly influenced by social values, are likely to be relevant in determining whether his or her sexual adjustment is regarded as dysfunctional.

General aspects of classifying sexual dysfunctions

One reasonable approach to the classification of sexual dysfunctions is to base it partly on the phase of sexual response which is affected. As a result of their pioneering laboratory studies of sexuality during the 1950s and 1960s Masters & Johnson (1966) identified three phases of sexual response: *excitement* (or arousal), *orgasm* and *resolution*. However, the use of sexual response alone as a means of classification will omit a very important aspect of sexuality, namely *sexual interest*. This refers to a person's sexual drive or willingness to engage in sexual behaviour. There are two further important factors to be taken into account when describing sexual dysfunctions. First, a problem may have been present from the onset of sexual activity (a *primary* dysfunction) or it may have occurred after a period of normal sexual functioning (*secondary*). Second, a dysfunction may occur in all sexual settings (*total*) or only in some settings but not others (*situational*).

The types of sexual dysfunctions

The more common sexual dysfunctions are listed in Table 14.1, using the general approach to classification outlined above. It is apparent that not all the dysfunctions can neatly be accommodated into the categories of sexual interest and response. The rest of this part of the chapter will be devoted to consideration of each of the dysfunctions shown in the table.

The sexual dysfunctions of women

Impaired sexual interest. Impaired sexual interest, which receives other labels such as 'inhibited sexual drive' and 'low libido', embraces a range of difficulties. These include a lack of spontaneous interest in sex but an

Table 14.1 The sexual dysfunctions

Category	Women	Men
Interest	Impaired sexual interest	Impaired sexual interest
Excitement/arousal	Impaired sexual arousal	Impaired sexual arousal
Orgasm	Orgasmic dysfunction	Premature ejaculation Retarded/absent ejaculation
Other	Vaginismus Dyspareunia Sexual phobias	Painful ejaculation

ability to respond to the partner's approaches with pleasurable arousal; a lack of interest in initiating sexual activity; and being totally averse to the sexual approaches of the partner. As is the case with men, levels of sexual interest vary greatly among women and therefore it is difficult to draw a clear distinction between normal and abnormal. The extent of a woman's interests in sex is not only reflected in her behaviour with a partner, but also in frequency of sexual thoughts and fantasies, attraction to other people, and masturbation.

Impaired sexual interest is the most common sexual dysfunction in women. In a Danish general population study of 40-year-old women a third reported they had never experienced 'spontaneous sexual drive' and 12% had not experienced 'libido' under any circumstances (Garde & Lunde 1980a). In a recent British general population study 16.7% of women with partners had impaired sexual interest according to specific criteria, although far fewer regarded this as a problem (Osborn et al 1987). The prevalence of this dysfunction increased with age, and, as in the Danish study (Garde & Lunde 1980b), was more common in lower than higher social class women.

Impaired sexual interest is also the most frequent sexual dysfunction among women referred to sexual dysfunction clinics. In one clinic, for example, this problem was identified as the principal difficulty in 52% of female presenters (Hawton 1985). As is discussed later in this chapter, female impaired sexual interest is often associated with other major problems, especially general relationship difficulties and depression.

Impaired sexual arousal. Impaired sexual arousal refers to failure of the normal physiological responses (e.g. vaginal engorgement and lubrication) to sexual stimulation, and lack of sensations usually associated with sexual excitement. It is a relatively uncommon problem in women with unimpaired sexual interest, except when sex hormone levels are disturbed, as occurs following the menopause and for a short time after childbirth.

Orgasmic dysfunction. The category of orgasmic dysfunction usually includes women who do not experience orgasm, or do so very rarely, in spite of adequate sexual interest, arousal and stimulation. It is important, especially for treatment purposes, to distinguish women with total orgasmic dysfunction from those who can experience orgasm through masturbation but not with their partner. Since women vary greatly in the frequency with which they reach orgasm during sexual activity, the extent to which a woman regards herself as having a problem concerning orgasm will depend on her and her partner's previous experience.

In their survey of American women, Kinsey et al (1953) found that the proportion of married women who had never experienced orgasm decreased steadily with age. From a more recent analysis of their data Gebhard & Johnson (1979) reported that overall almost 13% of married women had never experienced orgasm by any means. In a British general population survey almost 16% of women with partners had not experienced orgasm during sexual activity in the three months prior to interview (Osborn et al 1987). The prevalence of this dysfunction was greater in older than younger women. Among women referred to a sexual dysfunction clinic orgasmic dysfunction was identified in 18% of one series (Bancroft & Coles 1976) and 19% of another (Hawton 1985). Women now appear to present for help with this problem less often than previously, possibly as a result of the increased availability of self-help books and articles.

Vaginismus. For women with vaginismus sexual intercourse is either impossible or extremely painful, because attempts at vaginal penetration cause spasm of the muscles surrounding the entrance to the vagina. Vaginismus is nearly always the result of a specific phobia concerning vaginal penetration, the reaction of the vaginal muscles being an involuntary response to the conditioned fear. This is virtually always a primary problem, although it can occasionally occur as a secondary difficulty following a sexual trauma, such as rape, or a vaginal infection. Interestingly, in one study of women with vaginismus their sexual adjustment other than their difficulty in having sexual intercourse was found not to differ markedly from that of a control group of women attending a family planning clinic (Duddle 1977).

Because vaginismus is largely a primary problem it usually occurs in young women during their first sexual relationships. There is commonly a history of failed attempts at using tampons. Many women with vaginismus have distorted ideas about their genitals, believing their vagina to be far too small to accommodate a penis. Some women have additional beliefs that, for example, their genitals are unpleasant in some way.

No information is available about the prevalence of vaginismus in the general population. Women with this problem may present in gynaecology or infertility clinics. Vaginismus is a fairly common reason for referral to sexual dysfunction clinics, with between 12% (Bancroft & Coles 1976) and 18% (Hawton 1985) of presenting women having this problem.

Dyspareunia. Dyspareunia, or pain during sexual intercourse, can be of different types. The pain may be at the entrance to the vagina, in which case it is likely to be due to a physical cause (such as a vaginal infection), mild vaginismus or lack of arousal. If lack of arousal is the reason the pain will usually diminish during sexual intercourse. Dyspareunia can also occur on deep vaginal penetration. This often has a physical cause (such as pelvic infection or ovarian disease); however, it can also result from impaired sexual arousal, when the normal ballooning of the inner part of the vagina and elevation of the uterus that accompany sexual arousal (Masters & Johnson 1966) fail to occur. Consequently the cervix is buffeted during sexual intercourse and this causes the pain; and the pain may in turn impair arousal even further.

Hardly any information is available concerning the prevalence of dyspareunia, although this problem is often seen in women referred to gynaecology clinics. Four per cent of women assessed in a sexual dysfunction clinic had dyspareunia as their main problem (Hawton 1985).

Sexual phobias. Sometimes a woman will have a specific fear about sexual activity, although sexual phobias more often occur in the setting of other dysfunctions, especially impaired sexual interest or arousal. Examples include aversion to vaginal secretions or seminal fluid, or to some particular aspect of sexual activity. These latter types of phobia may be associated with an earlier traumatic sexual experience such as rape or incest (Feldman-Summers et al 1979, Becker et al 1982). It is not known how common sexual phobias are.

The sexual dysfunctions of men

Impaired sexual interest. While most people of either sex experience periods of loss of interest in sex, it is relatively rare in the UK for men to seek help because of prolonged impairment of sexual interest. This may in part be because men with this problem will often also experience erectile dysfunction or some other sexual difficulty and will seek help for this instead. However, clinics in the USA now report that this problem is relatively common among male attenders (Schreiner-Engel & Schiavi 1986). This may reflect changing attitudes, in that traditionally men have found it difficult to admit to lack of interest. Perhaps this is because of the myth that men always desire sexual activity. Interestingly, in a study of 'normal' American couples 35% of the wives and 16% of the husbands reported 'disinterest' in sex (Frank et al 1978). Other general population studies of male sexuality have largely neglected to ask about levels of sexual interest, but have focused entirely on problems of sexual performance, especially erectile difficulties.

Erectile dysfunction. Erectile dysfunction includes a wide range of difficulties, such as failure to get an erection under any circumstances, erections only being partial, full erections being possible but only in some circumstances (e.g. during masturbation but not with a partner), or the erection being lost whenever sexual intercourse is attempted. Erectile dysfunction is relatively rare in young men but becomes common after the age of 50. Thus, in their general population study, Kinsey and colleagues identified erectile difficulties in 0.1% of men at age 20, 1.9% at age 40, 6.7% at age 50, and 27% at age 70 (Kinsey et al 1948). In a study of Swedish married men aged between 22 and 55 years erectile dysfunction was reported by 7% (Nettelbladt & Uddenberg 1979), a very similar figure to that reported in a study of American husbands (Frank et al 1978).

Erectile dysfunction is the most common problem in men attending sexual dysfunction clinics, being the presenting problem in at least 50% (Bancroft 1983, Hawton 1985). As might be expected from the general population statistics, men seeking help with this problem are generally older than those with other types of sexual dysfunction (Bancroft & Coles 1976).

Premature ejaculation. While premature ejaculation obviously refers to rapid ejaculation, there is no satisfactory definition of this dysfunction. Some workers have defined premature ejaculation in terms of the extent to which ejaculation is delayed long enough for the partner's satisfaction (Masters & Johnson 1970), others in terms of the specific duration of sexual intercourse (Kilmann & Auerbach 1979). While ejaculation which occurs repeatedly and unintentionally before vaginal penetration is clearly abnormal, it is impossible to define precise limits of functional and dysfunctional performance in men who do not have such a severe problem. Most clinicians base their assessment on the extent to which a couple regard the man's ejaculatory control as being sufficient to allow sexual intercourse which is satisfactory for both of them. However, it is worth noting that Kinsey and colleagues reported that three-quarters of married men in their survey estimated that they ejaculated within two minutes of vaginal penetration (Kinsey et al 1948).

Rapid ejaculation is extremely common in young men in their initial sexual encounters, probably because of high arousal due to novelty, anxiety, and, perhaps, previous experience of rapid ejaculation during masturbation. Most men gradually develop control over their speed of ejaculation. Persistent premature ejaculation is very often a primary problem, control never having developed. However, premature ejaculation can begin as a secondary problem later in life, sometimes as a result of stress and sometimes accompanying the development of erectile dysfunction resulting from either psychological or organic causes.

Premature ejaculation was identified in 36% of husbands in the American study by Frank et al (1978) and in 38% of husbands in the Swedish study of Nettelbladt & Uddenberg (1979). In spite of these apparently high rates premature ejaculation is far less often a presenting problem of men in sexual dysfunction clinics, having been identified in 14.5% in one clinic (Bancroft 1983) and in 16% in another (Hawton 1985). This discrepancy is because the figures in the general population studies were based upon operational definitions of premature ejaculation, not upon whether the men, or their partners, regarded their speed of ejaculation as a problem.

Retarded or absent ejaculation. In men with retarded or absent ejaculation there is either absence of ejaculation or ejaculation is unusually delayed. Ejaculation may be absent under any circumstance (including masturbation and sleep), or occur during masturbation and/or sleep but not during sexual activity with a partner. The latter is the most common presentation. This problem affects both the experience of orgasm and ejaculation itself, and must be distinguished from 'dry orgasm', when there is an orgasmic experience but no ejaculation. This can result from a variety of physical factors, including some forms of medication (e.g. monoamine oxidase inhibitors and major tranquillizers) and surgery (e.g. prostatectomy). *Retrograde ejaculation* is a term used when ejaculate passes back into the bladder rather than along the penile urethra, and results from disturbed functioning of the bladder sphincter. In this case the orgasmic experience occurs but no external ejaculation.

Retarded or absent ejaculation is uncommon. Thus 'difficulty ejaculating' was reported by only 4% of men in Frank et al's (1978) American study, although by 10% of men in Nettelbladt & Uddenberg's (1979) study in Sweden. Retarded or absent ejaculation was identified in only 6% of men seen in a sexual dysfunction clinic (Hawton 1985).

Painful ejaculation. Painful ejaculation is usually caused by physical disorders (e.g. venereal infection) rather than psychological factors, and therefore will not be considered further here.

Sexual satisfaction and dissatisfaction

The current description of sexual disorders has so far concentrated on specific dysfunctions. Sometimes people ask for help not because they have a sexual dysfunction but because they find their sexual relationship unsatisfactory in a more general sense. Furthermore, whether or not couples seek help because of sexual dysfunction will in part depend on their overall satisfaction with their sexual relationship. Thus a sexual dysfunction is often tolerated by a couple if their relationship is happy in other respects. Such couples are also more likely to be able to solve their sexual difficulties without outside help (Chesney et al 1981). Other factors which contribute to sexual dissatisfaction include loss of attraction between partners, restricted foreplay, and lack of variety in sexual activity.

THE CAUSES OF SEXUAL DYSFUNCTIONS

Methods of investigating aetiology

Numerous causes of sexual dysfunctions have been proposed. Many of these are based largely on informed speculation. However, in recent years there have been attempts at investigating causes in a more systematic fashion. There are three broad methods of investigating the aetiology of sexual problems: clinical case studies; response to therapeutic interventions; and psychological and physiological studies.

Clinical studies

Many of the proposed causes of sexual dysfunctions are based on the unrigorous approach of weighing up the frequency with which particularly likely aetiological factors crop up in case material in routine clinical practice. While this is a highly unsatisfactory method from a scientific viewpoint, nonetheless most causal propositions which guide clinical management tend to be derived in this way.

A refinement of such a crude approach involves comparison of patient samples with normal samples (preferably matched for major demographic characteristics) with regard to possible aetiological factors. An alternative method is to compare the prevalence of sexual dysfunction in a group of individuals who have all experienced a particular stress with another group who have not had this experience. This type of approach has been used, for example, to investigate the possible association between childhood sexual abuse and adulthood sexual dysfunction.

Response to therapeutic interventions

Having identified likely causes, the effects of specific therapeutic measures aimed at modifying them can then be investigated. This approach is largely confined to assessing the role of current maintaining factors. An obvious example is that of anxiety, which is thought to be a major component in many sexual disorders. If specific measures which reduce anxiety also result in significant improvement in sexual function this will tend to support the idea that anxiety is an important aetiological or maintaining factor. Little attention has been paid to this approach to investigating causes of sexual dysfunctions. However, this is partly because it is usually extremely difficult to investigate a specific therapeutic intervention in isolation from other more general therapeutic strategies.

Psychological and physiological studies

The development of objective methods of assessing sexual arousal has opened up new approaches to investigating causality, although these are largely only of relevance to the study of current maintaining factors rather than historical factors. Sexual arousal can now be measured fairly reliably in men using penile plethysmography, in which a mercury-filled strain gauge, or some modification of this, is placed around the penis and connected up to a polygraph recorder (Bancroft & Bell 1985). Changes in penile circumference can then be recorded. Several measures have been developed for recording sexual arousal in women, most assessing changes in vaginal blood flow (Geer et al 1974). These means of assessment can be used, for example, to explore possible differences in arousability of dysfunctional and non-dysfunctional subjects when exposed to erotic stimuli, including films, slides, or fantasy. The individuals' subjective levels of arousal can be assessed using rating scales or by asking them to alter an indicator on an arousal scale.

These types of investigation, while having some major drawbacks, particularly those relating to the unusual demands of a laboratory situation, have enabled researchers to study several aspects of sexual dysfunctions. Such investigations have examined, for example, whether there are differences between dysfunctional and non-dysfunctional subjects in terms of the correlation between objective and subjective measures of arousal, and whether introducing an anxiety-provoking or distracting stimulus has a different effect on sexual arousal for each group of subjects. Laboratory studies of this kind have begun to yield information about sexual dysfunction which has potentially important treatment implications (see below).

A broad aetiological model

Sexual dysfunctions were until relatively recently regarded as symptoms of deep-seated disturbances of personality originating in early childhood or adolescent experiences. Thus Freud (1949) postulated that the roots of sexual problems lay in disturbed maturation through the various phases of childhood sexuality that he had described, resulting in interference of the normal development of child–parent relationships. While most clinicians accept the important impact that early experiences may have on adult sexuality, few would now subscribe to an aetiological theory almost entirely dependent on this viewpoint. Recent years have seen a shift to a much broader view of causality, with less emphasis on early experiences, and rather more on learning, stress, educational and cognitive factors.

Any consideration of aetiology of sexual dysfunctions must take account of the many physical causes of sexual problems. These will not be detailed here since they have been adequately described elsewhere (Bancroft 1983, Hawton 1985, 1987). Suffice to say that sexual function is highly vulnerable to a large number of physical influences, including many illnesses (e.g. diabetes, neurological disorders), surgical procedures (e.g. pelvic operations, mastectomy) and drugs, including medication (e.g. antihypertensives, psychotropic drugs), alcohol and illicit drugs. However, even in individuals whose sexual difficulties are primarily due to physical factors, psychological influences, especially a person's response to the difficulty, are often of considerable importance in determining the extent of the sexual problem.

The rest of this chapter will be confined to discussion of psychological and social causes of sexual dysfunctions. A useful approach to considering the aetiology of sexual dysfunctions, which has the advantage of emphasizing the interactive nature of contributory factors, is to differentiate the causes into three groups: *predisposing factors* — experiences and influences, including those early in life, which have made an individual vulnerable to developing sexual difficulties at a later stage; *precipitants* — events or experiences associated with the actual appearance of the sexual dysfunction; *maintaining factors* — which cause the dysfunction to persist. While some dysfunctions are determined by factors in all three categories, others, especially primary dysfunctions, may have no obvious precipitant. Others will occur against a background of normal early sexual development.

The specific causes of sexual dysfunctions

As noted earlier, there are numerous postulated causes for sexual disorders. In this discussion of specific causes an attempt has therefore been made to restrict the range of factors to those of greatest clinical relevance (Table 14.2).

Table 14.2 Psychological causes of sexual dysfunction

Predisposing factors	
Disturbed family relationships/environment	Traumatic early sexual experiences
Inadequate sex education	
Precipitants	
General relationship problems	Random failure
Childbirth	Dysfunction in the partner
Traumatic sexual experience	Psychiatric disorder
Maintaining factors	
Anxiety	Fear of emotional intimacy
Poor communication	Inadequate sexual information
General relationship problems	Psychiatric disorder

Predisposing factors

Disturbed family relationships/environment. Several features of the early family environment may have potential effects on sexual adjustment in adulthood, although these are not necessarily direct effects. How children or adolescents perceive their families' attitudes towards sexuality and personal relationships will be one factor. For example, sex is a taboo subject in many families, all mention of it being actively avoided, while in others there may be more overtly expressed negative attitudes towards sexuality. The conflict between this background and an adolescent's growing sexual interest can be a source of guilt which may persist into adulthood, especially if the family attitudes are not countered subsequently by more positive attitudes and experiences (e.g. in friends, school and partner relationships).

Such a background may contribute to subsequent poor sexual adjustment. For example, a boy who views sexual enjoyment by women as not in keeping with his parental model of a heterosexual relationship may develop a 'double-standard' attitude towards women. Thus, in later life he may differentiate between the type of woman who might make a suitable permanent partner because she appears relatively non-sexual, and the type of woman with whom a casual rather than permanent relationship is acceptable because she shows an active interest in sexual relations. Such a man may experience difficulty later if he discovers that his apparently sexually restrained permanent partner is in fact at least as interested in sexual activity as himself. Similarly, a woman who in adolescence was encouraged by her mother to regard sex as an unfortunate experience to which men subjected women may feel guilty when she discovers the strength of her own sexual desires.

The association between more general aspects of parent–child relationships and subsequent sexual adjustment have been investigated. Death or separation of parents, and poorer relationships with parents, especially the parent of the opposite sex, have all been identified more commonly in the histories of both men and women with sexual dysfunctions when compared with others with good sexual adjustment (O'Connor & Stern 1972, Fisher 1973, Uddenberg 1974, Nettelbladt & Uddenberg 1979). However, since such studies have been based on enquiry of adults themselves, one must be cautious in accepting the results at face value because of the possibility of distortion in retrospective accounts. Nevertheless, the weight of these findings, together with clinical experience, is impressive. It should not be assumed, however, that the effects of poor child–parental relationships are direct. It is more likely that the consequences for sexuality will be indirect, resulting from effects on self-esteem, trust, or the ability to cope with emotional intimacy (see below).

Inadequate sex education. Although difficult to demonstrate, it is a strong clinical impression that many people who present for professional help for sexual dysfunctions display poor knowledge about sexuality. This applies especially to those now of middle or older age whose schooling and home life characteristically lacked any education concerning sex. Information was often therefore acquired from friends, whose own level of knowledge may have been just as poor. As a consequence, sexual information is often particularly poor concerning the opposite sex. Male ignorance about the female clitoris is a common example. Sexual ignorance can be a major predisposing factor in the development of subsequent sexual dysfunction.

Traumatic early sexual experiences. It is becoming increasingly obvious that many children have sexual experiences, especially as a result of child sexual abuse or incest. Father–daughter sexual activity is by far the most common form of abuse. Relatively little information is available concerning how often such experiences are associated with subsequent sexual problems and what makes such an association more likely. One American study suggested that sexual dysfunction following sexual abuse was more likely if: (i) the abuse had occurred in late childhood and early adolescence rather than early childhood; (ii) the experience had powerful emotional consequences at the time, especially as a result of pressure to participate, pain, and dislike for the abuser; and (iii) sexual molestation happened relatively frequently and over a long period (Tsai et al 1979).

It also appears that child sexual abuse can act as an immediate precipitant of disturbed sexual adjustment. Some girls who had been sexually abused were reported to become sexually disinhibited at a very early age, relating to adults in an erotic fashion (Yates 1982). Promiscuity during adolescence and early adulthood can be another consequence (Browne & Finkelhor 1986), possibly because sexual behaviour has been learned as an apparently effective means of relating to the opposite sex and gaining affection, or because of the diminished sense of responsibility a victim of sexual abuse may have for her body.

Precipitants

General relationship problems. As noted earlier, sexual dysfunction is very often symptomatic of problems in a couple's general relationship. This is most likely when the dysfunction is one of impaired sexual interest and aversion to sex. The extent to which this is apparent in couples presenting for help with sexual difficulties is discussed below.

Childbirth. Sexual dysfunction, especially in women, often follows childbirth. There are several emotional and physical explanations for this. For many women interest in sex declines during late pregnancy and does not return until a few weeks or months after they have given birth (Robson et al 1981). This may partly be the result of the considerable hormonal changes that occur at this time, but other factors including tiredness and concern about physical appearance may also contribute. However, in some women childbirth results in chronic impairment of sexual interest. The most common reason is that depression has developed following the birth. This does not refer to 'post-partum blues', which is a brief episode of disturbed mood occurring in probably the majority of mothers during the week after giving birth, but rather post-natal depression, which occurs in 10–15% of mothers (Kumar 1982). This is typically characterized by lack of energy, anhedonia, sleep disturbance and, sometimes, self-neglect. Loss of sexual interest is also a major feature of this disorder, which may persist for many months or possibly even longer if unrecognized or not treated appropriately.

Childbirth may have other important psychological consequences for a couple's sexual adjustment. Some men, for example, become resentful of the attention their partners pay to the baby. Pressure may be put on the wife to engage in sex when she is not feeling like it. This can lead to resentment in both partners. The man may feel resentful because his wife is not now as responsive as she was earlier in their relationship. The woman may feel likewise because she is very aware of her partner's demands and yet feels he does not understand the changed nature of her needs at this time, which are often for affection rather than sex.

In the author's clinical experience childbirth is the most common precipitant of impaired female sexual interest (apart from cases in which the sexual problem is secondary to general relationship difficulties).

Traumatic sexual experience. It is a widely accepted view that sexual trauma can be a precipitant for sexual dysfunction, although evidence for this is surprisingly scant. Rape and other types of sexual assault are the most obvious examples. There is evidence from interview studies comparing groups of rape victims and control subjects that rape victims gain less satisfaction from sexual activity after the assault, have sexual intercourse less often, and are at risk of developing problems concerning sexual interest, sexual arousal and orgasm (Burgess & Holmstrom 1979, Feldman-Summers et al 1979, Becker et al 1982). Frank aversion to all sexual activity has also been reported as common among rape victims (Becker et al 1982). Other victims show aversion or decreased satisfaction with regard to specific sexual behaviours that occurred during the assault, such as sexual intercourse, touching the genitals, and visual exposure to male genitals, while behaviours not usually involved in rape (e.g. masturbation, showing and receiving affection) remain unaffected (Feldman-Summers et al 1979).

Random failure. Sometimes sexual dysfunction is precipitated by an isolated experience of failure during sexual activity. An often quoted example is of a middle-aged man who has erectile failure on one or a few occasions when he has been drinking heavily or subject to stress in his everyday life. Fear of failure and performance anxiety may then cause further failures such that a vicious circle is established, leading to persistent erectile dysfunction. The partner's response to occasional failures is likely to be an important determinant of subsequent sexual adjustment.

Dysfunction in the partner. It is not uncommon to find in couples presenting to sexual dysfunction clinics that both partners have sexual problems. This was the case in 29% of female and 31% of male presenters in one series (Bancroft 1983), and in 29% of presenters of either sex in another (Hawton & Catalan 1986). Very often one partner's sexual dysfunction has precipitated the problem in the other partner. The most frequent associations are between impaired female sexual interest or orgasmic dysfunction and premature ejaculation or erectile dysfunction.

Psychiatric disorder. Sexual dysfunctions are often symptoms of psychiatric disorder (see below). However, there is evidence that an episode of psychiatric illness can precipitate sexual difficulty which persists even though the psychiatric disorder has resolved. This applies particularly to problems concerning sexual interest. In a study of individuals of both sexes with 'inhibited sexual desire' (defined according to DSM III criteria), who at the time of assessment had relatively normal psychological profiles, the life-time prevalence of affective disorder was significantly higher than among control subjects who did not have sexual difficulties. Moreover, the onset of loss of sexual interest almost always coincided with or followed an initial episode of depression. As a result the authors of the study suggest that depression and inhibited sexual desire might have a common biological basis or that affective psychopathology may contribute to the development of the sexual dysfunction (Schreiner-Engel & Schiavi 1986).

Maintaining factors

Anxiety. Anxiety concerning performance, possible failure, and the partner's reaction to perceived sexual inadequacy are central problems in the majority of individuals with sexual dysfunction; and such concerns are a major focus of treatment. Sex therapy partly aims to help couples engage in sexual activity in an increasingly relaxed fashion. Gradually rebuilding the sexual relationship from a basis of relatively undemanding but relaxing physical caressing is one means of doing this. Communication of concerns is another integral focus of treatment.

Recent laboratory studies have helped to elucidate the nature of the contribution of anxiety to the maintenance of sexual dysfunction (reviewed by Barlow 1986). This research has focused particularly on men with erectile dysfunction, but there is evidence that the findings and their interpretation are also relevant to other dysfunctions, including those of women. In summary, the studies suggest that: (i) men with psychogenic erectile dysfunction experience negative affect (especially anxiety) in sexual situations; (ii) such men tend to underestimate their levels of sexual arousal and also experience little sense of control over how aroused they become; and (iii) exposure to erotic stimuli related to sexual performance results in cognitive distraction from the erotic stimuli because of anxiety and concern about sexual performance. Furthermore, whereas men without dysfunctions who were made mildly anxious showed increased sexual arousal to erotic stimuli, mild anxiety inhibited sexual arousal in dysfunctional subjects. The therapeutic implications of such work are twofold. First, treatment should not aim to obliterate all anxiety since this may facilitate sexual response; and second, and more important, treatment should concentrate particularly on helping dysfunctional individuals focus their attention on both erotic stimuli and thoughts, and subjective arousal. This is, to some degree, at variance with the traditional approach in sex therapy which has emphasized the necessity of allowing sexual arousal to occur in a relatively passive fashion while concentrating on relaxed exchange of pleasurable caressing.

Poor communication. The majority of couples with sexual dysfunction characteristically display poor communication concerning their sexual relationship, either because it has always been poor or because such communication deteriorated once the dysfunction became established. The inability to discuss sexual needs and concerns often compounds the sexual problem. For example, a woman who needs more affection and foreplay following childbirth before she becomes aroused may find it impossible to explain this to her partner, who may then mistake her reduced enthusiasm for sex as a personal rejection. Very often the result is that the man simply hurries sexual activity because he erroneously believes that his partner is not interested and only wants to get the act over as quickly as possible.

There is evidence that improvement in communication about sex is an important ingredient in successful therapy (Chesney et al 1981, Tullman et al 1981) and is one of the components of treatment most appreciated by couples (Hawton et al 1986).

General relationship problems. Just as discord in a relationship can precipitate a sexual dysfunction, so general relationship problems can lead to persistence of the sexual difficulty. In most couples, sexuality, harmony, affection and trust are closely intertwined, such that a disturbance in one aspect of the relationship is highly likely to affect the others. The degree of general discord in couples presenting to sexual dysfunction clinics varies greatly. For example, general relationship difficulties were judged definitely to be contributing to sexual dysfunction in 17% of men and 24% of women referred to a sexual dysfunction clinic in Edinburgh. However, for 47% of male presenters and 32% of female presenters the clinicians were uncertain whether or not sexual dysfunction was secondary to general relationship difficulties (Bancroft 1983). Treatment for sexual problems can include some degree of 'marital therapy', provided the relationship is not too discordant (Hawton 1985). Indeed, the effects of sex therapy on marital harmony can be considerable and are usually sustained (Hawton et al 1986). At the same time, however, the quality of the general relationship before treatment is an important predictor of how effective treatment will be, both in the short term (Mathews et al 1976, Hawton & Catalan 1986) and in the long term (Hawton et al 1986).

Fear of emotional intimacy. Kaplan (1979) defined intimacy as 'a special quality of emotional closeness between two people . . . an affectionate bond . . . composed of mutual caring, responsibility, trust, open communication of feelings and sensations, as well as the non-defended interchange of information about significant emotional events'. She and other workers believe that fear of emotional intimacy is seen quite often in individuals with sexual dysfunction. Typically such a person will have had a succession of relationships, each of which ends at a similar point in its development because further involvement appears to pose too much of a threat for the individual. While sexual adjustment may appear to be satisfactory early in the relationship it deteriorates rapidly once emotional closeness develops further. The consequent sexual dysfunction is usually impaired sexual interest. However, this can also be a factor in most of the other types of sexual problems. Fear of emotional intimacy is often found in people from family backgrounds characterized by lack of warmth and affection (Kaplan 1979), or physical or sexual abuse (Browne & Finkelhor 1986).

Inadequate sexual information. Just as poor sexual knowledge can be a vulnerability factor for sexual dysfunction it can, if it persists, also be a maintaining factor. Poor communication can compound the effects of ignorance because it prevents the capacity to learn from the partner. Sex education is an important component of sex therapy with many couples (Hawton 1985).

Psychiatric disorder. The contribution of psychiatric disorder to the onset of sexual dysfunction has already been discussed. Current psychiatric disorder is also an important factor in the maintenance of sexual difficulties. The major effect of depression on sexual functioning is on interest rather than performance (Beck 1967, Mathew & Weinman 1982). In a comparative study of depressed and non-depressed women, Weissman & Paykel (1974) found that while frequency of sexual intercourse was little reduced in the depressed women their interest in sex was markedly impaired. However, depression can also cause orgasmic dysfunction and erectile difficulties. Active treatment of depression will usually result in improved sexual adjustment although, as noted earlier, it can persist even following full resolution of the depressive symptomatology. Low self-esteem commonly occurs during depression (Beck et al 1979) and this may be reflected in negative attitudes concerning a person's own attractiveness, which may be a contributory factor in the sexual difficulties of many depressed individuals.

Reduced sexual interest is also often reported by people suffering from schizophrenia (Lyketsos et al 1983), although the medication (typically phenothiazines) used to treat this condition can be one reason, especially if there are also problems in sexual performance. Sexual interest and other sexual problems are often part of the clinical picture of anorexia nervosa (Kolodny et al 1979), which is not surprising, since anorexia is often attributed to fears concerning mature sexuality and is usually accompanied by considerable disturbances of sex hormone levels due to starvation (Crisp 1967, Beaumont et al 1972). Surprisingly, the deleterious effects of anorexia nervosa on sexuality are not reported by all sufferers (Beaumont et al 1981).

Lastly, but very importantly, alcoholism can have devastating effects on sexual adjustment. Jensen (1979) reported sexual dysfunction in 63% of male alcoholics, with all types of sexual dysfunction being common. Sexual difficulties are also frequently reported by females who abuse alcohol (Klassen & Wilsnack 1986). There are several reasons for this, including the deleterious effects of alcoholism on relationships, and the many physical consequences of alcoholism, such as nerve damage (including to the nerves involved in sexual response) and hormonal disturbances. Drug addiction has equally serious effects on sexuality (Kolodny et al 1979).

CONCLUSIONS

In recent years the nature of sexual dysfunctions has been more clearly understood and described. Development of reasonably effective treatment methods has not only helped many sufferers but also assisted in clarifying aetiology. While empirical studies of causal factors have not been extensive, they have nonetheless provided further clues about how sexual problems develop and especially helped elucidate the factors which maintain them. It is now apparent that clinical investigation of the psychogenesis of sexual pathology in most individuals requires that account be taken of historical factors, major stresses and current maintaining factors before a full understanding can be obtained.

REFERENCES

Bancroft J 1983 Human sexuality and its problems. Churchill Livingstone, Edinburgh
Bancroft J, Bell C 1985 Simultaneous recording of penile diameter and penile arterial pulse during laboratory-based erotic stimulation in normal subjects. Journal of Psychosomatic Research 29: 303–313

Bancroft J, Coles L 1976 Three-years experience in a sexual problem clinic. British Medical Journal 1: 1575–1577
Barlow D 1986 Causes of sexual dysfunction: the role of anxiety and cognitive interference. Journal of Consulting and Clinical Psychology 54: 140–148
Beaumont P J V, Beardwood C J, Russell G F M 1972 The occurrence of the syndrome of anorexia nervosa in male subjects. Psychological Medicine 2: 216–231
Beaumont P J V, Abraham S F, Simson K G 1981 The psychosexual histories of adolescent girls and young women with anorexia nervosa. Psychological Medicine 11: 131–140
Beck A T 1967 Depression: clinical, experimental, and theoretical aspects. Harper & Row, New York
Beck A T, Rush A J, Shaw B F, Emery G 1979 Cognitive therapy of depression. Guilford, New York
Becker J V, Skinner L J, Abel G G, Treaccy E C 1982 Incidence and types of sexual dysfunction in rape and incest victims. Journal of Sex and Marital Therapy 8: 65–74
Browne A, Finkelhor D 1986 Impact of child sexual abuse: a review of the literature. Psychological Bulletin 99: 66–77
Burgess A W, Holmstrom L L 1979 Rape: sexual disruption and recovery. American Journal of Orthopsychiatry 49: 648–657
Chesney A P, Blakeney P E, Chan F A, Coley C M 1981 The impact of sex therapy on sexual behaviors and marital communication. Journal of Sex and Marital Therapy 7: 70–79
Crisp A H 1967 Anorexia nervosa. British Journal of Hospital Medicine 1: 713–718
Duddle M 1977 Etiological factors in the unconsummated marriage. Journal of Psychosomatic Research 21: 157–160
Feldman-Summers S, Gordon P E, Meagher J R 1979 The impact of rape on sexual satisfaction. Journal of Abnormal Psychology 88: 101–105
Fisher S 1973 The female orgasm: psychology, physiology, fantasy. Allen Lane, London
Frank E, Anderson C, Rubinstein D 1978 Frequency of sexual dysfunction in 'normal' couples. New England Journal of Medicine 299: 111–115
Freud S 1949 Three essays on the theory of sexuality. Imago, London
Garde K, Lunde I 1980a Female sexual behaviour: a study in a random sample of 40-year-old women. Maturitas 2: 225–240
Garde K, Lunde I 1980b Social background and social status; influence on female sexual behaviour. A random sample study of 40-year-old Danish women. Maturitas 2: 241–246
Gebhard P H, Johnson A B 1979 The Kinsey data: Marginal tabulations of the 1938–1963 interviews conducted by the Institute for Sex Research. Saunders, Philadelphia
Geer J, Morokoff P, Greenwood P 1974 Sexual arousal in women: the development of a measurement device for vaginal blood volume. Archives of Sexual Behaviour 3: 559–564
Hawton K 1985 Sex therapy: a practical guide. Oxford University Press, Oxford
Hawton K 1987 Sexual problems associated with physical illness. In: Weatherall D J, Ledingham J G G, Warrell W A (eds) Oxford Textbook of Medicine, 2nd edn. Oxford University Press, Oxford
Hawton K, Catalan J 1986 Prognostic factors in sex therapy. Behaviour Research and Therapy 24: 377–385
Hawton K, Catalan J, Martin P, Fagg J 1986 Long-term outcome of sex therapy. Behaviour Research and Therapy 24: 665–675
Jensen S B 1979 Sexual customs and dysfunction in alcoholics: part I and part II. British Journal of Sexual Medicine 6(53): 29–32, 6(54): 30–34
Kaplan H S 1979 Disorders of sexual desire and other new concepts and techniques in sex therapy. Brunner/Mazel, New York
Kilmann P R, Auerbach R 1979 Treatments of premature ejaculation and psychogenic impotence: a critical review of the literature. Archives of Sexual Behavior 8: 81–100
Kinsey A C, Pomeroy W B, Martin C E 1948 Sexual behaviour in the human male. Saunders, Philadelphia
Kinsey A C, Pomeroy W B, Martin C E, Gebhard P H 1953 Sexual behaviour in the human female. Saunders, Philadelphia
Klassen A D, Wilsnack C 1986 Sexual experience and drinking among women in a US national survey. Archives of Sexual Behavior 15: 363–392
Kolodny R C, Masters W H, Johnson V E 1979 Textbook of sexual medicine. Little Brown, Boston

Kumar R 1982 Neurotic disorders. In: Kumar R, Brockington I F (eds) Motherhood and mental illness. p 101 Academic Press, London

Lyketsos G C, Sakka P, Mailis A 1983 The sexual adjustment of chronic schizophrenics: a preliminary study. British Journal of Psychiatry 143: 376–382

Masters W H, Johnson V E 1966 Human sexual response. Little, Brown, Boston

Masters W H, Johnson V E 1970 Human sexual inadequacy. Little, Brown, Boston

Mathew R J, Weinman M L 1982 Sexual dysfunctions in depression. Archives of Sexual Behavior 11: 323–328

Mathews A, Bancroft J, Whitehead A et al 1976 The behavioural treatment of sexual inadequacy; a comparative study. Behaviour Research and Therapy 14: 427–436

Nettelbladt P, Uddenberg N 1979 Sexual dysfunction and sexual satisfaction in 58 married Swedish men. Journal of Psychosomatic Research 23: 141–147

O'Connor J F, Stern L O 1972 Developmental factors in functional sexual disorders. New York State Journal of Medicine 72: 1838–1843

Osborn M, Hawton K, Gath D 1987 Sexual dysfunction among middle-aged women in the community. British Medical Journal (in press)

Robson K M, Brant H A, Kumar R 1981 Maternal sexuality during pregnancy and after childbirth. British Journal of Obstetrics and Gynaecology 88: 882–889

Schreiner-Engel P, Schiavi R C 1986 Lifetime psychopathology in individuals with low sexual desire. Journal of Nervous and Mental Disease 174: 646–651

Tsai M, Feldman-Summers S, Edgar M 1979 Childhood molestation: variables related to differential impacts on psychosexual functioning in adult women. Journal of Abnormal Psychology 88: 407–417

Tullman G M, Gilner F H, Kolodny R C, Dornbush R L, Tullman G D 1981 The pre- and post-therapy measurement of communication skills of couples undergoing sex-therapy at the Masters and Johnson Institute. Archives of Sexual Behavior 10: 95–109

Uddenberg N 1974 Psychological aspects of sexual inadequacy in women. Journal of Psychosomatic Research 18. 33–47

Weissman M M, Paykel E S 1974 The depressed woman: a study of social relationships. University of Chicago Press, Chicago

Yates A 1982 Children eroticized by incest. American Journal of Psychiatry 139:482–485

15

Peter G. Britton

Abnormalities in the elderly

INTRODUCTION

In recent years interest in the inter-relationships between normal and abnormal psychological processes and ageing has increased markedly. A measure of this interest is reflected in the growth of research activity in relation to any area involving the elderly and the vast rise in the number of publications that has occurred. General reviews of clinical psychology in relation to the elderly can be found in Hanley & Hodge (1984) and Woods & Britton (1985). The topic of mental health and ageing has been thoroughly explored in major texts such as those by Birren & Sloane (1980) and Levy & Post (1982).

The reasons for this expansion in work with the elderly have been complex. Amongst the most powerful is the need to be more aware of the processes of age-related change in order to direct economic resources to the best effect in the context of vastly increasing numbers of the very old. There are other reasons. One is that understanding of basic psychological processes such as memory and language can be greatly assisted by the analysis of abnormal states. The elderly, both normal and abnormal, provide a useful source of information in which psychological change may be related to findings from other disciplines, such as neurochemistry and neuropathology. Insights gained may generalize to other parts of the life-span. The work in relation to dementia and depression in the elderly, to be reviewed in this chapter, illustrates many of these points.

This chapter will concentrate on those aspects of abnormal psychology most relevant to the elderly, whilst drawing attention to specific facets of abnormality in the elderly in relation to other topics covered in the remainder of this book. Concern will be directed mainly to dementia, since it represents one of the most specific 'elderly related' abnormal processes. Other problem areas include depression and the particular effects of alcohol and drugs. Some interesting insights will be mentioned from work on older persons who have suffered trauma and physical illness as well as links with more neuropsychological disorders, particularly Parkinson's disease, although this chapter does not attempt to explore neuropsychology and mental handicap in the elderly in any detail.

METHODOLOGY AND COGNITIVE CHANGE

The adequate definition and understanding of age-related change has always been surrounded by complex methodological problems. Studies of changes in cognitive functioning in the normal elderly illustrate well the difficulties which may be encountered in any attempt to produce a research design which will allow clarity of inference. Without an adequate baseline of normal expectancy it is difficult to put studies of abnormal groups into context. A fuller account of these methodological issues in work with the elderly is given in Chapters 19 and 20 of Botwinick (1978) and Chapter 2 of Woods & Britton (1985).

Early studies, such as those reported in the book by Wechsler (1958), presented a model of inevitable cognitive decline as age advances, with decline accelerating in old age. This decline was taken to be global, crossing the spectrum of all cognitive abilities, and inevitable. Such was the pervasive influence of this position that it dominated texts for professionals working with the elderly until quite recently.

However, work employing increasingly sophisticated statistical and psychological models has led to very different conclusions (Schaie 1977). These reject the concept of global, inevitable decline and emphasize the plasticity of change within the individual. Global decline is seen as not being inevitable. Individual differences in the extent of decline are considerable and related to a number of factors in the individual and the environment. Medical and sensory factors influence performance, as do cultural and environmental changes. The capacity for the individual to adapt to these changes has been underestimated.

These findings emerged from studies which employed innovative designs. The initial cross-sectional studies *overemphasized* age-related decline. Longitudinal studies have other problems, the most severe of which is subject attrition, and these *underestimate* decline. Mixed models, cross-sequential and other designs, have improved the validity of the inferences drawn but it would seem that it is very difficult to find a statistical model which avoids some confounding of the variables (see Botwinick 1978).

Similar problems occur with the psychological models underlying the test materials or assessment procedures which have been employed. Most global intellectual tests were devised with the aim of emphasizing traditional psychometric virtues such as reliability. The quest for reliability may exclude material which best reflects individual variability and change. In addition, many test items do not 'mesh' with the culture and environment of the individuals being assessed. These issues are now increasingly well explored in the literature (Kendrick 1982, Rabbitt 1982) but many problems, like the influence of attitudinal and motivational factors, require further study (Volans & Woods 1983).

This brief overview of some of the methodological problems in adequately defining and assessing cognitive change with advancing age in normal groups gives a background and context for understanding work with abnormal subjects. Many of the same difficulties apply and must be taken into account in the statistical and psychological design of adequate research. A review of abnormal processes in the elderly can now be approached cautiously but, perhaps, rather more wisely after mature consideration of some of the pitfalls of design and inference involved in work on age-related change.

DEMENTIA

The complex of psychological changes which have been included within the scope of dementia are the most pervasive and problematical of the abnormalities in the elderly. An attempt will be made to explore some of the questions which arise in efforts to determine the nature of this disorder, or complex of disorders, in both medical and psychological terms. The importance of dementia may be judged by estimates of its prevalence, ranging from 5% to 15% of the population aged over 65, and increasing to 20–40% in those over 80 years (Levy & Post 1982). This importance is further seen in the intensive multidisciplinary efforts which have been made to clarify its nature in recent years, usefully summarized in a special issue of the *British Medical Bulletin* in 1986.

Research into the psychological sequelae of dementia has been conducted across a range of types and subtypes of dementia and a wide age range. 'Dementia-like' psychopathology may occur from an extremely early age in relation to renal failure. Groups of 'demented' patients are often extremely heterogeneous and ill-defined when research sample descriptions are considered in any detail. It may be difficult to compare findings across groups described as having 'dementia' without specific delineation of their characteristics. The next sections will explore some models of dementia and examine some of the characteristics which may be used to define groups of people for research purposes.

What is dementia?

Nobody is very sure of the answer to this question, either in medical or psychological terms (Wang 1977, Jorm 1985). The term dementia has had a variety of usage over the past century, from the general 'out of one's mind', to highly specific definitions of supposed subtypes. One of the major problems of the gross definitions, such as 'out of one's mind', is the danger of the professional inaction and apathy which may ensue. This was highlighted in the report of the Royal College of Physicians (1981), which produced a working definition as follows: 'the global impairment of higher cortical functions including memory, the capacity to solve the problems of day-to-day living, the performance of learned perceptuo-motor skills and the control of emotional reactions, in the absence of gross clouding of consciousness. The condition is irreversible and progressive.'

The problem of any definition is that it tends to encapsulate and ossify thought on the disorder. The earlier section on normal cognitive changes in the elderly has mentioned that inappropriate attitudes may arise from misinterpretation of 'global' changes. The above definition may be appropriate once the disorder has become well established in the individual. However, there may be substantial variability in both physical and psychological processes. The definition and analysis of such variability could be important for an optimal regime of care.

Within the overall, blanket diagnosis of dementia some investigators have argued for many subtypes. Lishman (1978) outlined 11 possible categories of dementia, some of which, such as Korsakoff's syndrome, have a known cause and may be treatable. Others have cautioned against delineating too many subgroups which may have little justification in themselves (Levy & Post 1982). Mild early dementia, especially in the community, may be difficult to define. The studies of Bergmann et al (1971) and Ron et al (1979) found that one-third of those initially diagnosed as dementing were not confirmed as having the disorder at follow-up.

Excluding the treatable disorders which can lead to dementia and avoiding excessive subdivision leaves two major groups. One is that of multi-infarct dementia, associated with raised blood pressure and characterized by a process of 'stepwise' deterioration arising from ischaemic lesions. The other, and most important group, is that commonly described as senile dementia of the Alzheimer type (SDAT), characterized by a more gradual process of deterioration. This review will concentrate on the latter, since multi-infarct dementia is more appropriately covered in the neuropsychological literature (Miller 1977).

Models of the causation of dementia

The causation of SDAT is unknown. Genetic influences have been suggested but not, as yet, proven (Breitner & Folstein 1984, Heyman et al 1983). Corsellis (1986) has repeated earlier suggestions that viral agents may be implicated. Perry (1986) has revisited the heavy metal deposition hypotheses of the 1970s initially raised in relation to dialysis encephalopathy (English et al 1978), which implicated increased aluminium levels in the water supply. As with many disorders a multifactorial aetiology may eventually be established with apparent subtypes related to the inter-relationships between 'causal' and 'contributory' agents.

Neuropathology and neurochemistry

The characteristic features of presenile dementia as described by Alzheimer (1907) were neuropathological changes. The neocortex and hippocampus were said to contain neuritic plaques and neurofibrillary tangles. The hippocampus might also show Hirano bodies and granulovascular degeneration. These features were first reliably demonstrated at post-mortem in demented elderly people by Roth et al (1967), and their presence and distribution have been confirmed by later studies (Perry 1986). However, the presence of these features is not unique to SDAT and similar changes may be found in both the brains of the normal elderly and those with multi-infarct dementia (Perry 1986).

It seems that abnormal protein structures are clearly present in SDAT in patterns which may be charcteristic. Unfortunately these patterns cannot readily be ascertained in vivo, which makes neuropathological markers rather less useful in research, particularly that concerned with the early stages of dementia.

Efforts have been made to relate in vivo non-invasive techniques of visualization of brain structure to the definition of dementia. Pneumoencephalography was originally used but has given way to the more sophisticated computerized axial tomography (CAT) and positron emission tomography (PET) scanning (McGreer 1986). These techniques confirm the presence of cerebral atrophy in SDAT and are able to suggest that temporal lobe atrophy may be a characteristic feature (Wilcock & Esiri 1983). However, in practice there are substantial problems in the method of using these techniques to define groups for research. Their use is extremely costly and until much better normative data on the normal elderly have been obtained, their use in defining subgroups of demented subjects remains doubtful.

Neurochemical changes in SDAT cover a wide range of possibilities, but undoubtedly the major focus has been on cholinergic deficiencies. These seem to be related to the severity of the disorder and may be a possible target for therapeutic intervention. Perry & Perry (1982) found deficiencies in hippocampal choline acetyltransferase and acetylcholinesterase in SDAT; and Wilcock & Esiri (1983) report similar deficiencies in the temporal lobe. These findings raise the possibility of replacement therapy to counteract psychological change (Hollander et al 1986). Other neurochemical evidence draws attention to additional changes in the noradrenergic system (Cross et al 1981) and somatostatin (Rossor et al 1984).

Implications for psychological studies

What implications do these models of SDAT have for psychological studies? In the near future it may be possible to use neuropathological and neurochemical markers to provide specific definition of groups and subgroups of demented individuals, preferably for longitudinal studies. In particular, cholinergic system markers and PET scanning may be the most useful.

At present caution is needed in interpreting studies which may relate to diffuse and ill-defined groups. It is also difficult to keep up with a rapidly changing situation with regard to the subdivision of dementia. The presenile and senile dementias were unified as one thing — senile dementia of the Alzheimer type — in the 1970s. The early 1980s saw two dementias advocated again with old-age onset (Alzheimer's disease I or ADI) and middle-age onset (ADII) varieties (Bondareff 1983). However, Jorm (1985) has concluded that 'although AD is a variable disorder, there is at this stage no evidence of qualitative subtypes'.

Morris (1981), taking some suggestions from Isaacs (1979) and Ron et al (1979), proposed the following criteria for selection of an elderly group of Alzheimer-type demented subjects:
1. A history of progressive dementia of at least three months duration.
2. No evidence of myocardial infarction, peripheral vascular or cerebrovascular disease.
3. No significant disease of renal, hepatic or endocrine systems.
4. No evidence of severe head injury, space-occupying lesion or intracranial infection.
5. No evidence of alcoholism or drug addiction.
6. No evidence of a history of previous affective illnesses.
7. No evidence of depressed mood on admission.

These criteria provide a basis for the evaluation of the adequacy of definition of the subject samples in studies under consideration.

Some recent work suggests that a close examination of the family history of dementia should be included in any investigation (Heyman et al 1983). The argument is that possible links with genetic or specific environmental agents may thus be more readily traced.

PSYCHOLOGICAL ABNORMALITY IN DEMENTIA

The previous sections have indicated that understanding of the neurochemical and neuropathological bases of dementia has developed significantly in recent years. The same is true of understanding of the psychological processes involved. In this, the core of the chapter, the themes which emerge from psychological research will be traced. It will be seen that there is a clear development from initial studies which looked at global aspects of cognitive functioning in ill-defined groups of patients with 'dementia' to recent, sophisticated attempts to define specific cognitive functions in rather more precisely defined groups. These features are seen most clearly in the work on memory, where confirmation of the gross clinical picture of memory loss in the early studies has developed into very specific investigations of subtle aspects of the memory process. Such studies will lead to a clearer understanding of the problems of demented individuals and assist those concerned with their management.

Cognitive change in dementia

Generalized cognitive impairment is one of the most obvious signs of dementia. Marsden (1978), in a chapter on the diagnosis of dementia, refers to 'the syndrome of global disturbance of higher cognitive functioning in an alert patient'. To the relative or care agent the impairment of cognitive ability may be obvious in a variety of practical ways long before the syndrome is established clinically. Many relatives have a clear understanding that 'something is wrong' from subtle changes in patterns of behaviour, idiosyncratic 'happenings' and memory lapses.

Psychologists initially approached the definition of these changes with the major psychometric tests of intelligence, such as those associated with the name of Wechsler (e.g. Wechsler 1955). The book by Savage et al (1973) reviews this literature and relates changes found in dementia to normal patterns of functioning. Miller's (1977) book deals with similar studies, with an emphasis on presenile dementia.

Amongst the most interesting of the findings from this period were those of Orme (1955, 1957). He used the combination of the Mill Hill Vocabulary Scale and Progressive Matrices. He found that whilst scores on the Progressive Matrices showed more decline in normal elderly subjects than the Vocabulary scores, both declined equally in dementia. A review by Inglis (1958) summarized findings to that date and concluded that there was evidence of a substantial decline in cognitive test performance in dementia. This generalized overall decline was further defined by evidence that verbal and performance abilities declined at rates different from those expected as a result of normal ageing. In particular, verbal abilities, especially vocabulary, showed substantial additional decline in dementia.

More recent work has taken up these themes as the reviews by Savage et al (1973) and Miller (1977) reported. Their general conclusions were that there is evidence in both 'presenile' and 'senile' dementia for a global loss of cognitive functioning and that there may be a pattern of change relating to deficits on particular subtests. Botwinick (1978) has argued that this global loss distinguishes the demented from normal elderly in that, with the exception of extreme old age or the pre-death period, the normal elderly do not show significant loss on long-term acquired abilities (e.g. vocabulary). However, Bolton et al (1966) and Whitehead (1973) found little difference between patterns of decline in normal old age and dementia. The use of so-called deterioration indices is thus questionable when based on an assumption of a pattern of change specific to dementia.

What conclusions may be drawn from these studies? They show that there is evidence of a global overall effect of dementia on cognitive ability. However, they give little information about the pattern of such change and its relationship to the progress of the disorder. This may not mean that no such patterns exist. The tests may be flawed in their ability to detect such changes. Most global cognitive tests, of necessity, contain material suitable for a wide range in both age and ability. The content of items may be inappropriate and insensitive for the elderly. It is also likely that the tests do not contain enough items in the lower range of ability to discriminate adequately at this level, thus resulting in a 'floor' effect.

A study by Loring & Largen (1985) used a broadly based selection of more appropriate tests with subjects having both senile and presenile dementia. They found that, overall, the two groups showed similar patterns of deficit with decrements in visuo-spatial tests, mental tracking and motor speed being less obvious in the senile group. The reported intention to follow up this sample over a year should produce longitudinal results which are currently lacking in the literature (mainly due to death reducing the viability of sample numbers). This study is an indication that there may be useful insights to be gained in the future from more sophisticated longitudinal global studies of cognitive functioning. These should use test material appropriate to age and ability levels, and perhaps contrast group data with the pattern of decline seen in the individual case. Such work would provide an interesting overall context in which to interpret the more specific studies on psychological functions, such as memory, which will be considered next.

Memory and dementia

Alongside global intellectual deterioration memory loss has traditionally been seen as closely associated with dementia. Again there is a history of early work with ill-defined groups and equally poorly specified models of memory. Work in this area has benefited in the past decade as a result of both the increasing sophistication of models of dementia and models of memory. Development has been aided by the way in which those mainly interested in developing models of memory have seen studying dementia as potentially assisting their endeavours, whilst also contributing to the understanding of psychological processes in dementia.

Models of memory

These have evolved substantially in the past thirty years. During the 1950s single-process models of memory were increasingly seen as inappropriate and alternative ideas emerged. This process has continued to the present with advancing sophistication of definition and analysis. There would appear to be three areas which need to be considered in relation to abnormalities in the elderly. These are: the input mechanisims; the process of analysis and storage; and the output mechanisms.

Sensory mechanisms

In order for a stimulus to be registered it must be recognized by some sensory process. In the elderly, and possibly particularly in those with dementia, these processes may be impaired. Hunt (1979) has drawn attention to the extent of problems of physical health in the elderly, and a review by Marsh (1980) emphasizes sensory losses. Visual acuity may decline substantially, especially in the very old, and other visual processes, such as tracking ability, may be seriously affected. Colour vision and response to changes in intensity of illumination are also subject to deterioration.

In the same way hearing is often impaired in a variety of ways. Loss may occur differentially over the auditory spectrum and alter the ability to discriminate and locate sounds. Other senses are also affected but age-related changes are much less well documented.

These changes suggest that considerable effort must be made in ensuring that sensory deficits are recognized and controlled for, especially in dealing with the elderly with dementia. Unfortunately, there is little evidence in most of the experimental literature that these factors have been taken seriously enough. Appropriate stimuli must be used which are within the sensory range of all subjects. Intermodality distraction and interference need to be recognized and controlled. These factors are liable to be underestimated and under-regarded in research workers unfamiliar with working with the normal elderly.

Memory mechanisms and storage

The model proposed by Broadbent of two basic memory processes, short- and long-term memory, has been subject to much elaboration. This model has been developed by Baddeley (1976) and seen in the context of information processing in the work of Atkinson & Shiffrin (1968, 1971). The Atkinson & Shiffrin model has been useful in the way in which it raises working hypotheses in relation to process and deficit in memory. Its influence has been behind many British studies on memory and dementia in the 1970s and 1980s. The model suggests that incoming 'raw' sensory material enters a series of *sensory registers* ('buffers' or 'iconic memory') which initially process material before transfer to a *short-term store* ('working memory' or 'primary memory'). Mechanisms within the short-term store control whether the information will be acted upon, retained by rehearsal, coded and/or fed into the *long-term store* ('secondary memory'), whence it may be retrieved via the short-term store by appropriate processes (recall and recognition). This model provides a useful basis for structuring an exploration of inter-relationships between memory and dementia. Many studies have used more specific forms of the model and these will be referred to as appropriate in the following discussion.

Short-term memory in dementia

This section will explore the operation of the sensory register in dementia, work on attention and encoding, and other factors relating to the efficiency of short-term memory. That there is a deficiency in short-term memory is widely reported (e.g. Kopelman 1985a, Miller 1977) and it is the nature of this deficit that provides the significant question.

Sensory memory has been regarded as an extremely short-term store which acts as the input buffer for the memory mechanism. Sperling (1960) identified such a store (iconic memory) for visual information lasting for a very short period utilizing tachistoscopically presented matrices of letters or numbers. He was able to trace a rate of decay using different stimulus characteristics such as intensity and duration. Research with the elderly and in dementia using this task has been surrounded by methodological problems. Walsh (1982) suggested that the technique of partial recall was not appropriate with the elderly and is confounded by deficits in recognition and attention. Walsh & Thompson (1978), using critical flicker-fusion methodology, suggested that younger people had a duration of iconic memory 15% longer than the elderly.

In presenile dementia the backward masking technique has been used by Miller (1977). He reported that increased exposure time was necessary for the demented group to identify the original stimulus correctly. Schlotterer et al (1984) used a similar task with SDAT patients with two types of mask. In the first experiment a mask was used which had a pattern of segments similar to the task stimulus, and SDAT patients required increased exposure times. When the mask was a light flash demented subjects performed at a similar level to age-matched controls.

Experiments of this type are susceptible to problems of ocular functioning. Bronstein & Kennard (1985) have drawn attention to eye movement factors in tracking experiments in Parkinson's disease. These issues were also reflected in a paper by Coyne et al (1984), who questioned the sensitivity of the retina in SDAT. They replicated the studies of Miller and Schlotterer et al referred to earlier and found that an SDAT group were less impaired by a random visual noise mask than a pattern mask after controlling very carefully for intensity. An explanation was offered in terms of two hypotheses. The first suggested that the light flash mask may be processed peripherally, the random noise mask both centrally and peripherally, and the pattern mask centrally. Alternatively, the pattern mask might interfere more because of increased similarity between the original stimulus and the pattern mask, thus requiring more from central processing mechanisms as compared with the random noise mask.

These recent papers raise interesting possibilities. SDAT patients clearly show an impairment of sensory memory, but further research is required to clarify the mechanisms involved. It would also be interesting to see these experiments (or suitable alternatives) repeated with both older normal subjects and those in a more advanced stage of the dementing process.

As far as short-term memory (STM) is concerned, the digit span test has traditionally been used to examine the capacity and efficiency of STM. A similar verbal test, the immediate recall of an address, forms part of the usual 'bedside cognitive assessment' of the medical practitioner. Studies of the normal elderly reflect little decrement in performance of these tasks until well into old age (Craik 1977). In SDAT there is evidence of a marked decline in STM when various materials and modalities are used (Kopelman 1985a, Miller 1977).

The verbal digit span test was used by Miller (1973), Corkin (1982) and Kopelman (1985a), with a non-verbal analogue (tapping a series of blocks in a predetermined order) also being used by Corkin (1982). Both tasks showed a decline in SDAT, suggesting a decrement in STM. A contrary finding is that of Weingartner et al (1981), who found no substantial change in their group of 'progressive ideopathic dements'. However, this group may not be comparable with other SDAT groups in either severity or type of dementia. A rather better defined group was employed by Kaszniak et al (1979) and gave results showing a consistent digit span deficit. This study also used CAT scan evidence to confirm the disorder as SDAT.

Miller (1973) reported a deficit in dementing patients in word-span (direct recall of word lists). Wilson et al (1983) used a technique which was developed by Tulving and showed marked interference effects in word recall in SDAT which was related to STM deficits. Many studies in the 1970s also explored the recency effect in STM in dementia. When word (or similar) lists are presented and recall requested, a recency effect normally operates, indicated by better recall of the most recent material. Whilst Miller (1971) reported an increased deficit in presenile dementia. Gibson (1981) found little difference between older subjects with dementia and normal controls. It may well be that, as Glanzer (1972) has suggested, the methodology is flawed in that factors other than an STM deficit may be in operation.

Other techniques have explored the possibility of accelerated forgetting in SDAT. The Brown-Peterson task, in which a consonant trigram is recalled following a distractor task, has been extensively used. Studies by Corkin (1982) and by Kopelman (1985a) both reported that SDAT groups showed more rapid forgetting than controls. Kopelman suggested that this 'indicates a severe impairment of short-term memory in Alzheimer patients'.

Morris (1986) has presented two experiments which attempt to clarify the locus in the memory process of deficits on this task. He used 'patients in the early stages of SDAT' and elderly controls. In the first study three distractor tasks were used, placing different demands on central processing. Simple articulation caused 'substantial forgetting' in the SDAT group and had little effect on the controls. Digit reversal and digit addition as distractor tasks produced increased forgetting in both SDAT and normal controls, with the SDAT group showing the greater impairment. These findings using verbal tasks were supplemented in a second experiment, when a simple non-verbal task (tapping) was found to produce effects similar to articulation in the first study. Taken together it would appear that these studies suggest that in SDAT the abnormal forgetting may well be explained by an impairment in the central executive system of the working memory model (Baddeley 1983).

Kopelman (1985a, b) reviews links between the neurochemistry and neuropathology of SDAT and the psychological findings, suggesting that many of the STM and LTM deficits which have been observed are explicable by, and consistent with, neurochemical predictions. An example cited is work on attentional mechanisms. Deficits found by Wilson et al (1983) in the capacity of STM were related to an attentional deficit. Such deficits may be linked to the noradrenergic system disorders commonly found in SDAT.

Miller (1977) has argued for a more detailed analysis of the basic psychological processes underlying the STM deficit of the presenile dementias. One area which has been the subject of much effort is the process of encoding. Miller (1972) proposed that encoding mechanisms may be selectively impaired in dementia. If encoding processes are disabled or inefficient then overload of the limited-capacity STM may occur. Miller's study showed the predicted effect with control subjects being more confused by acoustic similarities between words than demented patients, which suggests reduced efficiency of coding in the latter. However, this finding has been criticized by Morris (1984), who suggested that the material used may have led to 'floor' effects in the demented group and spurious findings.

Morris has explored this area in recent years in a series of systematic and detailed studies. He used an elaboration of the memory model which Baddeley (1983) has outlined. In this model a unitary STM store is replaced by 'working memory'. This consists of a limited-capacity central executive processor with both a verbal and visuo-spatial slave system (the 'articulatory loop' and 'visuo-spatial scratch pad'). Although little direct work has been done on the visuo-spatial scratch pad, the studies previously cited on sensory or inconic memory may have some relevance.

Most reported work has concerned the articulatory loop, which potentially accounts for many phenomena in verbal STM. It has two possible components: a phonological input store and a rehearsal process involving subvocal speech. In this model phonological similarity may lead to confusable memory traces and impair STM. Similarly, increased word length may reduce the ability to rehearse words subvocally when these are presented visually, and hence STM may be impaired.

The results reported by Morris (1984) suggested that the functioning of the articulatory loop was relatively unimpaired in SDAT. Both the phonological similarity effect and word length were comparable to age-matched controls. He therefore concluded that the locus of the reported STM deficit in dementia was in the central executive mechanism of the Baddeley model. Morris further suggested that this explanation is consistent with the findings of experiments on dichotic listening tasks (Caird & Inglis 1961), in which demented patients showed excessive impairment.

In conclusion, it is apparent from this brief review that STM is impaired in SDAT compared to normal elderly subjects. Overall capacity of STM is reduced (Kopelman 1985a, Morris 1984) and the rate of forgetting is increased (Kopelman 1985a). The locus of these deficits in the psychological and medical models of dementia awaits further clarification. Morris has indicated that the central executive may be substantially impaired, and this is supported by the reported work on attentional deficits and difficulties on the Brown–Peterson task. This area is the subject of much ongoing research of considerable methodological sophistication, and future developments should be interesting and informative.

Long-term memory

Problems with long-term memory (LTM) in dementia are one of the most evident signs of the disorder. At a very early stage awareness of the location of common features of the environment, names of people and places, etc., becomes affected. Research has attempted to define the extent and depth of this loss and to look for models of memory functioning which may assist in the analysis and understanding of the deficits observed. Deficits have been found across a wide range of aspects of LTM, including both verbal (Corkin 1982, Kopelman 1985a) and non-verbal (Corkin 1982, Muramoto 1984).

Possible links between LTM deficit and abnormalities in STM processes have been extensively investigated. Many studies have used the serial position effect referred to earlier in the section on STM. In presenile dementia the work of Miller (1971, 1973) showed little in the way of a 'primacy effect' (i.e. enhanced recall of the earlier words in the list) using verbal material as compared with controls. Gibson (1981) used both verbal and non-verbal material and found that SDAT patients were impaired on both tasks. However, Kirschner et al (1984) found a greater impairment in LTM when using non-verbal material (line drawings of common objects).

These studies are interesting in that they raise many theoretical issues. It would seem that STM and LTM may be inter-related. LTM deficits may be caused by a failure to cope with material in the crucial processing stages of STM, resulting in problems of information transfer to LTM. Morris (1986) has suggested that central processor deficits may inhibit effective LTM processing. Kopelman (1985a) has linked the LTM deficit to a problem in acquisition into LTM from STM, which he suggests may be associated with cholinergic depletion.

One of the most productive themes in research on LTM has been that of exploring the episodic–semantic memory distinction proposed by Tulving (1972). Episodic memory refers to the diary type record of events unique to the individual and organized around temporal and spatial contexts. Semantic memory is largely concerned with the individual's language system, i.e. words and their meaning and use in interpreting the environment.

Many studies have shown episodic memory deficits in SDAT, but the possible effects of the disorder on semantic memory were less clear initially.

At a simple level SDAT groups have been found to have difficulties in object naming. These may imply word-finding difficulties, suggesting an impairment in either access to the lexicon or disorganization of the lexicon in semantic memory (Skelton-Robinson & Jones 1984). Clarke (1980) used a task which required SDAT patients to recognize letter strings as words within the English language. SDAT patients were slower than controls at this task but accuracy was little impaired. This experiment suggests that the basic lexicon may be relatively unimpaired in SDAT. However, she suggests that access to the lexicon may be less fluent and that this may cause problems in the encoding processes of episodic memory.

Support for this view is given by the work of Weingartner et al (1981), who used 'ideopathic dements'. They found that demented patients were not facilitated by semantically similar words or clusters of words in a free recall paradigm, even with repeated trials. The demented group were able to structure word lists but unable to use this structure to facilitate memory. They concluded that their patient group had difficulty is accessing semantic memory, leading to less well-structured memory traces which, being weaker, were more susceptible to disruption or forgetting.

One problem with these studies is possible contamination from the differing attentional loads. Nebes et al (1984) used tasks with varying attentional demands to explore this issue. Their first task involved a comparison between processing time for semantically similar and unrelated words. Both SDAT and normal control subjects showed comparable facilitation for semantically similar words, suggesting that, at this simple level, semantic memory appeared intact in SDAT. In their second task strings of letters of increasing approximation to English were used, with the hypothesis being that recall would be facilitated by closer approximation. In the third task word sequencing of increasing approximation to English sentences was used, again with the expectation that closer approximation would facilitate performance. On both the latter tasks SDAT subjects again performed similarly to controls, indicating that semantic structure remained largely intact.

It would seem that the problem in SDAT in relation to semantic memory is in access to the lexicon which produces encoding variability and impairing episodic memory. This finding links well with neurochemical and neurophysiological evidence and with the STM findings, as discussed above. These tend to implicate central processor rather than specific function deficits as the primary locus of the memory problems which are encountered.

A review by Warrington (1986) brings together interesting insights from studies on memory processes in neuropsychology and old age. She proposes a 'memory for events' (cf. episodic memory) and 'memory for facts' (cf. semantic memory). The former have cognitively mediated schemata, with the latter being organized categorically. These categories fit well with the deficits observed in amnesic and other neuropsychologically impaired groups. Their implication in dementia is that inter-relations between the two systems must be fluent for efficient memory. The gross disconnections between the systems seen in severely amnesic patients may not be found in SDAT. However, the evidence cited earlier on episodic and semantic memory and their interaction would seem to inter-relate well with Warrington's model.

Craik & Lockhart (1972) suggested that processing of material in memory might proceed at a variety of levels, from a surface to a deep and complex level. Retention might then be related to an increased depth of processing. Corkin (1982) found that SDAT patients showed no substantial facilitation with increased depth of processing, suggesting that they were not effectively coding the material.

Encoding deficits in verbal material have been studied by Larner (1977) and Wilson et al (1983). Normal subjects showed a word frequency effect, with high-frequency (common) words being less reliably recognized than low-frequency words. This process depends on the efficiency of the mechanisms for word analysis, with rarer words being easier to encode distinctively. Both studies found that the word frequency effect was less marked in SDAT, with the latter study suggesting more effective recognition for *common* words (i.e. the reverse of the expected effect). It was concluded that the explanation for this lay in poor initial coding of the material.

However, Diesfeldt (1984) reported an interesting study linking encoding and retrieval. This indicated deficits in both encoding and retrieval processes for SDAT. The findings were that *when cued to do so* SDAT subjects used categorizations which were not used spontaneously. However, even so they were not as efficient as normal controls, thus impairing SDAT performance in a free recall situation. Buschke (1984) found similar effects using non-verbal material with a very small sample ($N = 4$). There are suggestions in this work that non-verbal material may not be encoded in the same way as verbal. Further research in this area is required to clarify the issue.

Much controversy has surrounded the nature and extent of possible retrieval deficits in SDAT. Initially it was thought by many that this crucial 'output' stage of the memory process was little affected by dementia. For example, Miller (1973) used the apparent stability of remote memory in presenile dementia to suggest that the retrieval mechanisms must be reasonably intact. He further explored this area in an interesting series of experiments (Miller 1975) in which, using a paradigm adapted from Warrington & Weiskrantz (1970), he explored the contrast between free and cued recall and recognition in presenile dementia.

The task used presented a list of ten words, repeated three times, and followed by a distractor task to avoid rehearsal. Retention was then assessed using free recall, recognition from a list of ten correct and ten incorrect words, and a cued recall task in which the initial letters of each stimulus word were presented. Patients with presenile dementia performed less well than controls on the free recall and recognition tests, but at a similar level to controls on cued recall. Morris et al (1983) used subjects with early SDAT in a similar experiment and obtained comparable results. Memory impairments in SDAT were evident in recognition but not cued recall tests.

One possible explanation for this effect is that dementia may produce interference effects. Stored information may not be appropriately encoded or processed, allowing abnormal interference in free recall or recognition modes. The partial information in cued recall circumvents this problem and facilitates recall. Wilson et al (1983) found that SDAT patients had fewer intrusions from prior lists in free recall tasks but a similar total number of intrusions. Thus the interference was coming from items not contained in the experimental task. It would seem that there is evidence of adequate encoding of material in both presenile dementia and SDAT, but that the information is difficult to retrieve without the appropriate cue.

A recent study by Bowles & Poon (1985), comparing aspects of memory in old and young adults, may raise some useful points for this discussion. They suggested a division of semantic memory into a semantic network, conceptually organized and containing information about word meanings, as well as a lexical network, organized orthographically and phonetically, which contains word names. They found that in a primed condition (similar to cued recall) their elderly group were able to perform as well as younger subjects. They argued that retrieval deficits may arise from impaired access to the lexical network from the semantic network. This model may be a useful basis for exploration of some of the findings of retrieval deficits in SDAT and of problems in access between semantic and episodic memory systems.

Summary

There can be no doubt that memory mechanisms are impaired in SDAT. All stages of the memory process seem to be impaired — sensory memory, short-term and long-term memory. Sensory memory may be impaired due to attentional deficits (Schlotterer et al 1984). Short-term memory is reduced in capacity and shows an increased loss rate or 'forgetting' (Kopelman 1985a, Morris 1986). Morris suggests an explanation in terms of an impairment of the 'central executive' processor in SDAT. Long-term memory is impaired in both the quality and quantity of information retained. Input (encoding) and retrieval deficits are widely reported and have been explained by a variety of models. The distinction between episodic and semantic memory, proposed by Tulving (1972), has led to a clearer understanding of the processes involved.

The 1980s have seen a vast increase in publications in this area. The most hopeful sign is the increased cooperation between those studying the memory process as a basic process in animals and man, and those interested in memory deficits in abnormal states. The literature of the 1960s and 1970s gives many examples of the poor interface between these groups, whereas recent work shows more evidence that the common problems and potential solutions are being recognized. The future should bring clearer insights, particularly when it is possible to follow the natural history of dementia from normal state to death with appropriate neurochemical and brain-imaging techniques, coupled with sophisticated psychological assessment of specific facets of the memory process.

Language in dementia

Language processes in dementia have been increasingly studied in recent years. Miller (1977) reviewed earlier work in this area and Bayles (1982) has presented a specific review of language function in SDAT. These reviews pointed to certain areas sensitive to the effects of dementia, particularly in moderate or severe cases. They suggested that, whilst some language functions such as syntax, correct oral reading and phonology may be preserved, the semantic aspects (i.e. use of words, object naming and verbal fluency) may be more affected by an evolving dementia. It may well be that gross impairment of language processes is not easily seen in the mild cases of presenile and senile dementia which form the population studied in the majority of investigations.

Impairments in conversational speech have been of interest in that they may provide initial cues to the onset of dementia in the general clinical situation. Binks & Davies (1984) presented insights from work with a group of individuals in community settings and referred to disturbances of semantic and conversational expectancies. Words were used inappropriately and out of context, with conversational content lacking form and fluency. An analysis of a 45-minute conversation with five SDAT and five control patients was reported by Hutchinson & Jensen (1980). Their SDAT group tended to develop topics or utterances with much less depth than controls, although analysis of types of speech suggested that the content of utterances was similar to that of the control subjects. The progress of conversation was more often interrupted in the SDAT group by irrelevant tangential topics.

This work using the analysis of real conversations from day-to-day settings of the individuals concerned seems to have promise. Obviously when contrasted with the methodological sophistication of the memory work just considered there are potential problems. However, it should be possible with increased sophistication of analysis of speech and conversational patterns to obtain insights into the pattern of conversation at various stages of the dementing process. This should give information about the underlying psychological processes and also provide valuable material for those caring for the dementing individual.

Specific aspects of the language process have been studied in detail. Dysphasia has been one of the targets of this activity and a variety of aphasia tests has been used. Skelton-Robinson & Jones (1984) used a group of 20 SDAT patients and administered a confrontation naming test which included words of a variety of types as well as of differing frequences of usage. The degree of dementia was assessed behaviourally and cognitively. A 'striking finding . . . is that there is a significant relationship between the degree of senile dementia and naming difficulties'. Although Rochford (1971) had suggested earlier that naming errors were largely due to impaired visual recognition, this paper concluded that the major problem lay in language processes. The authors argue for caution in the use of tests with demented subjects which 'depend upon correct naming by subjects in order to test subsequent recall'.

Many studies in this area have used the Schuell Minnesota test (e g. Walker 1980, 1981). SDAT patients performed much less well than elderly controls on the test as a whole as well as on specific subsections. They made more errors of a semantic and phonological nature, but Walker cautions that many of the subtests of this battery involve cognitive factors other than language abilities. The results may thus be confounded by such things as poor memory.

A similar caution was advanced by Semple et al (1982) in the interpretation of their results from the administration of three aphasia tests to a dementing group. Their subjects performed poorly on both simple tests of language understanding and expression, as well as on more complex tests where the ability to integrate descriptive language was assessed. The authors suggested that memory difficulties and apraxia may have influenced their findings.

More specific measures seem necessary to define and isolate the locus and extent of dysphasic phenomena. Such an attempt to analyse word-naming difficulties in dementia is seen in the work of Kirschner et al (1984). They proposed a three-stage process in object naming. The first is object recognition — a perceptual task. Secondly, there is word identification — a semantic task; and, finally, encoding into a motor response. Their study indicated that both the first and second stages are impaired in dementia. Real objects were more successfully named than photographs or line drawings, suggesting a problem at the first or perceptual stage. In addition high-frequency objects were more easily named than low-frequency, implying a semantic difficulty. Both deficits were related to the assessed severity of dementia.

Verbal fluency has been widely reported to be substantially impaired. Experiments typically ask the individual to generate words with a given initial letter or belonging to a set category (e.g. items of furniture). Both have been found to be affected in more severe SDAT by Rosen (1980), whilst milder SDAT patients were more competent at the category version of the task. The latter result was not supported by Weingartner et al (1981), who found a younger demented group to be less able to generate words within a given category. Miller (1984) contrasted a variety of clinical groups on measures of verbal fluency and concluded that in SDAT there may be a close relationship between verbal fluency and general verbal intelligence.

Reading ability has been considered to be relatively well preserved in SDAT until the later stages of the disorder, although understanding of the material read may be absent. Nelson & McKenna (1975) used a mixed group of demented subjects and showed that their performance on the Schonell reading test remained reasonably intact when other functions were seriously impaired. However, the Schonell test had problems with item content. This led Nelson & O'Connell (1978) to develop the National Adult Reading Test. They concluded that the reading ability of demented subjects was unimpaired on this test when compared with controls and that, in dementia, this test may give a useful estimate of premorbid intelligence. Nebes et al (1984) found similar results when comparing 20 demented patients (DSM III primary progressive dementia) with age-matched controls. The National Adult Reading Test scores were little different in the two groups.

Language ability in dementia may appear relatively intact, with little effect on fluency, grammar and articulation until the disorder is severe. Reading may appear unimpaired but naming is affected at an early stage. There are problems in isolating language and its effects from a more general consideration of deficits in cognitive functioning.

Psychological change in dementia: an overview

There have been many attempts to produce a psychological model of the dementing process. A descriptive model would be useful if it led to the integration of the diffuse findings and encouraged more effective research, as well as raising possible avenues for help and remediation. Attempts have been made to produce such models and some will be examined next.

One of the earliest was the 'accelerated ageing' model, which views dementia as an acceleration and extension of the normal ageing process. At a superficial level some of the physiological and psychological changes seen in dementia might support this model. However, increased knowledge of both normal and abnormal processes has greatly reduced support for this view. On the physiological side, whilst some of the changes seen in SDAT also occur in normal ageing, the nature and extent of the changes found in SDAT are not seen in normal ageing. The same is true also for most psychological functions.

Other models have postulated a 'developmental reversal' of the processes of cognitive growth in childhood (Rosen & Mohs 1982). The model of childhood development proposed by Piaget has been suggested as a basis for this reversal. The evidence available offers little support for such models, and indeed their relevance to child development is increasingly questioned. Sensory deprivation and arousal deficit models have also been proposed. The former relates the psychological phenomena of dementia to losses from lack of stimulation due to sensory loss and withdrawal from stimulation. The latter (Kendrick 1972) suggests that reduced levels of cerebral excitation may inhibit cognitive performance in dementia. Neither of these models has sustained support.

It would seem that neuropsychological models which allow for the perceived variability and heterogeneity of performance as dementia develops may have the most promise (Moscovitch 1982, Rosen & Mohs 1982). These relate specific pathological changes to psychological dysfunctions and exploit the more recent developments in neurochemical, neuropathological and psychological research. However, there may be problems due to the diffuse nature of the changes observed in brain functioning in dementia. It is likely, nevertheless, that the coming years will see more adequate descriptive models appearing as the sophistication of knowledge about the underlying processes reduces dependence on simplistic notions developed from extremely heterogeneous and ill-defined groups of 'demented' subjects.

DEPRESSION IN THE ELDERLY

Various aspects of this psychological abnormality have been explored elsewhere in this book (see Chapters 5 and 1). This discussion will be confined to some issues of particular relevance to the elderly. Depending upon the specificity of the definition of depression employed, estimates of the prevalence of depression range from 2% to 30% of the elderly population. It would seem that up to the age of 75 years depression is the most common psychogeriatric problem (Post 1982). Depression in the elderly remains especially difficult to identify and treat. Its presentation may be confused with normal ageing or dementia and its treatment complicated by idiosyncratic reactions to antidepressant drugs.

Factors influencing the onset of depression in the elderly are similar to those in younger people. Social problems, stressful life events and stress due to impaired physical health all play their part in causation (Murphy 1982) and may affect outcome and prognosis (Murphy 1983). The effect of problems in physical health in the development of depression is much more apparent than with younger people (Bergmann 1982).

Changes in cognitive ability in elderly depressed patients have been given much attention in the past, perhaps stimulated by the often sterile request to attempt to provide evidence to distinguish depression from dementia. Gross changes in intellectual ability have been investigated using global IQ tests (Savage et al 1973). Hospitalized depressed patients were found to have a range of dysfunctions with some examples of severe retardation and with the degree of intellectual loss being related to the degree of depression. The same group also reported community studies of less severely depressed individuals, who also showed an overall decline on most subtests of a global IQ test. Nunn et al (1974) also found that those with lower IQs were more susceptible to depression and more resistant to treatment.

Attempts to assess the nature and extent of memory dysfunction in elderly depressives do not remotely approach the levels of psychological sophistication seen in work on dementia. Work by Savage et al (1973) suggested that digit span was impaired in severe hospitalized depressed patients, whereas Whitehead (1973) did not find a significant impairment. This latter study compared performance in depressed subjects before and after treatment on a number of memory tests (mainly of LTM). A recognition test, memory passages and paired associate learning did not change with remission of symptoms, but a serial learning test and a synonym-learning test did show improvement.

Conflicting results have been obtained from work by Irving et al (1970), who found depressed elderly patients to be impaired on paired associate learning. Neville & Folstein (1979) found that recall of pictorially presented material was preserved in a similar group. In contrast Kendrick et al (1979) found impairments in object-learning test performance in elderly depressed subjects as compared with matched controls.

Explanations for these results have varied. In comparison with SDAT, depressed patients seem to make fewer random errors or do not respond at all rather than responding in an idiosyncratic or random way. This slowing down or lack of response has been compared to the 'retardation' described in the psychiatric literature on depression (Neville & Folstein 1979). Medication and treatment may have influenced the results in many studies. Depressed patients may have been maintained on psychoactive drugs for extended periods and may have received eletroconvulsive therapy (ECT). There is evidence that tricyclic drugs can improve intellectual performance in such conditions as tardive dyskinesia (Collerton et al 1985) and that ECT may impair memory.

Depression in the elderly may affect both overall intellectual functioning and specific cognitive abilities. There is, as yet, no clear guidance from the literature on the nature and extent of the deficits that may occur. When compared with the increasing methodological sophistication of work on dementia this area leaves a lot to be desired. This is surprising since clarification of some of the issues should greatly assist treatment.

Models of depression in the elderly

The need to provide some form of effective therapy for the depressed elderly and the problems with drug treatment have led to recent attempts to clarify the applicability of psychological models of depression to the elderly. These models have ranged from the behavioural, through cognitive-behavioural notions, to psychodynamic approaches (see Hanley & Baikie 1984).

The behavioural model of Lewinsohn (1975) raised the possibility that depression might be related to a number of aspects of reinforcement such as the loss of reinforcement (both environmental and social), the emission of less reinforceable behaviour, and reduced reinforcer effectiveness. On the surface it is not unreasonable to feel that these factors may be especially powerful in the elderly for a combination of reasons. However, a simple relationship between quantity of reinforcement and depression in the elderly may not be relevant and the quality of reinforcers (both overt and covert) needs to be considered. Similarly a simple relationship between activity and depression is not likely to account for depression in the elderly.

Models involving a combination of cognitive and behavioural insights, such as that of Beck (1973), are beginning to be applied to depression in old age. These models combine ideas from the behavioural models (e.g. reinforcement loss and learned helplessness) with a component related to the individual's interpretation of events. Vezina & Bourque (1984) explored links between cognitive structures and depression as well as looking at cognitive coping strategies. The depressed elderly had substantially more dysfunctional attitudes and negative cognitions than normal elderly subjects. The authors suggested that the cognitive abnormalities found in the depressed elderly did not differ from those of younger depressed patients and they encouraged the use of related cognitive therapies.

It is evident that, whilst there have been advances in the application of these psychological models to depression in the elderly, much remains to be clarified with regard to their practical use. The changes seen in intellectual processes in normal ageing may affect both the causation of depression and the way that it can be treated.

OTHER DISORDERS IN THE ELDERLY

The importance of dementia and depression in terms of their prevalence and impact have absorbed most of the effort made by psychologists in relation to abnormalities in the elderly. Some disorders of the elderly lie largely outside the scope of this book. Neuropsychological dysfunction and ageing in the mentally handicapped are two examples. A brief attempt will now be made to introduce some important smaller topics concerning the effects of alcohol and drugs, Parkinson's disease, the effects of cerebral trauma and physical illness.

Alcohol is a pervasive substance in Western cultures and its effects are well documented, even in the elderly (Mishara & Kastenbaum 1980, James 1983). The problems posed by excessive alcohol use lie largely in the possibility of confusion between disorders such as dementia and specifically alcohol related problems like the Korsakoff syndrome. The latter can present initially with many of the memory problems associated with SDAT but lacks the global intellectual deficit or the progressive nature of SDAT (Cutting 1978). These has been little detailed research into memory processes in alcohol-related disorders of the elderly. Neville & Folstein (1979) showed differences between SDAT and Korsakoff patients, with the latter performing better than the former on an object recognition task.

However, this is a small contribution to a real understanding of the phenomena.

The literature on the psychological effects of illicit drugs or substance abuse contains evidence that these problems exist in the elderly, but there is very little comment, and even less evidence, on specific psychological effects. What is known is that prescribed drugs may produce unexpected and bizarre psychological sequelae (Evans 1982). The literature on delirium in the elderly is evidence of the need to clarify the psychological effects of drugs. Drugs may produce few problems in younger subjects yet interact adversely with the neurochemistry of the elderly, producing a profound effect on psychological processes. Similar problems may be seen as a result of physical illnesses or trauma. Again these effects are noted in the literature as 'intellectual confusion', 'memory loss', etc., with little information as to the extent or nature of the loss of function.

Parkinson's disease has recently become much better understood from both neurological and psychological standpoints. Parkinson (1817) in his original definition of the disorder commented on the lack of intellectual deficit, yet most investigators have found both general and specific impairments. A review by Rosin (1982) summarized the neurochemistry and neuropathology of the disorder. Although there is clear evidence of a neurotransmitter deficit in the dopaminergic system this may not be the only mechanism involved. The administration of the drug L-dopa may reduce symptomatology but not affect the progress of Parkinson's disease.

Brown & Marsden (1984) reviewed the relevant literature and concluded that previous estimates suggesting a 25–30% prevalence of dementia in Parkinson's disease were grossly exaggerated. They suggest a more realistic estimate of 15%. Some psychological studies have found an overall decline in intellectual abilities (e.g. Loranger et al 1982). The deficits found on a global intellectual test (WAIS) were spread over a range of subtests. However, Lees & Smith (1983), with a sample of early Parkinsonian patients, found no gross abnormalities of cognitive functioning on a wide range of tests but some evidence of subtle and specific memory impairments. These were most apparent on tests such as the Wisconsin Card Sorting Test and the Benton Fluency Test. They related these deficits to damage to the 'dopamine-containing mesocorticolimbic pathway' in Parkinson's disease.

Motor deficits have been extensively studied, indicating impairments in perceptuo-motor tasks. Flowers (1978) suggested that it was useful to look at the separation of automatic 'ballistic' movements from fine-controlled movements within a task. Parkinsonian patients were thought to show considerable impairment of the initial large-scale movement in a motor task. Recent studies, like that of Oyebode et al (1986), have confirmed this finding.

Research in Parkinson's disease has been surrounded by methodological problems in the definition of patient groups and in separating out the effects of ageing, other disorders and drug treatment on psychological functioning. This is now an active research area for experimental psychologists and their work should start to clarify some of the problems associated with Parkinson's disease.

CONCLUSIONS AND COMMENT

The psychological study of abnormality in the elderly reviewed in this chapter reflects considerable advances that have been made over the past few years. In the 1960s the 'blunderbuss' study was in vogue, throwing global tests of intellectual functioning and personality at ill-defined subject groups and using inappropriate research designs. Perhaps this stage of development had to be passed through in order to delineate more specific problems. However, the areas that were explored tended to remain poorly developed until there were links established between those interested in normal and abnormal ageing and between neuropsychology and psychogeriatrics. Current research models seem much more productive and appropriate, with clear links to 'pure' experimental psychology whilst also remaining of an applied and applicable nature.

Of the aspects that have been discussed, research on dementia is now particularly well developed. If current efforts can be sustained, a level of understanding of psychological processes is being approached, particularly with regard to memory and language, which should offer specific assistance in understanding and caring for the individual sufferer. The psychological treatment of depression in the elderly has potential value, alongside pharmacological interventions, given advances in understanding the age-specific aspects of the disorder.

The least well developed and under-investigated areas are those concerning psychological changes associated with physical illness in old age. Disorders such as diabetes, and those of the cardiovascular and respiratory systems, produce a range of psychological problems which remain largely unexplored. A similar comment can be made about the effects of drugs in the elderly, whether properly prescribed or not.

In the introduction to this chapter the need for an improved understanding of psychological abnormality in the elderly was justified in terms of an increasing demand for knowledge to assist health care and promote a better quality of life. There is now a firm basis of knowledge with regard to the range of psychological factors that are important and an enhanced awareness of appropriate methodology with which to pursue their understanding.

REFERENCES

Alzheimer A 1907 Uber eine eigenarte Erzkrankung der Hirnrinde. Allgemaine Zeitschrift fur Psychiatrie 64: 146–148
Atkinson R C, Shiffrin R M 1968 Human memory: a proposed system and its control

processes. In: Spence K W, Spence J T (eds) The psychology of learning and motivation: advances in research and theory. Academic Press, New York
Atkinson R C, Shiffrin R M 1971 The control of short-term memory. Scientific American 225: 82–90
Baddeley A D 1976 The psychology of memory. Harper & Row, London
Baddeley A D 1983 Working memory. Philosophical Transactions of the Royal Society of London B302: 311–324
Bayles K A 1982 Language function in senile dementia. Brain and Language 16: 265–280
Beck A T 1973 The diagnosis and management of depression. University of Pennsylvania Press, Philadelphia
Bergmann K 1982 Depression in the elderly. In: Isaacs B (ed) Recent advances in geriatric medicine. Churchill Livingstone, Edinburgh
Bergmann K, Kay D W K, Foster E M, McKechnie A A, Roth M 1971 A follow-up study of randomly selected community residents to assess the effects of chronic brain syndrome and cerebrovascular disease. In: Psychiatry Part II: Exerpta Medica International Congress Series No 274. Excerpta Medica, Amsterdam
Binks M C, Davies M G 1984 The early detection of dementia: a baseline from healthy community dwelling old people. In: Bromley D B (ed) Gerontology: social and behavioural aspects. Croom-Helm, London
Birren J E, Sloane R B 1980 Handbook of mental health and aging. Prentice-Hall, Englewood Cliffs, NJ
Bondareff W 1983 Age and Alzheimer's disease. Lancet 1: 1477
Botwinick J 1978 Aging and Behavior. Springer, New York
Bowles N L, Poon L W 1985 Ageing and retrieval in semantic memory. Journal of Gerontology 40: 71–77
Brietner J C S, Folstein M F 1984 Familial Alzheimer dementia: a prevalent disorder with specific clinical features. Psychological Medicine 14: 63–80
British Medical Bulletin 1986 Dementia. 42(1)
Broadbent D E 1958 Perception and communication. Pergamon, London
Brody M B 1942 The measurement of dementia. Journal of Mental Science 88: 317–327
Bronstein A M, Kennard C 1985 Predictive ocular motor control in Parkinson's disease. Brain 108: 925–940
Brown R G, Marsden C D 1984 How common is dementia in Parkinson's disease? Lancet 1: 1263–1265
Buschke H 1984 Cued recall in amnesia. Journal of Clinical Neuropsychology 6: 433–440
Caird W K, Inglis J 1961 The short-term storage of auditory and visual two channel digits by elderly patients with memory disorders. Journal of Mental Science 107: 358–370
Clarke E O 1980 Semantic and episodic memory impairment in normal and cognitively impaired elderly adults. In: Obler L K, Albert M L (eds) Language and communication in the elderly: clinical, therapeutic and experimental issues. Lexington Books, Lexington, Mass
Collerton D, Fairbairn A, Britton P G 1985 Cognitive performance of medicated schizophrenics. Psychological Medicine 15: 311–315
Corkin S 1982 Some relationships between global amnesias and the memory impairments in Alzheimer's disease. In: Corkin S, Davies K L, Groudon J H (eds) Alzheimer's disease: a report of progress in research. Raven Press, New York
Corsellis J A N 1986 The transmissibility of dementia. British Medical Bulletin 42: 111–114
Coyne A C, Liss L, Geckler C 1984 The relationship between cognitive status and visual information processing. Journal of Gerontology 39: 711–717
Craik F I M 1977 Age differences in human memory. In: Birren J E, Schaie W K (eds) Handbook of the psychology of aging. Van Nostrand Rheinhold, New York
Craik F I M, Lockhart R S 1972 Levels of processing: a framework for memory research. Journal of Verbal Learning and Verbal Behavior 11: 671–684
Cross A J, Crow T J, Perry E K 1981 Reduced dopamine-beta-hydroxylase activity in Alzheimer's disease. British Medical Journal 282: 93–94
Cutting J 1978 The relationship between Korsakoff's syndrome and 'alcoholic dementia'. British Journal of Psychiatry 132: 240–251
Davies A D M, Gledhill K J 1983 Engagement and depressive symptoms in a community sample of elderly people. British Journal of Clinical Psychology 22: 95–106
Diesfeldt H F A 1984 The importance of encoding instructions and retrieval cues in the

assessment of memory in senile dementia. Archives of Gerontology and Geriatrics 3: 51–57
English A, Savage R D, Britton P G, Ward M K, Kerr D N S 1978 Intellectual impairment in chronic renal failure. British Medical Journal 1: 888–890
Evans J C 1982 The psychiatric aspects of physical disease. In: Levy R, Post P (eds) The psychiatry of late life. Blackwell, Oxford
Eysenck M D 1945 A study of certain qualitative aspects of problem solving in senile dementia patients. Journal of Mental Science 91: 337–345
Flowers K 1978 Some frequency response characteristics of Parkinsonism in pursuit tracking. Brain 101: 19–34
Gibson A J 1981 A further analysis of memory loss in dementia and depression in the elderly. British Journal of Clinical Psychology 20: 179–186
Glanzer M 1972 Storage mechanisms in recall. In: Bower G H (ed) The psychology of learning and motivation: advances in research and theory, Vol 5. Academic Press, New York
Hanley I, Baikie E 1984 Understanding and treating depression in the elderly. In: Hanley I, Hodge J (eds) Psychological approaches to the care of the elderly. Croom-Helm, London
Hanley I, Hodge J 1984 Psychological approaches to the care of the elderly. Croom-Helm, London
Heyman A, Wilkinson W E, Hurwitz B J et al 1983 Alzheimer's disease: genetic aspects and associated clinical disorders. Annals of Neurology 14: 507–515
Hollander E, Mohs R C, Davies K L 1986 Cholinergic approaches to the treatment of Alzheimer's disease. British Medical Bulletin 42: 97–100
Hunt A 1979 Some aspects of the health of elderly people in England. Health Trends 11: 21–23
Hutchinson J M, Jensen M 1980 A pragmatic evaluation of discourse communication in normal and senile elderly in a nursing home. In: Obler L K, Albert M L (eds) Language and communication in the elderly: clinical, therapeutic and experimental issues. Lexington Books, Lexington, Mass
Inglis J 1958 Psychological investigations of cognitive deficit in elderly psychiatric patients. Psychological Bulletin 54: 197–214
Irving G, Robinson R A, McAdam W 1970 The validity of some cognitive tests in the diagnosis of dementia. British Journal of Psychiatry 117: 149–156
Isaacs B 1979 The evaluation of drugs in Alzheimer's disease. Age and Ageing 8: 1–7
James O F W 1983 Alcoholism in the elderly. In: Krasner N, Madin S, Walker R (eds) Alcohol related problems: room for manoeuvre. Wiley, Chichester
Jorm A F 1985 Subtypes of Alzheimer's dementia: a conceptual analysis and critical review. Psychological Medicine 15: 543–553
Kaszniak A W, Garron D C, Fox J 1979 Differential effects of age and cerebral atrophy upon spans of immediate recall and paired associate learning in older patients suspected of dementia. Cortex 15: 285–295
Kendrick D C 1972 The Kendrick battery of tests: theoretical assumptions and clinical uses. British Journal of Social and Clinical Psychology 4: 63–71
Kendrick D C 1982 Why assess the aged? A clinical psychologist's view. British Journal of Clinical Psychology 21: 47–54
Kendrick, D C, Gibson A J, Moyes I C 1979 The revised Kendrick Battery: clinical studies. British Journal of Social and Clinical Psychology 18: 329–340
Kirschner H S, Webb W C, Kelly M P 1984 The naming disorder of dementia. Neuropsychologia 22: 23–30
Kopelman M D 1985a Rates of forgetting in Alzheimer type dementia and Korsakoff's syndrome. Neuropsychologia 23: 623–638
Kopelman M D 1985b Multiple memory deficits in Alzheimer type dementia: implications for pharmacotherapy. Psychological Medicine 15: 527–541
Larner S 1977 Encoding in senile dementia and elderly depressives: a preliminary study. British Journal of Social and Clinical Psychology 16: 379–390
Lees A J, Smith E 1983 Cognitive deficits in the early stages of Parkinson's disease. Brain 106: 257–270
Levy R, Post F 1982 The psychiatry of late life. Blackwell, Oxford
Lewinsohn P M 1975 The behavioral study and treatment of depression. In: Hersen M,

Eisler R, Miller P (eds) Progress in behavior modification. Academic Press, London
Lishman W A 1978 Organic psychiatry. Blackwell, Oxford
Loranger A W, Goodell H, McDowell F H, Lee J E, Sweet R D 1982 Intellectual impairment in Parkinson's syndrome. Brain 95: 405–412
Loring D W, Largen J W 1986 Neuropsychological patterns of presenile and senile dementia of the Alzheimer type. Neuropsychologia 23: 351–357
McGreer P L 1986 Brain imaging in Alzheimer's disease. British Medical Bulletin 42: 24–28
Marsden C D 1978 The diagnosis of dementia. In: Isaacs B, Post F (eds) Studies in geriatric psychiatry. Wiley, Chichester
Marsh C 1980 Perceptual changes with aging. In: Busse E W, Blazer D C (eds) Handbook of geriatric psychiatry. Van Nostrand Rheinhold, New York
Miller E 1971 On the nature of the memory disorder in presenile dementia. Neuropsychologia 9: 75–80
Miller E 1972 Efficiency of coding and the short-term memory deficit in presenile dementia. Neuropsychologia 10: 221–224
Miller E 1973 Short- and long-term memory in presenile dementia. Psychological Medicine 3: 221–224
Miller E 1975 Impaired recall and the memory disturbance in presenile dementia. British Journal of Social and Clinical Psychology 14: 73–79
Miller E 1977 Abnormal ageing. Wiley, Chichester
Miller E 1984 Psychological aspects of dementia. In: Pearce J M S (ed) Dementia: a clinical approach. Blackwell, Oxford
Mishara B L, Kastenbaum R 1980 Alcohol and old age. Grune & Stratton, New York
Morris R G 1981 Memory and information processing dysfunction in dementia. Unpublished MSc thesis, University of Newcastle upon Tyne
Morris R G 1984 Dementia and the functioning of the articulatory loop system. Cognitive Neuropsychology 1: 143–197.
Morris R G 1986 Short-term forgetting in senile dementia of the Alzheimer type. Cognitive Neuropsychology 3: 77–97.
Morris R G, Wheatley J, Britton P G 1983 Retrieval from long term memory in senile dementia: cued recall revisited. British Journal of Clinical Psychology 22: 141–142
Moscovitch M 1982 A neuropsychological approach to perception and memory in normal and pathological aging. In: Craik F I M, Trehub S (eds) Aging and cognitive processes. Plenum Press, New York
Muramoto D 1984 Selective reminding in normal and demented aged people: auditory–verbal versus visual–spatial tasks. Cortex 20: 461–478
Murphy E 1982 Social origins of depression in old age. British Journal of Psychiatry 141: 135–142
Murphy E 1983 The prognosis of depression in old age. British Journal of Psychiatry 142: 111–119
Nebes R D, Martin D C, Horn L C 1984 Sparing of semantic memory in Alzheimer's disease. Journal of Abnormal Psychology 93: 321–330
Nelson H E, McKenna P 1978 The use of current reading ability in the assessment of dementia. British Journal of Social and Clinical Psychology 14: 259–267
Nelson H E, O'Connell A 1978 Dementia: the estimation of premorbid intelligence levels using the New Adult Reading Test. Cortex 14: 234–244
Neville H J, Folstein M F 1979 Performance on three cognitive tasks by patients with dementia, depression or Korsakoff's syndrome. Gerontology 25: 285–290
Nunn C, Bergmann K, Britton P C, Foster E M, Hall E H, Kay D W K 1974 Intelligence and neurosis in old age. British Journal of Psychiatry 124: 446–452
Orme J E 1955 Intellectual and Rorschach test performance of a group of senile dementia patients and a group of elderly depressives. Journal of Mental Science 101: 863–870
Orme J E 1957 Non-verbal and verbal performance in normal old age, senile dementia and elderly depressives. Journal of Gerontology 12: 408–413
Oyebode J R, Barker W A, Blessed G, Dick D J, Britton P G 1986 Cognitive functioning in Parkinson's disease: in relation to prevalence of dementia and psychiatric diagnosis. British Journal of Psychiatry 149: 720–725
Parkinson J 1817 An essay on the shaking palsy. Sherwood, Neely & Jones, London
Perry E K 1986 The cholinergic hypothesis — ten years on. British Medical Bulletin 42: 63–69

Perry R, Perry E K 1982 The ageing brain and its pathology. In: Levy R, Post F (eds) The psychiatry of late life. Blackwell, Oxford

Post F 1982 Functional disorders. In: Levy R, Post F (eds) The psychiatry of late life. Blackwell, Oxford

Rabbitt P M 1982 How to assess the aged: an experimental psychologist's view. British Journal of Clinical Psychology 21: 55–59

Rochford G 1971 A study of naming errors in dysphasic and demented patients. Neuropsychologia 9: 437–443

Ron M A, Toone B K, Garralda M E, Lishman W A 1979 Diagnostic accuracy in presenile dementia. British Journal of Psychiatry 134: 161–168

Rosen W G 1980 Verbal fluency in ageing and dementia. Journal of Clinical Neuropsychology 2: 135–146

Rosen W G, Mohs R C 1982 Evolution of cognitive decline in dementia. In: Corkin S, Davis K L, Crowdon E (eds) Alzheimer's disease: a report of progress in research. Raven Press, New York

Rosin A J 1982 Parkinsonism. In: Isaacs B (ed) Recent advances in geriatric medicine, Vol 2. Churchill Livingstone, Edinburgh

Rossor M N, Iverson L L, Johnson A J, Mountjoy C Q, Roth M 1984 Cholinergic deficit in frontal cerebral cortex in Alzheimer's disease is age dependent. Lancet 2: 1422

Roth M, Tomlinson B E, Blessed G 1967 The relationship between quantitative measures of dementia and of degenerative changes in the cerebral grey matter of elderly subjects. Proceedings of the Royal Society of Medicine 60: 254–260

Royal College of Physicians, Committee on Geriatrics 1981 Organic mental impairment in the elderly. Journal of the Royal College of Physicians 15: 141–147

Savage R D, Britton P G, Bolton N, Hall E H 1973 Intellectual functioning in the aged. Methuen, London

Schaie K W 1977 Towards a stage theory of adult cognitive development. Journal of Ageing and Human Development 8: 129–138

Schlotterer G, Moscovitch M, Crapper-McLachlan D 1984 Visual processing deficits as assessed by spatial frequency contrast sensitivity and backward masking. Brain 107: 309–325

Semple S E, Smith C M, Swash M 1982 The Alzheimer disease syndrome. In: Corkin S, Davis K L, Growdon E (eds) Alzheimer's disease: a report of progress in research. Raven Press, New York

Simpson S, Woods R T, Britton P G 1981 Depression and engagement in a residential home for the elderly. Behaviour Research and Therapy 19: 435–438

Skelton-Robinson M, Jones S 1984 Nominal dysphasia and the severity of senile dementia. British Journal of Psychiatry 145: 168–171

Sperling G 1960 The information available in brief visual presentation. Psychological Monographs 74: Whole No 498

Tulving E 1972 Episodic and semantic memory. In: Tulving E, Donaldson W (eds) Organisation of memory. Academic Press, New York

Vezina J, Bourque P 1984 The relationship between cognitive structure and symptoms of depression in the elderly. Cognitive Therapy and Research 8: 29–36

Volans J, Woods R T 1983 Why do we assess the aged? British Journal of Clinical Psychology 22: 213–214

Walker S A 1980 Application of a test for aphasia to normal old people. Journal of Clinical and Experimental Gerontology 2: 185–198

Walker S A 1981 Communication as a changing function of age. In: Communication problems of the elderly. College of Speech Therapists, London

Walsh D A 1982 The development of visual information processes in adulthood and old age. In: Craik F I M, Trehub S (eds) Aging and cognitive processes. Plenum Press, New York

Walsh D A, Thompson L W 1978 Age differences in visual sensory memory. Journal of Gerontology 33: 383–387

Wang H S 1977 Dementia of old age. In: Smith K L, Kinsbourne M (eds) Aging and dementia. Spectrum, New York

Warrington E K 1986 Memory for facts and memory for events. British Journal of Clinical Psychology 25: 1–12

Warrington E K, Weiskrantz L 1970 Amnesic syndrome: consolidation or retrieval? Nature 228: 628–630

Wechsler D 1955 Manual for the Wechsler Adult Intelligence Scale. Psychological Corporation, New York

Wechsler D 1958 The measurement and appraisal of adult intelligence. Williams & Wilkins, Baltimore

Weingartner H, Kaye W, Smallberg S, Ebert M H, Gillin J C, Sitaram N 1981 Memory failures in progressive ideopathic dementia. Journal of Abnormal Psychology 90: 187–196

Whitehead A 1973 The pattern of WAIS performance in elderly psychaitric patients. British Journal of Social and Clinical Psychology 12: 435–436

Wilcock G K, Esiri M M 1983 Age and Alzheimer's disease. Lancet 2: 346

Wilson S, Bacon L D, Fox J H, Kramer R L, Kaszniak A W 1983 Word frequency effect and recognition memory in dementia of the Alzheimer type. Journal of Clinical Neuropsychology 5: 97–104

Woods R T, Britton P G 1985 Clinical psychology with the elderly. Croom-Helm, London

Name Index

Abbagnano, N, 32, 43, 46
Abraham, K, 128, 138, 159
Abraham, S F, 277, 291, 292
Abrams, D B, 302, 314
Abramson, L Y, 141, 143, 154, 156–158, 159, 160, 162
Ackernecht, E H, 28, 46
Adams, H E, 232, 240
Adams, W J, 305, 314
Agras, S, 177, 190
Agras, W S, 281, 288, 292
Ajuriaguerra, J, de, 45, 47
Ajzen, I, 303, 315
Akhtar, S, 194, 200, 214
Akiskal, H S, 157, 158, 160
Albarracin, T A, 28, 47
Albrecht, F M, 28, 47
Alexander, J, 231, 233, 244
Alkhani, M, 86, 93
Alloy, L B, 143, 160
Allport, G W, 220, 240
Alpher, V S, 220, 244
Alston, W P, 220, 240
Alzheimer, A, 339, 358
Amenson, C S, 69, 93, 149, 164
Anderson, J R, 174, 190
Andreasen, N C, 102, 124
Andrew, R J, 91, 93
Andrews, G, 76, 77, 93
Aneshensel, C S, 93
Angrist, B M, 122, 124
Aplin, D Y, 262, 264
Arthur, A Z, 40, 47
Asberg, M, 196, 279
Ashworth, C M, 144, 145, 160
Astrup, C, 138, 160
Atkinson, R C, 344, 358
Auerbach, R, 323, 334
Azrin, N H, 308, 313, 314

Babcock, H, 131, 160
Babor, T F, 303, 315
Baddeley, A D, 344, 346, 347, 360
Badger, L W, 69, 95

Baikie, E, 356, 361
Bain, A, 43, 47
Baker, M, 157, 160
Baker, R, 313, 315
Balagura, S, 269, 297
Ball, B, 40, 47
Ballinger, J C, 132, 165
Bancroft, J, 146, 152, 321–323, 325, 326, 334
Bandura, A, 128, 160, 179, 180, 182, 190, 221, 240, 300, 301, 303, 315
Banks, M H, 78, 93
Bannister, D, 144, 162
Barlow, D, 331, 334
Barlow, D H, 54, 66
Barrett, E S, 170, 190
Barrowclough, C, 87, 93
Barthes, R, 27, 28, 47
Bartis, S P, 259, 260, 267
Bastian, H C, 43, 47
Bateson, G, 80, 93
Bauman, K E, 303, 315
Bayles, K A, 352, 360
Beaumont, P J V, 277, 291, 292, 333, 334
Bean, L L, 70, 97
Bebbington, P E, 71–75, 93
Beck, A T, 17, 24, 67, 93, 131, 133, 140, 141, 151, 152, 154, 158, 160, 163, 166, 167, 182, 183, 190, 209, 214, 289, 292, 332–334, 357, 360
Becker, J, 139, 160
Becker, J V, 322, 330, 334
Becker, M H, 303, 315
Beech, H R, 198, 207, 208, 214
Beels, C C, 82, 94
Beinhart, H, 291, 298
Beiser, M, 78, 94,
Bell, C, 325, 333
Bellak, A S, 222, 240
Bemis, K, 288, 290, 294
Benjamin, L S, 222, 223, 234, 242
Bennett, D, 90, 99
Bentall, R P, 117, 124
Bentley, M, 34, 47

365

NAME INDEX

Bergmann, K, 339, 354, 360
Berkman, P L, 71, 94
Bernstein, D A, 59, 66
Berrios, G E, 26, 28–30, 35–37, 39–44, 47
Beyth-Marom, R, 118, 124
Bianchi, G N, 231, 240
Billings, A G, 78, 79, 94, 308, 315
Billod, T, 32, 47
Binks, M C, 352, 360
Birchwood, M, 85, 89, 92, 94, 98
Birley, J L T, 81, 82, 94
Birren, J E, 336, 360
Bishop, D V M, 22, 24, 103, 124
Black, A, 194, 201, 214
Blackburn, I M, 133, 139–142, 145, 152–154, 160, 164, 167
Blackburn, R, 221, 225, 226, 233–236, 238–241, 244
Blakey, R, 313, 315
Blanchard, F A, 292, 293
Blaney, P H, 140, 143, 150, 160
Blashfield, R K, 231, 232, 241
Blasius, D, 26, 47
Bleuler, E, 102, 124, 201, 214
Block, J, 220, 241
Bobrow, D G, 107, 109, 126
Bollote, G, 37, 47
Bondareff, W, 341, 360
Bondy, M, 34, 35, 47
Bonham, K G, 145, 146, 152, 160
Borkovec, T D, 58, 66, 179, 191
Boskind-Lodahl, M, 270, 293
Boring, E G, 26, 34, 37, 47
Botwinick, J, 337, 342, 360
Bourque, P, 357, 363
Bower, E, 230, 241
Bower, G H, 136, 154, 155, 160, 181, 184, 186, 190
Bowman, I A, 29, 48
Bowlby, J, 157, 160
Bowles, N L, 351, 360
Bowskill, 277, 291
Boyd, J H, 69, 94, 128, 160
Braff, D L, 112, 126
Bregman, E, 175, 190
Brennan, H J, 110, 124
Breuer, J, 257, 265
Brewer, W F, 180, 190
Bridgman, P W, 8, 24
Brietner, J C S, 339, 360
Britton, P G, 336, 337, 364
Broadbent, D E, 107, 108, 112, 117, 124, 344, 360
Brockington, I F, 20, 24
Brody, M B, 341, 360
Bromet, E, 72, 77, 307, 315
Bronstein, A M, 345, 360
Brooks, G P, 28, 48
Brown, G W, 68, 70, 71, 74–77, 81–86, 128, 149, 157, 160, 170, 172, 191

Brown, R G, 358, 360
Brown, S A, 302, 315
Browne, A, 328, 332, 334
Brownfell, K D, 269, 293, 312, 315
Bruch, H, 270, 272, 276, 278, 281, 293
Buchsbaum, M S, 147, 158, 160
Bucknill, J C, 32, 48
Buhrich, N A. 252, 255, 266
Buranen, C, 249, 251, 267
Burgess, A W, 330, 334
Burt, C, 43, 48
Burvill, P W, 75, 95
Buschke, H, 350, 360
Buss, A H, 170, 190
Buss, A R, 35, 48
Butler, G, 183, 190
Byrne, D G, 69, 94, 120, 124, 145, 160

Caird, W K, 347, 360
Calloway, E, 111, 124
Cameron, N, 124, 223, 241
Campbell, E A, 70, 74. 77, 94, 144, 145, 154, 161
Campbell, D T, 52, 54, 60, 61, 66
Cameron, N, 118, 124
Canguilhem, G, 29, 48
Cannon, W B, 169, 191
Canton, G, 82, 94
Cantor, G N, 34, 48, 232, 241
Cantwell, D P, 284, 293
Caplan, G, 74, 94
Carey, G, 203, 204, 214
Carle, N, 86, 94
Carmichael, H T, 17, 25
Carr, A, 195, 208, 214
Carr, D B, 172, 191
Carroll, B J, 158, 161
Carroll, J B, 133, 134, 162
Carson, R C, 222, 234, 240, 241
Casper, R C, 276, 293
Castel, R, 26, 48
Catalan, J, 330, 332, 334
Catalano, R, 73, 95
Cattell, R B, 139, 161
Chambard, E, 40, 47
Chaney, E F, 308, 311, 315
Chapman, J P, 103, 105–107, 111, 124, 125
Chapman, L J, 103, 106, 124
Chaslin, P, 43, 48
Charcot, J M, 33, 48
Chave, S, 172, 193
Chesney, A P, 324, 331, 334
Chick, J, 230, 244
Chodoff, P, 248, 254, 265
Christie, M J, 145, 161
Claridge, G S, 103, 119, 120, 124
Clark, D M, 136, 161, 187, 191
Clarke, E O, 349, 360
Clarke, M G, 275, 293
Clarkin, J F, 230, 241

Cleary, R, 71, 96
Cleckley, H, 224, 235, 237, 241
Clement, P F, 291, 295
Cloninger, C R, 255, 267
Cobb, J P, 199, 216
Cochrane, R, 72, 74, 94
Coffey, H S, 228, 234, 242
Cohen, A, 43, 48
Cohen, J E, 11, 12, 24
Cohen, M B, 134, 161
Cohen, P R, 182, 190
Coben, R M, 137, 138, 161
Cohen, S, 79, 94
Coleman, R E, 152, 161
Coles, C, 321, 322, 334
Collerton, D, 356, 360
Collicutt, J R, 117, 124
Collins, A M, 155, 161
Comstock, G W, 71, 75, 95
Condiotti, M M, 303, 315
Cook, M, 180, 191
Cook, T D, 52, 54, 60, 61, 66
Cooke, D J, 76, 95
Cooper, J E, 18, 24, 195, 202, 214
Cooper, P J, 272, 273, 275–279, 281, 286, 290, 291, 293, 298
Cooper, Z, 272, 293
Cooter, R J, 34, 48
Coppen, A, 19, 24, 139, 158, 161
Corkin, S, 346, 348, 350, 360
Cornblatt, B A, 121, 124
Corsellis, J A N, 339, 360
Costello, C G, 2, 5, 74, 77, 95, 149, 156, 161
Coyne, A C, 345, 360
Coyne, J C, 154, 161
Cowie, V, 203, 216
Craigen, D, 238, 242
Craighead, 142, 161, 165,
Craik, F I M, 345, 350, 360
Creer, C, 90, 95
Crisp, A H, 270, 272, 274, 276, 281, 293, 333, 334
Cromwell, R L, 105, 124
Cronkite, R C, 307, 315
Cross, A J, 340, 360
Cutting, J, 114, 124, 357, 360

Dagonet, H, 32, 37, 48
Dalbo, A, 258, 266
Danzinger, K, 37, 48
Darwin, C, 36, 48
Daston, L J, 45, 48
Daumezon, G, 38, 48
Davenport, P R, 78, 95
Davies, A D M, 356, 360
Davies, M G, 352, 360
Davis, K L, 157, 158, 166
Davis, R, 291, 293
Dawson, M E, 111, 123, 124, 126, 145, 161

Dean, A, 71, 75, 94
Deaux, K, 70, 94
D'Elia, G, 146, 161
De Monbreun, B G, 142, 161
Denny, R, 179, 191
De Silva, P, 171, 177, 191, 195, 196, 200, 201, 203, 206, 212, 214
Despine, P, 32, 48
Diamond, B L, 30, 50
Diesfeldt, H F A, 350, 360
Di Scipio, W J, 140, 163, 279, 295
Doane, J E, 88, 94
Dodd, D K, 269, 293
Dohrenwend, B P, 72, 94
Dohrenwend, B S, 72, 94
Dole, V P, 310, 315
Dollard, J, 205, 206, 214
Donnelly, M, 26, 48
Dooley, D, 73, 94
Dorner, K, 26, 48
Dowson, J H, 200, 214
Draguns, J G, 231, 232, 241
Dressler, W W, 69, 94
Drevet, A, 26, 48
Drewnowski, A, 292, 293
Drinka, G F, 28, 39, 48
Dubbert, P M, 269, 293
Duddle, M, 321, 334
Dumas, G, 26, 48

Eastman, C, 181, 191
Eaves, G, 141, 161
Eber, H W, 139, 160
Ebert, M H, 158, 161
Eckert, E D, 279, 286, 293
Eckhardt, B, 73, 95
Eddy, N B, 299, 315
Edwards, G, 303, 308, 315
Eisler, R, 43, 48
Ellenberger, H F, 32, 48
Ellis, A, 140, 141, 161
Emery, G, 182, 190
Emmelkamp, P M G, 194, 203, 206, 208, 214
Endicott, J, 18, 24
Endler, N S, 220, 243
English, A, 339, 361
English, H B, 175, 191
Epstein, S, 220, 221, 241
Erdelyi, M, 221, 241
Erlenmeyer-Kimling, L, 121, 124
Esiri, M M, 340, 364
Esquirol, J E, 39, 41, 48
Esterson, A, 80, 97
Evans, J C, 358, 361
Evans, R W, 229, 241
Everitt, B J, 23, 24
Ey, H, 37, 48
Eysenck, H J, 2, 5, 11, 21, 22, 24, 116, 124, 128, 139, 161, 172, 191, 206, 214, 233, 234, 241

NAME INDEX

Eysenck, M, 183, 191
Eysenck, M D, 354, 361
Eysenck, S B G, 110, 124, 234, 241

Fairburn, C G, 272, 273, 275–277, 279, 286, 289, 290, 291, 293
Falloon, I R H, 88, 95
Falret, J P, 30, 31, 48
Faure, H, 41, 48
Feather, N T, 78, 95
Fechner, G T, 35, 48
Feighner, J P, 18, 28, 271, 294
Feldman-Summers, S, 322, 330, 334
Fenichel, O, 204, 214
Fennell, M J V, 144, 145, 154, 161, 167
Ferguson, D M, 231, 240
Ferster, C B, 147, 161
Finkelhor, D, 328, 332, 334
Finlay-Jones, R A, 75, 95, 170, 172, 191
Fischoff, B, 118, 124
Fishbein, M, 303, 315
Fisher, K A, 132, 162
Fisher, S, 328, 334
Fleminger, J J, 257, 266
Flor-Henry, P, 146, 147, 162
Flowers, K, 358, 361
Foa, E B, 201, 203, 206, 209, 210, 213–215
Fogarty, S J, 136, 167
Folstein, M F, 339, 349, 352, 360, 363
Foucalt, M, 26, 29, 48
Foulds, G A, 132, 162, 219, 232, 241
Fowles, D C, 238, 241
Fraccon, I G, 82, 94
Frances, A, 233, 241
Frank, E, 322–324, 334
Frankenhaeuser, M, 158, 162
Fransella, F, 144, 162
Fremouw, W J, 291, 296
Freud, S, 48, 128, 138, 162, 204, 215, 257, 265, 326, 334
Friedman, A S, 131, 137, 162
Friedman, S, 237, 243
Frith, C D, 111, 115, 116, 118, 125
Frost, R O, 202, 215, 292, 293
Frydman, M D, 77, 95
Fuchs, C Z, 151, 162
Furneaux, W D, 132, 162

Galin, D, 257, 266
Garcia, J, 177, 191
Garde, K, 320, 334
Gardiner, H M, 44, 48
Garety, P A, 90, 95, 118, 125
Garfinkel, P E, 270–274, 276–278, 281–283, 294
Garner, D M, 270–274, 276, 278, 281, 289, 290, 294
Garner, W R, 114, 125
Garrow, J S, 271, 294
Gebhard, P H, 320, 334

Geer, J, 325, 334
Gelder, M, 19, 25
Georget, E, 39, 48
Germer, C K, 107, 127
Gerner, R H, 285, 294
Gershon, E S, 157, 162, 282, 294
Gibson, A J, 346, 361
Gibson, H B, 133, 162
Gift, T E, 78, 95
Gilbert, P, 157, 158, 162
Giles, D E, 154, 166
Gillespie, R D, 138, 162
Gilmore, G C, 110, 113, 126
Gilman, S L, 36, 49
Glanzer, M, 346, 361
Gledhill, K J, 356, 360
Glithero, E, 251, 252, 255, 266
Goffman, E, 81, 95
Gold, P W, 285, 295
Goldberg, D P, 78, 96
Golden, R, 230, 241
Goldstein, M, 81, 87, 95
Golin, S, 143, 154, 162
Goorny, A B, 176, 191
Gordon, J R, 301, 307, 316
Gorenstein, E E, 239, 241
Gotlib, I H 154, 161
Gottesmen, I I, 203, 204, 214
Gottheil, E, 229, 244
Gottlieb, G, 146, 165
Gough, H G, 236, 237, 241
Gove, W R, 70, 95
Graf, M, 149, 164
Grannick, S, 131, 162
Granville-Grossman, K L, 157, 162
Gray, J A, 172, 189, 191, 206, 210–212, 215, 238, 241
Greden, J F, 133, 134, 162
Greene, S M, 140, 162
Greenfield, N S, 253, 266
Greenley, J R, 86, 95
Greenway, A P, 26, 45, 49
Greiz, E, 187, 188, 191, 193
Griesinger, W, 29, 49
Groat, R, 288, 296
Gross, M M, 301, 315
Grosz, H J, 252, 262, 266
Gruzelier, J H, 119, 125, 146, 162
Gunderson, J, 229, 241
Guze, S B, 261, 266
Gwirtsman, H E, 275, 285, 295

Haber, J D, 232, 240
Haber, R N, 106, 125
Hagnell, O, 69, 71, 95, 96
Hale, W D, 152, 162
Haleym J, 81, 96
Halldin, J, 72, 96
Halmi, K A, 287, 295
Hamilton, E W, 141, 154, 162

NAME INDEX

Hamilton, W, 43, 49
Hammen, C M, 140, 141, 162
Hammer, M, 82, 96
Hammond, W A, 270, 295
Hanley, I, 336, 356, 361
Hare, E, 194, 215
Hare, R D, 225, 233, 234, 236, 238, 239, 241
Harris, T, 70, 71, 74–77, 94, 128, 149, 157, 160
Harrison, J, 201, 212, 216
Hartmann, E L, 116, 125, 146, 162
Hashmi, F, 72, 96
Hauri, P, 141, 162
Hauser, R, 38, 49
Hawkins, R C, 291, 295
Hawton, K, 316, 320–324, 326, 330–332, 334
Heather, N, 303, 315
Heider, F, 156, 162, 179, 191
Heilbrun, A B, 237, 242
Helsing, K J, 71, 75, 95
Hempel, C G, 7–9, 21, 25, 226, 232, 242
Hemsley, D R, 86, 91, 96, 103, 106, 108, 110, 115, 117, 118, 124, 125, 187, 191
Henderson, D, 138, 162
Henderson, M, 235, 242
Henderson, S, 76, 77, 82, 96
Henry, G M, 134, 162
Herman, C P, 291, 292, 295
Hersen, M, 54, 66, 222, 244
Hershenson, M, 106, 125
Hertzog, D B, 275, 270, 295
Hewlett, J H G, 132, 165
Heyman, A, 339, 341, 361
Hibbert, G A, 182, 191
Hibscher, J A, 291, 295
Hilgard, E R, 38, 49, 259, 266
Hill, A B, 229, 242
Hill, S W, 269, 295
Hink, R F, 120, 125
Hiroto, D S, 156, 163
Hirsch, S R, 19, 25, 80, 96
Hirschfeld, R M A, 70, 96
Hoberman, H M, 79, 94
Hodge, J, 336, 361
Hodgson, R J, 19, 25, 169, 191, 194–196, 199–203, 205, 206, 215, 300, 301, 309, 312, 313, 315, 316
Hoeldtke, R, 28, 49
Hoffman, R E, 17, 125
Hogan, R, 220, 242
Hogarty, G E, 85, 89, 96
Holden, N L, 275, 296
Holland, A J, 282, 295
Hollander, E, 340, 361
Hollender, M H, 250, 266
Hollingshead, A B, 70, 96
Hollon, S D, 140, 141, 152

Holmstrom, L L, 320, 334
Hooley, J M, 83, 96
Hope, R A, 279, 294
Horowitz, M, 201, 212, 215
House, B J, 55, 66
Howard, R C, 239, 242
Hsu, L K, 274, 279, 284, 295
Huang, 173, 192
Hudson, J I, 283–285, 295
Hudson, M S, 285, 295
Hugdahl, K, 176, 192
Hughes, P L, 285, 288
Humphrey, L L, 282, 295
Hunt, A, 343, 361
Hunt, G M, 313, 316
Hutchings, B, 237, 243
Hutchinson, J M, 352, 361
Huxley, P J, 78, 96

Ilfeld, F W, 71, 72, 75, 96
Imboden, J B, 236, 267
Ingham, J G, 76, 77, 97, 98, 263, 266
Inglis, J, 342, 347, 361
Irving, G, 356, 361
Isaacs, B, 341, 361
Isnard, C A, 103, 125
Iyanaga, S, 34, 49

Jackson, P R, 73, 78, 93, 99
Jackson, S W, 29, 49
Jacobs, S, 82, 96
Jacyna, K, 33, 49
Jakes, S, 116, 125
Jalley, M, 30, 49
James, O F W, 357, 361
James, W, 117, 125
Janet, P, 194, 215, 246, 259, 266
Jensen, M, 352, 361
Jaspers, K, 32, 49, 194, 215
Jensen, S B, 333, 334
Jastak, J, 132, 163
Jerremalm, A, 170, 191
Johnson, A B, 320, 334
Johnson, C, 277, 295
Johnson, J S, 71, 75, 98
Johnson, V E, 316, 317, 321, 323, 335
Jones, D J, 274, 295
Jones, K, 30, 49
Jones, R G, 141, 163
Jones, S, 349, 352, 363
Jorm, A F, 338, 341, 361
Joseph, M H, 122, 125

Kalant, H, 301, 316
Kane, J M, 262, 265
Kanfer, F H, 11, 14, 25, 150, 163
Kaplan, D, 269, 296
Kaplan, H S, 277, 294, 332, 334
Karpman, B, 224, 242
Kass, F, 227, 242

NAME INDEX

Kastenbaum, R, 357, 362
Kaszniak, A W, 346, 361
Katz, J, 283, 286, 287, 296
Kavanagh, D J, 181, 191
Kawada, Y, 34, 49
Kazdin, A E, 54, 55, 57–59, 66
Kellner, R, 256, 266
Kelly, D H W, 145, 163
Kelly, G A, 144, 163
Kelso, K, 233, 244
Kennard, C, 345, 360
Kendall, P C, 141, 163
Kendell, R E, 6, 10, 11–13, 15, 20, 22, 23, 25, 128, 140, 163, 246, 263, 264, 266, 273, 279, 295
Kendrick, D C, 134, 163, 337, 354, 356, 361
Kenyon, F E, 247, 266
Kernberg, O, 228, 229, 242
Kessler, R C, 70, 71, 96
Keys, A, 286, 295
Killen, J D, 303, 316
Kilmann, P R, 323, 334
Kiloh, L G, 146, 163
Kimble, G A, 45, 49
King, L S, 37, 49
King, R D, 90, 96
Kinsey, A C, 254, 266, 317, 320, 322, 323, 334
Kiriike, N, 285, 295
Kirkley, B G, 281, 290, 295
Kirschner, H S, 348, 353, 361
Kiser, R S, 173, 191
Klassen, A D, 333, 334
Klein, D B, 26, 49
Klein, D C, 143, 163
Kline, P, 227, 242
Klinger, E, 150, 163
Klerman, G L, 68–70, 99
Knight, R A, 112–114, 125
Knight, R G, 109, 125
Kolodny, R C, 333, 334
Kopelman, M D, 344, 346–348, 351, 361
Kosten, T R, 226, 229, 232, 242
Kottgen, C, 89, 97
Kovacs, M, 152, 163
Kozak, M J, 209, 210, 213, 214
Kraepelin, F, 35, 49, 105, 125, 129, 138, 163
Krantz, S, 140, 141, 162, 163
Kreitman, N, 18, 25
Kretschmer, E, 138, 163
Kringlen, E, 203, 215
Kriss, M R, 152, 163
Kuipers, L, 83, 86, 90, 97
Kumar, R, 329, 335
Kuper, A, 44, 49
Kupfer, D J, 133, 146, 163

Lader, M H, 145, 163, 170, 191, 252, 253, 258, 266

Lain Etralgo, P, 28, 30, 49
Laing, R D, 80, 97
Lair, C V, 249, 266
Lane, T W, 181, 191
Lang, A R, 302, 316
Lang, P J, 186, 191, 210, 215
Langner, T S, 71, 97
Lanteri-Laura, G, 27, 31, 34, 36, 37, 49
Lapidus, L B, 119, 126
Largen, J W, 343, 362
Larner, S, 350, 361
Larson, R, 277, 295
Laufer, R S, 201, 215
Lawson, D M, 302, 317
Layard, R, 70, 97
Lazare, A, 227, 242
Lazarus, A A, 149, 163
Leary, D E, 32, 34, 38, 49
Leary, T, 228, 234, 242
Le Blanc, J, 158, 163
Ledley, R S, 11, 25
Lee, W F, 283, 296
Lee-Evans, J M, 239, 241
Lees, A J, 358, 361
Lefebvre, M F, 143, 163
Leff, J P, 80, 83–88, 92, 97, 116, 125
Lehrer, P M, 169, 192
Leitenberg, A, 284, 296
Leitenberg, H, 283, 284, 296
Leon, G R, 230, 242
Leonard, C, 254, 267
Lesch, J E, 28, 49
Lesky, E, 34, 49
Levene, M, 144, 163
Levin, R A, 221, 244
Levy, R, 336, 338, 339, 361
Lewinsohn, P M, 69, 93, 138, 148, 119, 154, 158, 163, 164, 356, 361
Lewis, A, 37, 40, 49, 194, 202, 215, 245, 266
Ley, P, 60, 66
Liberman, R P, 82, 97
Libet, J, 149, 164
Lichtenstein, E, 303, 315
Liddell, A, 208, 214
Lidz, T, 80, 97
Liem, J, 71, 72, 79, 97
Liem, R, 71, 72, 79, 97
Likierman, H, 205, 215
Lindy, D C, 285, 296
Lion, J R, 219, 242
Lishman, W A, 135, 164, 339, 362
Litman, G, 301, 316
Lloyd, G G, 135, 164
Locke, J, 39, 49
Lockhart, R S, 350, 360
Loftus, E F, 156, 161
Lopez Pinero, J M, 28, 29, 39, 49
Loranger, A W, 358, 362

NAME INDEX

Loring, D W, 343, 362
Lorr, M, 227, 242
Losserand, J, 26, 50
Lowry, R, 26, 50
Lubow, R E, 122, 123, 125
Ludwig, A M, 261, 266, 309, 316
Lunde, I, 320, 334
Lusted, L B, 11, 25
Lyketsos, G C, 333, 335
Lykken, D T, 236, 238, 242
Lyons, H, 248, 254, 265

MacCarthy, B, 91, 97, 120, 125
Macht, M L, 135, 164
McClelland, D C, 139, 164
McClure, J N, 172, 192
McCord, J, 225, 235, 237, 242
McCord, W, 225, 235, 237, 242
McCutcheon, N, 269, 295
McFall, M G, 208, 215
MoGhie, A, 105, 107, 111, 125
McGreer, P L, 340, 362
McIver, D, 232, 242
Mack, D, 291, 292, 295
McKenna, P, 354, 362
Mackenzie, B, 44, 50
McKeon, J, 171, 192
McKinney, W T, 157, 158, 160
McLemore, C W, 222-234, 242
McLeod, C, 172, 184, 192
McManus, M, 226, 242
MacMillan, J F, 84, 97
McPherson, L M, 239, 242
MacPhillamy, D J, 149, 164
MacRae, J R, 305, 306, 316
Magaro, P A, 110, 120, 125
Magnusson, D, 220, 242
Maher, B A, 25, 26, 50, 104, 109, 115, 118, 126
Maher, W B, 26, 50
Mahoney, M J, 269, 296
Maier, N R F, 207, 215
Maier, S F, 155, 166
Mandler, G, 172, 192
Manly, P C, 143, 164
Mann, A H, 78, 97, 274, 296
Margaret, A, 223, 241
Margo, A, 116, 126
Marks, I M, 170, 178, 191, 192, 206, 215
Marlatt, G A, 301, 302, 307, 309, 316
Marsden, C D, 248, 249, 266, 341, 358, 362
Marsh, C, 343, 362
Marshall, M E, 34, 50
Marshall, W L, 222, 234, 239, 242
Martin, I, 145, 164
Marzillier, J S, 181, 191
Masserman, J H, 17, 25
Masters, W H, 316, 317, 321, 323, 335
Matarazzo. J D, 18, 25

Mathew, R J, 332, 335
Mathews, A, 172, 178, 182-184, 192, 332, 335
Maughs, S, 223, 243
Mausner, B, 302, 316
Maxwell, A E, 23, 25, 57, 66
May, R, 180, 192
Maybury, C, 225, 233, 234, 236, 241
Mayou, R, 263, 264, 266
Mechanic, D, 263, 266
Mednick, S A, 121, 126, 237, 243
Meehl, P, 230, 241
Mendels, J, 146, 158, 167
Menninger, K, 11, 14, 25
Menon, D K, 87, 97
Merry, J, 309, 316
Merskey, H, 252-255, 257, 266
Messick, S, 292, 297
Metalsky, G I, 143, 164
Metcalfe, M, 139, 140, 164
Michael, S T, 71, 97
Michelson, L, 208, 217
Mignot, H, 37, 48
Miklowitz, D J, 86, 97
Mill, J S, 32, 50
Miller, E, 58, 59, 63, 66, 252, 257, 266, 339, 342, 344-348, 350, 352, 353, 362
Miller, H, 250, 266
Miller, I W, 143, 164
Miller, N E, 205, 206, 214
Miller, P M, 76, 77, 97, 263, 266
Miller, W R, 59, 66, 128, 132, 134, 137, 143, 156, 164
Millon, T, 219, 223, 226, 231, 233, 235, 240, 243
Mills, I H, 287, 296
Milner, A D, 208, 215
Milner, P, 150, 158, 165
Mineka, S, 176, 180, 192
Minkoff, K, 140, 164
Mischel, W, 220, 221, 243
Mishara, B L, 357, 362
Mitchell, J E, 276, 280, 285, 288, 291
Mohs, R C, 355, 363
Monroe, S M, 79, 97
Montgomery, S A, 279, 296
Moos, R H, 78, 79, 94, 307, 308, 315
Mora, G, 26, 30, 50
Morales-Meseguer, J M, 29, 39, 49
Moravia, S, 33, 50
Morley, S, 58, 59, 66
Morris, I, 90, 95
Morris, R G, 341, 346-348, 351, 362
Moscovitch, M, 355, 362
Mowbray, R M, 223, 243
Mowrer, O H, 196, 192, 155, 164, 204, 205, 215, 300, 316
Mullen, P E, 285, 296
Munford, P R, 264, 266

NAME INDEX

Muramoto, D, 348, 362
Murphy, G, 26, 50
Murphy, D L, 134, 135, 158, 164, 167
Murphy, E, 358, 362
Murphy, T D, 33, 50
Murray, L G, 139, 164
Murray, R M, 204, 215
Myers, J K, 70, 82, 97, 98, 194, 215

Naghdi, S, 111, 124
Natale, M, 152, 164, 165
Nebes, R D, 349, 354, 362
Neale, J M, 101, 106, 112, 126
Needleman, H L, 287, 296
Neisser, U, 152, 165, 176, 192
Neitzel, M T, 59, 66
Nekanda-Trepka, C J S, 140, 165
Nelson, H E, 354, 362
Nelson, R E, 141, 165
Nettelbladt, P, 322–324, 335
Neville, H J, 356, 357, 362
Nicholi, M, 256, 267
Nichols, K A, 230, 243
Noble, P, 145, 165
Norman, D A, 107, 109, 126
Nuechterlein, K H, 111, 123, 126
Nunes, J S, 178, 192
Nunn, C, 355, 362
Nyswander, M E, 310, 315

Oberg, B B, 28, 50
O'Brien, E J, 220, 221, 241
O'Brien, G E, 74, 98
O'Connell, A, 354, 362
O'Connor, J F, 328, 335
O'Connor, P J, 176, 191
Ohman, A, 119, 126, 177, 188, 192
Olds, J, 150, 158, 165
Oltman, J, 237, 243
Oltmanns, T F, 101, 106, 107, 119, 126
Olweus, D, 220, 221, 243
Orford, J, 301, 308, 316
Orme, J E, 342, 362
Osborn, M, 320, 321, 335
Osselton, J W, 146, 163
Ost, L G, 170, 176, 192
Overall, J E, 20, 25
Overmeir, J B, 155, 165
Owen, A R G, 33, 50
Oyebode, J R, 358, 362

Palmer, R L, 270, 275, 296
Parchappe, M J B, 33, 50
Parkinson, L, 212, 215
Parkinson, J, 358, 362
Parry, G, 73, 74, 99
Parsons, J, 36, 50
Parsons, T, 263, 266
Partridge, G E, 224, 243
Passamanick, B, 17, 25

Patkai, P, 158, 162
Pattison, E M, 82, 98
Paulson, G W, 146, 165
Paykel, E S, 20, 25, 76, 79, 98, 157, 165, 234, 243, 272, 288, 296, 332, 335
Payne, R, 73, 98
Payne, R W, 132, 165
Pearlin, L I, 71, 75, 98
Peck, D F, 54, 57, 66
Pederson, J, 88, 95
Perigault, J, 207, 208, 214
Perlmuter, L C, 45, 49
Perris, C, 139, 146, 147, 157, 165
Perry, E K, 339, 340, 362, 363
Perry, R, 340, 363
Persons, J B, 209, 215
Peterson, C, 143, 154, 165
Petijean, F, 30, 50
Philips, C, 11, 13, 14, 16, 25
Piaget, J, 152, 165
Pichot, P, 223, 243
Pilowsky, I, 263, 264, 266
Pinsent, R J P H, 72, 98
Piran, N, 283, 296
Pistoia, L, 36, 50
Pitts, F N, 172, 192
Platman, S R, 234, 243
Platt, A M 30, 50
Platt, E S, 302, 316
Plutchik, R, 234, 243
Pogue-Geile, M F, 107, 126
Polich, J M, 308, 316
Polivy, J, 291, 296
Pollack, J M, 202, 215, 229, 243
Polyakov, V F, 109, 126
Poon, L W, 351, 360
Pope, H G, 288, 296
Porter, T M, 33, 35, 50
Post F, 131, 134, 165, 336, 338, 339, 355, 363
Post, R M, 136, 165
Poulton, E C, 64, 66
Prudo, R, 73, 77, 94
Putnam, H, 8, 25
Presley, A S, 227, 232, 233, 242, 243
Prusoff, B A, 234, 243
Pyle, R L, 273, 275, 276, 296
Pylyshyn, Z W, 186, 192

Quay, H C, 236, 237, 239, 243
Quinn, M, 238, 242

Rabbitt, C P, 112, 126
Rabbitt, P M, 337, 363
Rachman, S J, 11, 13, 14, 16, 19, 25, 58, 66, 154, 165, 169, 171, 172, 177, 180, 191, 192, 194–196, 199–203, 205, 206, 209, 212, 215, 216, 312, 316
Rack, P, 202, 216

Radloff, L S, 69, 70, 98
Ramul, K, 33, 50
Rance, L, 78, 98
Rankin, H J, 312, 313, 316
Rapaport, D, 132, 165
Raps, C S, 143, 153, 165
Rasmussen, S A, 194, 195, 199, 200, 216
Rath, G, 29, 50
Raush, H L, 221, 243
Ravaisson, F, 26, 50
Rayner, R, 175, 193
Raynes, N V, 90, 98
Razran, G, 179, 192
Reda, M A, 142, 154, 165
Redlich, F C, 70, 96
Redmond, D E, 193, 192
Reed, G F, 195, 196, 200, 208, 216
Regis, E, 36, 50
Rehm, L P, 150, 151, 161, 165, 167
Reiman, E M, 172, 192
Reisman, J M, 26, 50
Renaudin, E, 34, 50
Reus, V I, 135, 166
Rezin, V, 146, 153, 167
Ribot, T, 26, 34, 44, 50
Rice, D G, 253, 266
Richards, R J, 44, 50
Richardson, A, 90, 98
Richardson, P M, 108, 125
Ricks, D M, 81, 99
Riese, W, 29, 50
Rimm, D, 176, 192
Rist, F, 303, 316
Roberts, C R, 74, 75, 98
Robins, N L, 198, 216
Robinson, D N, 34, 50
Robinson, P H, 275, 296
Robson, K M, 329, 334
Roocatagliata, G, 35, 51
Rochford, G, 353, 363
Rochoux, T, 26, 51
Rodin, J, 268, 269, 296
Roemer, R A, 147, 166
Romanes, G J, 44, 51
Ron, M, 341, 363
Roper, G, 205, 216
Rosch, E, 232, 243
Rosen, H, 254, 267
Rosen, J C, 283, 284, 297
Rosen, W G, 353, 355, 363
Rosenberg, C, 202, 203, 216
Rosenhan, D L, 19, 25
Rosenow, D, 302, 316
Rosin, A J, 358, 363
Ross, J S, 118, 126
Rossor, M N, 340, 363
Roth, M, 340, 363
Rothschuh, K E, 34, 51
Rotter, J B, 156, 166
Routtenberg, A, 150, 166

Roy, A, 254–256, 267
Royer-Collard, A A, 26, 51
Rubens, R L, 119, 126
Ruderman, A J, 291, 292, 297
Rush, A J, 140, 141, 143, 154, 166, 167
Russell, G F M, 20, 25, 270–272, 275, 276, 280, 284, 287, 288, 297
Russell, M A H, 310, 316
Russell, M L, 136, 167
Russell, P N, 112, 126
Rutter, M L, 83, 84, 98
Ryle, G, 251, 260, 267

Sabine, E J, 288, 297
Saccuzzo, D P, 112, 126
Salkovskis, P M, 188, 192, 201, 209, 212, 216
Sanavio, E, 202, 216
Sanders, A F, 112, 126
Sartorius, N, 252, 262, 266
Saslow, G, 11, 14, 15
Savage, R D, 342, 355, 356, 363
Scadding, J G, 25
Scarr, S, 230, 243
Schacter, S, 269, 297
Schaie, K W, 337, 363
Schalling, D, 237, 243
Scheff, T J, 81, 98
Schiavi, R C, 322, 330, 335
Schildkraut, J, 158, 166
Schlotterer, G, 351, 363
Schmauk, F J, 236, 238, 243
Schneider, K, 9, 25, 224, 243
Schneider, W, 107, 111, 126
Schreiner-Engel, P, 322, 330, 335
Schulsinger, F, 237, 243
Schultz, D, 26, 51
Schwartz, G E, 146, 166, 170, 193
Schwartz, I K, 232, 243
Schwartz, R A, 232, 243
Schwartz, S, 108, 109, 126
Schwartz-Place, E J, 110, 113, 126
Schweder, R A, 220, 243
Schweitzer, I, 285, 297
Scull, A, 26, 30, 51
Seamon, J G, 188, 193
Seligman, M E P, 59, 66, 128, 143, 151, 155, 156, 158, 162–166, 172, 176, 177, 193, 200, 216, 301, 316
Semple, S E, 353, 363
Shagass, C, 146, 147, 166
Shakow, D, 81, 98
Shapiro, M B, 54, 66, 133, 166
Shaw, P, 182, 192
Sheehan, D V, 172, 191
Sheffield, B F, 256, 266
Shepherd, G, 90, 98
Sher, K J, 209, 216
Shiffrin, R M, 107, 111, 126, 344, 359
Shryock, R H, 33, 51

NAME INDEX

Shweder, R A, 221, 243
Sidman, M, 206, 216
Siegel, R A, 239, 243
Siegel, S, 305, 306, 313, 316
Siever, L J, 157, 158, 166
Silberman, E K, 144, 166, 262, 267
Silverman, J S, 147, 166
Simon, B, 35, 51
Simons, A D, 141, 142, 166
Simpson, S, 350, 363
Singer, M, 229, 241
Sirois, F, 249, 267
Skelton-Robinson, M, 349, 352, 363
Skinner, B F, 147, 166
Slade, P D, 116, 117, 124, 126, 278, 281, 297
Slater, E T O, 203, 216, 250–252, 255, 267
Sloane, R B, 336, 360
Slochower, J, 269, 297
Small, I F, 229, 244
Small, G W, 256, 267
Smart, D E, 279, 297
Smith, E, 358, 361
Smith, J, 89, 98
Snaith, R P, 255, 267
Snyder, M, 222, 244
Sokal, M M, 34, 51
Solomon, R, 207, 216, 301, 316
Solomon, Z, 74, 77, 98
Solyom, L, 279, 297
Spanos, N P, 260, 262, 267
Spencer, J A. 291, 297
Sperling, G, 345, 363
Spitzer, L, 129, 166, 230, 244, 268, 297
Spitzer, R L, 3, 5, 69, 98, 166, 244
Spoerl, H D, 34, 51
Spohn, H E, 114, 126
Spring, B, 104, 107, 122, 126, 127
Srole, L, 71, 98
Staum, M S, 26, 30, 51
Stangl, D, 231, 232, 244
Steele, R E, 72, 98
Stefanis, C, 252, 267
Steketee, G, 210, 216
Stern, L O, 328, 335
Stern, R S, 199, 216
Sternberg, S, 107, 112, 127
Stevens, H, 262, 267
Stockwell, T R, 300, 309, 312, 316
Stone, G C, 229, 244
Stopes-Roe, M, 72, 74, 94
Storey, R, 227, 242
Straube, E R, 107, 119, 127
Strauss, M E, 106, 127
Strauss, J S, 233, 244
Strickland, B R, 152, 166
Striegel-Moore, R H, 268, 269, 283, 297
Strober, M, 270, 276, 282, 283, 286, 287, 297
Stunkard, A J, 268, 269, 292, 297, 298

Sturgeon, D, 91, 98, 120, 127
Sturgis, E, 195, 203, 217
Subkov, A A, 305, 317
Surtees, P G, 71, 74, 76–78, 98
Sutherland, G, 212, 217
Sutton, S, 303, 317
Swift, W J, 285, 298
Szabadi, E, 133, 166
Szasz, T S, 11, 14, 25, 245, 250, 257, 267
Szmukler, G I, 274, 275, 284, 288, 298

Tamburini, N, 33, 41, 51
Tanner, J, 79, 98
Tarrier, N, 87, 91, 93, 98, 120, 127
Taylor, L, 172, 193
Taylor, M J, 278, 298
Taylor, R, 136, 167
Teasdale, J D, 136, 146, 152–155, 167, 206, 217
Tennant, C, 77, 79, 98, 99
Ternes, J W, 306, 317
Thompson, L W, 345, 363
Thomson, J D, 29, 51
Torrey, E F, 83, 99
Trapp, P, 249, 266
Trasler, G B, 237, 244
Triesman, A M, 108, 127
Trimble, M R, 254, 264, 267
Trower, P, 222, 244
Trudel, G, 59, 66
Tsai, M, 328, 335
Tsuang, M T, 194, 195, 199, 200, 216
Tucker, D M, 146, 167
Tuke, D M, 32, 51
Tullman, G M, 331, 335
Tulving, E, 348, 351, 363
Turkat, I D, 220, 221, 244
Turnbull, J D, 277, 298
Turner, S M, 208, 217, 222, 244
Turpin, G, 91, 99
Tyrer, P, 231, 233, 244

Uddenberg, N, 322–324, 328, 335
Underwood, G, 106, 127

Van den Hout, M A, 187, 188, 193
Van Praag, H M, 131, 167
Vaughn, C E, 83–85, 87, 89, 97
Velten, E, 136, 167
Venables, P H, 80, 111, 119, 125, 127, 146, 162
Vezina, J, 357, 363
Vidotte, G, 202, 216
Viek, P, 155, 163
Volans, P J, 208, 217, 337, 363
von Feuchtersleben, E, 39, 51

Yates, A, 328, 335

Zajonc, R B, 154, 168

Zamansky, H S, 259, 260, 267
Zawada, S L, 108, 125
Zeaman, D, 55, 63, 64, 66
Zeeman, E C, 103, 125
Ziegler, F J, 252, 255, 258, 263, 267

Zilov, G N, 305, 317
Zimmerman, J, 252, 262, 266
Zoccolillo, M, 256, 267
Zubin, J, 82, 86, 91, 104, 100
Zupan, M L, 34, 51

Subject Index

Addiction, see Dependence
Alcohol, 299–317, 358
  in the elderly, 358
Anorexia nervosa, 269–292
  antidepressant medication in, 287, 288
  beliefs, 278, 289, 290
  depression history, 283
  depressive symptoms, 279, 285, 286
  dexamethosone, 285
  diagnostic criteria, 271, 272
  eating habits, 276, 277
  epidemiology, 273, 274
  familial aggregation, 282
  family affective disorder, 283, 287
  family interaction, 282
  history of concept, 270
  neurotic symptoms, 279
  outcome, 284
  personality, 281
  starvation effects, 280
Anxiety, 169–190
  biological basis, 171–175
    behavioural inhibition system, 173–175
    limbic system, 172, 173
  cognitive models, 182–185
    cognitive schemata, 182, 183
    mood & memory, 184, 185
    processing biases, 183, 184
  conditioning models, 175–179
    incubation, 178, 179
    preparedness, 177, 178
    two-factor learning theory, 176, 177
  nature, 169–171
    anxiety disorders, 170, 171
      agoraphobia, 170
      generalised anxiety, 170
      panic attacks, 171
      phobias, 170
  panic attacks, 187, 188
  self-efficacy, 180-182
  sexual, 330, 331
Arousal
  in schizophrenia, 188–121
  sexual, 320

Attention, 107–110
Attitudes, 141, 142
Automatic vs controlled processing, 110–113
Avoidance learning, 173, 206, 207, 238

Beck's model of depression, 151–155, 357
Behavioural inhibition system, 173–175, 210, 211
Biological models, 122, 123
Briquet's syndrome, 249
Bulimia nervosa, 269–292
  antidepressant medication, 298
  anxiety reduction, 283, 284
  beliefs, 278, 289, 290
  depression history, 283
  depressive symptoms, 279, 286, 287
  dexamethasone, 285
  diagnostic criteria, 271–273
  eating habits, 277, 278
  epidemiology, 273–276
  family affective disorder, 283, 287
  neurotic symptoms, 279
  physical complications

Classification and diagnosis, 2–4, 6–24
  categorical vs dimensional, 20–23
  definition of diagnosis, 7
  multivariate techniques, 20
  of dementia, 238, 239
  of depression, 129–131
  of personality disorders, 223–235
  operational definitions, 8
  reliability, 16–19
  sexual dysfunction, 319
  validity, 19, 20
Cognitive change
  in dementia, 341–343
  in depression, 131, 132
Cognitive style, 140–145
Cognitive theories, 182–185, 151–157, 357
  of anxiety, 182–185
  of depression, 151–157, 357
Compensation neurosis, 250

SUBJECT INDEX

Conditioning, 147–151, 175–177, 205, 237, 238
　classical, 176, 177, 205, 237, 238
　instrumental/operant, 147–151, 176, 177, 205
Consciousness, disorders of, 42–44
Conversion, 257, 258
Craving, 311, 312

Decision making, 208
Delusions, 39, 40, 101, 102, 116, 117
　explanations of, 116, 117
　historical background, 39, 40
Dementia, 338–355
　cognitive change, 341–343
　definition, 338, 339
　language, 352–354
　　fluency, 353
　　naming, 352, 353
　　reading, 354
　memory, 343–352
　　long-term, 348–351
　　short-term, 345–348
　multi-infarct, 339
　neurochemistry, 339, 340
　neuropathology, 339, 340
Dependence, 299–317, 358
　associative learning, 304–306
　　tolerance, 304, 305
　cognitive factors, 302–304
　definition, 299–300
　general psychological model, 300–302
　in the elderly, 358
　relapse, 306–310
　　priming, 309
　　withdrawal, 306, 307
　treatment, 310–314
　　coping with craving, 311, 312
　　cue exposure, 312, 313
　　drug substitution, 310, 311
　　social interventions, 313–314
Depression, 128–159, 355–357
　classification, 129–131
　　bipolar, 129, 130
　　endogenous, 129–131
　　manic-depressive, 129
　　psychotic, 129, 130
　　unipolar, 129, 130
　cognitive style, 140–147
　　thought processes, 142–145
　　content of thought and attitudes, 140–142
　definition, 128–131
　　functional analysis, 130, 131
　　Research Diagnostic Criteria, 129–130
　in anorexia nervosa, 277, 285, 286
　in the elderly, 355–357
　　behavioural models, 356, 357
　　Beck's model, 357

psychophysiology, 145–147
psychological processes, 131–147
　intellectual level, 131–132
　learning and memory, 134–137
　motivation, 137, 138
　personality, 138–140
　speed, 132–134
psychological theories, 147–157
　behavioural, 147–151
　cognitive, 151–157
　　Beck, 151–155
　　learned helplessness, 155–157
social factors in, 68–79
Delusions, 39, 40, 101, 102, 115, 117, 118
　explanations of, 117, 118
Diagnosis, *see* Classification
Dichotic listening, 107, 108
Dietary restraint, 290–292
Dissociation, 259, 260
Drug dependence, 299–317
DSM III
　hysteria, 245
　obsessions & compulsions, 194–196
　personality disorder, 218, 219, 225–227, 231, 232
　schizophrenia, 101, 102
Dyspareunia, 321

Ejaculatory dysfunction, 323–324
Elderly, disorders of, 336–364
Electro-convulsive therapy, 132, 133
Emotion (see also: Anxiety & Depression, Expressed emotion), 170
Epidemiology, 122, 128, 273–276, 338
　of anorexia nervosa, 273, 274
　of bulimia nervosa, 273–276
　of dementia, 338
　of depression, 122
Erectile dysfunction, 322
Expressed emotion, 84–86, 91, 92
　physiological correlates, 91, 92, 120

Factitious disorders, 250
Faking, 262, 263
Family influences, 83, 86, 121, 122, 282
Fluency, 353

Ganser syndrome, 250
Gender, 68–70, 78, 252, 253
　in depression, 68–70, 78
　in hysteria, 252, 253
Genetics
　obesity, 268
　obsessive-compulsive disorder, 203, 204
　psychopathy, 237

Hallucinations, 40, 41, 102, 115, 116, 117
　explanations of, 116, 117
　history of, 40, 41

Historical aspects, 26–51
 definitions, 27, 28
 descriptive psychopathology, 28–37
  anatomoclinical view, 29
  asylums, 30, 31
  concepts, 31–37
   form vs content, 31–33
   non-verbal manifestations, 35, 36
   numerical representation, 33–35
   temporal dimension, 36, 37
 of personality disorders, 223–226
 signs of madness, 37–45
  affect, 44
  delusions, 39, 40
  disorders of consciousness, 42–44
  hallucinations, 40, 41
  motility, 45
  obsessions & compulsions, 41, 42
  volition, 44, 45
Hopelessness, 140
Hypochondriasis, 247, 248
Hysteria, 28, 245–267
 anxiety in, 253, 254
 Briquet's syndrome (or St. Louis hysteria), 249, 256
 childhood disturbance and, 256
 concepts of, 245–252
 depression in, 255
 gender, 252
 laterality of symptoms, 257
 mass or epidemic hysteria, 249
 models of, 257–265
  conversion, 246, 257, 258
  dissociation, 246, 259, 260
  faking, 262, 263
  illness behaviour, 263–265
  neurobiological, 260, 261
 physical disorder in, 255, 256
 sexual adjustment in, 254
Hysterical (or histrionic) personality, 226, 227, 248, 249

Illusions, 40, 41
Incubation of fear, 178, 179
Information processing, 106, 112, 113
 slowness in, 112, 113
Intelligence, 131, 132

Korsakoff syndrome, 357

Language, 133, 134, 352–354
 in dementia, 352–354
 in depression, 133, 134
Learned helplessness, 155–157
Learning, see Memory
Life events, 68, 77, 81, 82, 86, 87
 in depression, 68, 77
 in schizophrenia, 81, 82, 86, 87
Limbic system, 172, 173

Malingering, 247, 248, 262
Manic-depressive psychosis (see also Depression), 129
Medical model, 11–16
Memory
 in dementia, 343–352
  sensory loss and, 343, 344
  long-term, 348–351
  short-term, 344–348
 in depression, 134–137
Methodological issues, 4, 52–66, 104, 105
 analogue research, 57–60, 65
 demand characteristics in, 59
 control, 52, 61–64
 experimental validity, 53–56, 59, 61, 65
  external, 53, 54, 59, 65
  internal, 53, 56, 61
  statistical conclusion, 53, 55
 in ageing, 337, 338
 in schizophrenia, 104, 105
 measurement, 53
 quasi-experimental designs, 60, 61, 65
 single-case/small N designs, 53–57
  statistical analysis in, 57
 within subject designs, 64
Mood see Anxiety, Depression
Motivation, 131, 137, 138, 239
 in depression, 137, 138
 in personality disorders, 239
Munchausen's syndrome, 249

Naming, 352–353
Neurochemistry, 339, 340
Neuropathology, 339, 340
Neuropsychology of anxiety, 172, 173
Normal behaviour – in relation to abnormal, 26, 103, 104, 200–202
 historical aspects, 26
 obsessions & compulsions, 200–202
 schizophrenia, 103, 104

Obesity, 268, 269
 genetics, 268
 psychological factors, 268, 269
Obsessive-compulsive disorder, 194–217
 definition description, 194–202
  compulsions, 195–197, 200
  constituent elements, 197–199
  DSM III definition, 194–196
  obsessions, 195, 196, 200
  personality, 202
  relation to normal behaviour, 200–202
  resistance, 199
  rituals, 199
  ruminations, 199, 200
 historical background, 41, 42
 theories, 202–214
  Beech & Perigault, 207, 208
  cognitive deficit models, 208, 209

SUBJECT INDEX   379

learning, 204–207
  difficulties with, 206
  relation to animal avoidance learning, 206, 207
new anxiety theories, 209–212
  Foa & Kozak, 209–210
  Gray, 210–212
of obsessions, 212, 213
possible aetiological factors, 203, 204
psychoanalytic, 204
Orgasmic dysfunction, 320, 321

Panic Attacks, 187, 188
Parkinson's disease, 358, 359
Perceptual organisation, 113, 114
Personality (*see also* Personality disorders)
  in anorexia nervosa, 281
  in depression, 138–140
  obsessional, 202
Personality disorders (*see also* Psychopathic personality), 218–244, 248, 249
  classification, 223–235
    categories, 227–231
      borderline, 228–230
      compulsive, 228–230
      hysterical, (histrionic) 226, 227, 248, 249
      narcissistic, 227, 228
      obsessional, 202
      paranoid, 227, 228
      passive aggressive, 228–230
      schizoid, 230, 231
    categories vs dimensions, 233–235
    historical perspective, 223–226
      moral insanity, 223, 224
    value of present systems, 231, 232
  in relation to views of personality, 218–223
    behavioural view, 222
    interpersonal theories, 222
    psychiatric conceptions, 218, 219
    social learning theory, 222
    trait theories, 220, 221
Phobias, 170, 322
  sexual, 322
Preparedness, 177, 178
Priming, 309
Psychoanalysis, 204, 246, 257, 258
  and hysteria, 246, 257, 258
  and obsessive compulsive disorder, 204
Psychopathic personality, 235–240
  Cleckley's criteria, 233
  primary vs secondary, 224, 225, 235, 238
  theoretical approaches, 237–240
    conditioning studies, 238
    genetics, 237
    socialization, 239, 240
  validity of the concept, 235, 236

Psychophysiology
  of anxiety, 171–175
  of depression, 145–147
  of schizophrenia, 118–121

Reading, 354
Research Diagnostic Criteria, 3, 129, 130
  for depression, 129, 130
Resistance, 199
Retardation, 132–134
Rituals, 199
Ruminations, 199

Schizophrenia, 101–127
  definition and diagnosis, 101–104
    continuity with normality, 103, 104
    DSM-III criteria, 101, 102
    fundamental disturbances, 102, 103
  delusions, 101, 117–118
  hallucinations, 102, 116–117
  methodological problems, 104, 105
  models of perceptual/cognitive abnormality, 114–116
  perceptual/cognitive abnormalities, 105–114
    attention, 107–110
    automatic vs controlled processing, 110–113
  positive vs negative symptoms, 102
  psychophysiological abnormalities, 118–121
    arousal, 118–120
    in relation to expressed emotion, 120–121
  social factors in, 79–93
Self efficacy, 180–182
Sexual dysfunctions, 318–333
  causes, 324–333
    maintaining factors, 330–333
      anxiety, 330, 331
      fear of intimacy, 332
      inadequate sexual information, 332
      poor communication, 331
      psychiatric disorder, 332
      relationship problems, 331, 332
    precipitants, 329–330
      childbirth, 329
      dysfunction in partner, 330
      psychiatric disorder, 330
      random failure, 330
      relationship problems, 329
      traumatic experiences, 329, 330
    predisposing factors, 327–329
      disturbed family background, 327, 328
      early traumatic experiences, 328, 329
  classification of dysfunctions, 319

Sexual dysfunctions (contd)
  definition, 318, 319
  in hysteria, 254
  in men, 322–324
    erectile dysfunction, 322
    impaired interest, 322
    painful ejaculation, 324
    premature ejaculation, 323
    retarded or absent ejaculation, 323, 324
  in women, 319–322
    dyspareunia, 321
    impaired arousal, 320
    impaired interest, 319, 320
    orgasmic dysfunction, 320–321
    sexual phobias, 322
    vaginismus, 321
Shadowing, 107–109
Slowness, 112, 113, 200
  in information processing, 112, 113
Social influences, 67–99
  in depresssion, 68–79
    maintenance & remission, 78, 79
      gender, 78
      material circumstances, 78
      race, 78
      stressors, 78, 79
    onset factors, 68–78
      gender, 68–70
      race & migration, 72
      social class, 70–72
      social support, 74–77
      unemployment, 73, 74
  in schizophrenia, 79–93
    maintenance & remission, 83–87
      culture, 87
      expressed emotion, 84–86
      family influences, 83–86
      life events, 86, 87
      societal influences, 86
    onset, 80–83
      culture, 83
      family influences, 80, 81
      social networks, 82
      societal influences, 81
    social treatment, 87–92
      environmental influences, 90–92
      expressed emotion, 88, 89
      family interventions, 87–90
Socialization, 239, 240
Sociopath, see Psychopathy
Speed, 132
Symbolic learning, 179, 180

Thought disorder, 102, 103
Thought processes, 142, 145
Treatment, 87–93, 170, 310–314
  of anxiety, 170
  of dependency, 310–314
  social, 87–93

Vaginismus, 321

WHO International Classification of
    Diseases, 67, 218, 219, 225, 227,
    232
  depression, 67
  personality disorders, 218, 219, 225, 227,
    232
WHO Committee on Dependence, 299, 300
Withdrawal from drugs, 306, 307